PRACTICAL
BIOETHICS

PRACTICAL BIOETHICS

Ethics for Patients and Providers

J.K. Miles

broadview press

BROADVIEW PRESS – www.broadviewpress.com
Peterborough, Ontario, Canada

Founded in 1985, Broadview Press remains a wholly independent publishing house. Broadview's focus is on academic publishing; our titles are accessible to university and college students as well as scholars and general readers. With over 800 titles in print, Broadview has become a leading international publisher in the humanities, with world-wide distribution. Broadview is committed to environmentally responsible publishing and fair business practices.

© 2023 J.K. Miles

Library and Archives Canada Cataloguing in Publication

Title: Practical bioethics : ethics for patients and providers / J.K. Miles.
Names: Miles, J. K., author.
Description: Includes bibliographical references and index.
Identifiers: Canadiana (print) 20230212107 | Canadiana (ebook) 2023021214X | ISBN 9781554813711 (softcover) | ISBN 9781770488809 (PDF) | ISBN 9781460408162 (EPUB)
Subjects: LCSH: Bioethics—Textbooks. | LCGFT: Textbooks.
Classification: LCC QH332 .M55 2023 | DDC 174.2—dc23

Broadview Press handles its own distribution in North America:
PO Box 1243, Peterborough, Ontario K9J 7H5, Canada
555 Riverwalk Parkway, Tonawanda, NY 14150, USA
Tel: (705) 743-8990; Fax: (705) 743-8353
email: customerservice@broadviewpress.com

For all territories outside of North America, distribution is handled by Eurospan Group.

 Broadview Press acknowledges the financial support of the Government of Canada for our publishing activities.

Edited by Martin R. Boyne
Book Design by Em Dash Design

PRINTED IN CANADA

Contents

CHAPTER 1

Ethical Dilemmas in Medicine   23

CHAPTER 2

Ethical Principles for Resolving Dilemmas   61

CHAPTER 3

Dilemmas in the Patient–Provider Relationship 107

CHAPTER 4

Dilemmas in Medical Research 149

CHAPTER 5

Dilemmas at the End of Life   205

CHAPTER 6

Dilemmas with Scarce Medical Resources   247

CHAPTER 7

Dilemmas in Genetic and Reproductive Technology 293

CHAPTER 8

Dilemmas for Patients and Families 339

CHAPTER 9

Dilemmas with Abortion 383

J.K. Miles is also author of the Substack newsletter *Miles to Go*, which offers commentary and case studies that can be used to supplement this book.

jkmiles.substack.com

Acknowledgments

I wish to acknowledge the following people who helped make this text possible:

Dr. William Lawhead, Dr. Neil Manson, Jeri Conboy LCSW, Jessica Goetz FP-C, Rob Johnson M.D., Wayland Mutter CNP-BC, and Sam Deters read portions of this text and offered valuable feedback. Special commendation to all the bioethics students who suffered through drafts of this text and pointed out many, many grammatical errors. (Including the nameless student who gifted me the real-life case study "Billy Likes to Eat Mud." If you read this, contact me. I owe you.) Michalea Moore made many of the passages less obtuse.

Dr. William Lawhead gave me the guidance to get this text off the ground. It would likely not exist without his input. Dr. Dennis Ozment let me rattle on about bioethics during our visits. I learned a lot from the ethics committee at Blessing Hospital, who welcomed an outsider and allowed me to contribute to ethics consults.

Dr. Heloise Robinson worked as my research assistant, long distance, from Oxford, England, on a generous grant from the Institute for Humane Studies. Her insights and investigation were invaluable. Quincy University provided a sabbatical semester during which I could work on this draft. Thanks also to Christopher W. Suprenant, Director of the University Honors Program and Director of the Urban Entrepreneurship and Policy Institute at University of New Orleans, for providing research space during my sabbatical.

This text would have been considerably more difficult and delayed without support from the Institute for Humane Studies. My colleagues Dr. Teresa Reed, Dr. Matthew Bates, and Dr. Daniel Strudwick encouraged me to take on this project and kept me motivated whenever I grew discouraged. Stephen Latta rendered editorial duties with patience and detail, which makes me glad he was my first editor.

Nothing I do makes any sense without the tireless support of Stacie Botsay Miles, my wife. Judy Kennedy has to like this book because she is my mother, but I hope she likes it all the same.

This book is dedicated to my children: Wesley, Gloria, and Caroline. *esse virtuosum, pium et amandum.*

A Note to Readers

What makes this textbook different from other bioethics textbooks? In a word, practicality. My goal is to focus primarily on issues of practical relevance to medical providers and patients.

There are two approaches to bioethics. One we might call "academic bioethics" or "policy bioethics," because its subject matter is policy. For instance, what should those in authority do, given a particular advancement in biotechnology? If we can edit genes, should we do so? Policy questions can also revolve around moral status. Is the fetus a person? If so, is abortion always immoral? Many bioethics books focus primarily on these issues of policy, and there is nothing wrong with that. These are important debates for policymakers to have. It is worthwhile to know about them, for we should engage morally with the processes and policies that affect large numbers of people, even those that do not directly affect us.

However, the majority of us have little say in the determination of health-care regulations. Those policies may affect us, but even those of us who work in the health-care professions will rarely be faced with decisions concerning, say, the general moral permissibility of euthanasia or the social role of gene-editing technologies. We might advocate and react to such policies, and we might express our beliefs through protests and political actions, but most of us will not have the opportunity to alter decisions on these issues.

Every student of bioethics will, however, at some point get sick and need a medical provider. Most of us will eventually be in a situation where we have to make difficult medical decisions in partnership with health-care providers, whether concerning our own health or the health of our loved ones. For those of us who move on to careers in the health professions, it will most definitely be necessary to confront ethical dilemmas and make difficult decisions in complicated and morally complex situations. In light of these facts, *Practical Bioethics* gives priority to the provider–patient relationship first, and policy decisions second.

If we focus on the provider–patient relationship, then what sort of foundation should we have? Both patients and providers need a grounding in moral reasoning. Moral reasoning can help us to make decisions ethically (in this book, I use the terms *ethics* and *morals* interchangeably, as is typical in public discourse). Before we delve into the practical, thorny questions of end-of-life decisions or the treatment of research subjects, we have to have a core in the basic elements of morality: ethical dilemmas, principles, and theories. Chapters 1 and 2 do this. Chapter 1 addresses the nature of moral dilemmas and the need to resolve them. Chapter 2 covers moral principles in health care, as well as moral theories. I have tried to break up this deep dive into moral philosophy with some practical case studies and descriptions that will show how all this moral theory is valuable for the day-to-day decisions of medical providers, patients, and family members.

Once we have that core, we can start delving into issues that spring from the patient–provider relationship. For example, respecting patient autonomy is a given for most medical professionals. Patients have rights that limit what medical personnel can do to them; providers have duties with regard to due care and disclosure. These obligations may be listed in a patient bill of rights, but such lists do not tell us what it means to exercise a right or what sorts of duties flow from those rights. Questions about the implementation of rights and duties pervade the patient–provider relationship, often leading to moral dilemmas. Throughout this book, we will examine these and other dilemmas and moral quandaries that arise in the practice of health care.

My hope is that when you finish using this book, you will be a better patient. If you are a medical provider (or a future one), my hope is that you will have a better understanding of how to evaluate your decisions morally in order to do your job well.

Each of this book's chapters contains four parts:

1. OPENING GAMBIT (CASE STUDY)

Each chapter begins with a case study based on actual events. These cases have a clear dilemma that forces the reader to choose the lesser of two evils. Each dilemma will end with a choice between options to resolve the dilemma. You are encouraged to form a preliminary opinion and then test that opinion once you understand the conceptual issues in the rest of the chapter. Each case study and its ethical dilemma allow you to practice applying the principles and theories of bioethics.

2. WHAT'S AT STAKE? (CONCEPTUAL ISSUES)

These sections give a formal presentation of the questions or topics under consideration. Often, terms in bioethics are defined and reinforced by referring back to the Opening Gambit, revisiting the opening dilemma with new conceptual tools.

3. WHAT'S THE DEBATE? (READINGS)

With few exceptions, philosophical readings are difficult for the average student and are written in a style and vocabulary unfamiliar to health-care majors. *Practical Bioethics* borrows a successful feature from William Lawhead's *Philosophical Journey* (McGraw-Hill, 2011). Instead of short editorial comments at the beginning of each reading and questions at the end, the text frequently "interrupts" each reading with an explanation of the argument or a discussion question. These interjections are designed to make otherwise-difficult texts accessible to those not already immersed in academic bioethics.

4. ETHICS COMMITTEE (GROUP DELIBERATION ASSIGNMENTS)

Each chapter ends with a second case study that is geared toward a small-group discussion, as if the group were an ethics committee facing a dilemma. As a hospital ethics committee member, I know that clinical ethical decisions are rarely made in isolation. Ethical decisions are usually a group affair, with a consultant making recommendations to a care team including family members. Furthermore, medical providers often serve on hospital ethics committees, where dilemmas are discussed and resolved in groups. Students are encouraged to search for a consensus (or at least a majority decision) on how to resolve a dilemma and perhaps to let a majority vote decide their recommendation (ethics committees rarely have decisional authority, as they can only advise).

How Bioethics Journal Articles Work

Most of the readings in this book are from bioethics journals, and they can be difficult to navigate if you do not know the terrain. This short section gives you an orientation to bioethics journals and explains some of their customs.

Identifying Arguments

Academics publish in journals to debate with each other. Someone will write an article asserting something like "People should be able to sell their organs." Someone else will write another article saying, "Respectfully, selling your organs is immoral." Think of it as a sort of slower, long-distance instant message. By and large, the writers are professional ethicists or philosophers. A few are medical providers like doctors, nurses, or administrators. When you read these articles, you are listening in on a conversation between professionals on issues they care about.

These bioethics articles are almost always argumentative. The writer or writers (sometimes they collaborate to write an article) have an agenda. They have something they want you, the reader, to buy into or accept. They want to convince you of some conclusion.

Arguments of the rational kind (as opposed to the Twitter kind) are always composed of premises and conclusions. Premises are statements that support (i.e., give evidence for, give reasons for you to accept) the conclusion. The conclusion, also called the thesis, is just the statement that the authors want everyone to agree with.

The good news is that ethicists usually like to make their theses explicit early in their articles. Authors will lay out a general problem they are interested in by saying something like "Studies show that doctors give the least honest answers to the patients with the worst chances of survival." They will then signal their conclusion to the problem by saying, often in first person, "I want to argue this is paternalism, and it's wrong." This is the thesis. If you look back at the start of this section, I stated the general problem and my thesis in the first three sentences.

Responding to Arguments

So once you have found the thesis, what do you look for? You look for the argument, the premises. You should be able to pick out the evidence or statements the author uses to get you to agree with their thesis. It is important to pick out those sentences and be able to summarize them because this is the first step in critiquing them. That is right; I want you to disagree with the authors. Analyze their reasons and find holes in their arguments, if there are any. The good news is that arguments can go wrong in only a few ways:

1) The conclusion doesn't follow from the premises
An argument goes wrong if you cannot get to the conclusion from the premises given. It is a very real possibility that the premises will be all true and the conclusion just doesn't follow from them. You could also agree with all the author's premises and still not buy the conclusion. For instance, consider the following argument:

1. All medical providers are licensed.
2. All nurses are licensed.
3. Therefore, all nurses are medical providers.

Every one of these premises and the conclusion are true, but the conclusion does not follow from the premises. The conclusion just happens to be true. That isn't good enough to show there is a connection.

To see why the conclusion doesn't follow from the premises just replace "medical providers," "licensed," and "nurses" with "dogs," "cats," and "mammals":

1. All dogs are mammals.
2. All cats are mammals.
3. Therefore, all cats are dogs.

This argument looks quite a bit like the earlier one, and premises 1 and 2 are also true. Yet its conclusion is most definitely false, which just goes to show that arguments of this form don't work.

2) One or more of the premises are false
This one seems self-explanatory, doesn't it? Suppose the author makes an argument like the following:

1. Persons have a right to not be harmed.
2. Embryos are persons.
3. Therefore, embryos have a right not to be harmed.

This argument is valid. If 1 and 2 are true, the conclusion *has* to be true.

Are the premises true? If you had to go after a premise, which one seems the most problematic? Probably 2. It is not obviously true that embryos are persons. After all, we do not treat them like persons, they are not able to speak or reason, and they cannot feel pain like a person. This does not mean that it is obviously false that embryos are persons. After all, an embryo will become a full-grown person in time. So, if it is not already a person, when does a fetus become a person? At what stage of development? In addition, there are persons in vegetative states who cannot reason or feel pain, so it seems as though these things are not *necessary* in order to qualify as a person. Now we have ourselves a debate.

The argument above may or may not succeed, but its success hinges on whether its second premise is true. When you're reading through the articles included in this book, be sure to ask yourself which premises the author is using to support their conclusion, and try to determine whether any of them are false or contentious.

3) A term in the argument is ambiguous or misused
One of the ways in which arguments often go wrong is when someone uses a term in two different ways without explaining the difference. For example, consider this argument:

1. We all agree that the fundamental rights, such as the right to practice religion, must be enforced by law.
2. People also have a right to affordable health care.
3. Therefore, the right to affordable health care must be enforced by law.

This argument equates the right to practice religion with the right to affordable health care. But are those two rights that similar?

Most things we consider "rights" are claims on other people's behavior. If I have a right, it means I claim that you must treat me in a certain way. The right to practice my religion means you cannot interfere with my practice (provided it does not interfere with anyone else's rights). All that is required of you is not to interfere. Is the right to affordable health care the same species of right? It may or may not be a right (that is a matter for debate), but the claim on behavior is certainly different from that of the right to practice religion. In this case, the strength of the argument depends at least in part on the similarity and dissimilarity between these two rights.

When assessing an argument, always check to see whether important terms are being used in different ways from one premise to the next (or from premises to the conclusion). If there are important differences between how the terms are being used, it may be that the connection between the premises and the conclusion is not as strong as it first appears.

Academic Conversations

Academic articles are conversations that you are listening in on. This means that often you are hearing only one part of the conversation. The debate in journals about end-of-life decision making has been going on for over thirty years. That is a lot of chats. When you read an article about euthanasia or withdrawing treatment, the authors are going to reference something said in some other journal article. They might even be responding to an article published earlier just so they can argue that the conclusion of that article was wrong. So expect that the articles you read may refer back to some other article you have not read. It is not a big deal if you have not read that other article. The writers expect that not everyone can be privy to the entire discussion for the last thirty years. The writers will usually summarize enough of the other arguments so that you can follow along. Pay attention to these summaries.

If the writer only name-drops, "Like Professor X, I hold that ...," this just lets other academics know that the writer is situating themself within a group of like-minded thinkers and is hoping that if you associate them with Professor X, and you admire Professor X, you will not *totally* dismiss the writer's ideas as crazy. Writers do this to get you interested in what they have to say. It is just like when you are at a gathering and someone says just a little too loudly, "Well, you know, Dr. Smith and I agree on this." However, if your writer goes so far as to summarize Smith's argument or quotes from his argument, you know they are not just name dropping. This writer wants to engage with Smith's argument, usually to criticize it in some way or to take Smith's ideas and use them to solve another general problem.

Thought Experiments

Writers who do not engage with another author might just argue with themselves! That's right. If you are reading an article and suddenly an author seems to contradict themself, then check to make sure they aren't just entertaining an argument or position so that they can criticize it. A sign this is going on is when authors start a paragraph with phrases like "Suppose that ...," "You might think ...," "What if one were to say ...," or "Imagine the following...."

You might even see what philosophers call a "thought experiment." This is an imaginary story designed to make an analogy between some fake or fantastical situation and a very real, very serious issue. For instance, one of the most famous thought experiments in bioethics is about waking up in a hospital bed attached to a world-famous violinist who is using your kidneys because his are failing and you just happen to have the only kidneys that will keep him alive. Even though he has a right to life, does he have a right to use your kidneys while he waits for a transplant?

The author of this thought experiment, Judith Jarvis Thomson, is not suggesting anyone would ever do this. Rather, she is making an analogy between discovering that one is connected to the violinist and discovering that one is pregnant. Thomson bypasses all the arguments about the right to the life of the fetus. Like the violinist, the fetus may have a right to live, but it is depending on your own organs for survival. Thomson wants to convince you that even if the fetus has a right to life, aborting the fetus is morally permissible, just as unhooking yourself from the violinist is morally permissible. She's hoping to convince you that what's good for the violinist fantasy is good for the very real and serious reality of permitting or criminalizing abortion. Is she successful? (Take a look at Chapter 9 to see Thomson's article and a critique by Francis Beckwith.)

CHAPTER 1

Ethical Dilemmas in Medicine

The Transposition of the Great Arteries

Death is never easy, but the death of an infant is particularly traumatic for everyone involved. Infants born with transposition of the great arteries die lethargic, blue-tinged, and gasping for breath because the artery that sends blood to the lungs to receive oxygen bypasses the lungs altogether, sending oxygen-poor blood back into the body. For a long time there was only one way to save the infants: a complex surgery called the Senning procedure. The Senning procedure wasn't all that risky (infants died in only about 5 to 10 per cent of the cases), but survivors of the procedure were at a much greater risk for heart defects later in life; because their hearts were compromised, most never made it to old age.

The surgeons of the Great Ormond Street Hospital in London wanted to switch from the Senning procedure to something called the Jatene procedure. In the Jatene procedure, the arteries are surgically removed and reattached. The new procedure increases quality of life, and those who get the surgery can live full and active lives. There was a cost, however: Surgeons had to gain experience with the new procedure because surgeons learn on the job.

A study done twenty years after the fact showed that, in the beginning, infant deaths rose sharply for a few years but then declined rapidly so that almost no infant dies of transposition of the great arteries today. If the hospital had stuck with the traditional procedure, there would have been less risk to infants during surgery, but those infants would have had a poor quality of life. Since the hospital offered patients a new procedure, there was a greater risk in the short term, until the surgeons learned the new procedure. In the long run, however, the quality of life for the patients was much better. The choice to switch from an older, reliable procedure to a new one was a choice "between expertise and progress," according to author and surgeon Atul Gawande.[*]

Imagine that now you are in a similar position, as either a surgeon or someone else who weighs in on a similar change in procedure. In a hypothetical hospital, surgeons are faced with learning a new procedure for treating infants. If surgeons do not perform the procedure enough, they will never get good at it, but if they do develop the expertise, the overall good for patients will be significant.

However, if we allow surgeons to practice, there is a greater risk of complications or death. Assume, for the sake of the exercise, that there is no way to learn the procedure without operating on actual humans (often the case in real life). Would you vote for allowing the new procedure, knowing that it will almost certainly be better in the long run but at the price of increased risk of infants dying in the short term? In addition, just how much should surgeons tell the parents about their inexperience with the new procedure? Should they mention just the increased risk of dying or their inexperience with the procedure as well?

WHAT'S AT STAKE?

The medical providers at the London hospital faced an ethical dilemma. There are two choices, and neither choice is ideal. Technically, if there were three choices, our case would represent a trilemma. However, the term "dilemma" has come to mean a situation where there are at least two choices. Both choices seem unethical somehow. In addition, doing nothing isn't really an option, as a dilemma requires that one of the two possible outcomes occur.

When it comes to the choice of implementing a new surgical procedure, the staff at the hospital might feel like they are damned if they do and damned if they don't. Such dilemmas force us to weigh the costs and benefits of a particular action, but not just in terms of number of lives saved, or protecting patient rights, but also in terms of what we think is right and good for interactions between patients, medical providers (doctors/nurses/administrators), and the public.

These sorts of ethical clashes are what make bioethics interesting, vitally important, and uniquely relevant. The fact is that if you have any dealings with

---

[*] Atul Gawande, *Complications: A Surgeon's Notes on an Imperfect Science* (New York: Picador, 2002). Elements of this case study were taken from Gawande's description.

medicine or biotechnology as either provider or patient, you will probably face a dilemma where you are damned if you do and damned if you don't.

We begin our study of bioethics with dilemmas because this is where the study of ethics becomes practical. Most moral decisions are not moral dilemmas. Everyday we are faced with situations where it would be better for us to lie, cheat, or steal, but common-sense morality says we should not. There is no damned if you don't. You are wrong and morally blameworthy if you lie, cheat, or steal. However, most ethical concerns occur when there are reasons to do something that otherwise would be unethical. That's a moral dilemma.

It is possible to face dilemmas head on and come out with a resolution that meets three criteria: clear, coherent, and justified. Note that we say "resolution" rather than "answer" because an ethical dilemma might allow for more than one permissible option. If we are lucky, there will be several good resolutions to a dilemma. However, when it comes to bioethics, it is more likely we will face a decision that may not be ideal but one we can live with. Let's look at each of these claims:

- *Clear*: everyone involved—patients, family members, and providers—can understand not only what decision was made but also why it was made.

- *Coherent*: a decision that is consistent with other, similar ethical decisions.

- *Justified*: all those involved will be able to point to reasons that the decision makers used to make the decision, and whether they agree with the decision or not, any reasonable person would agree it was a reasonable decision.

Why is "justified" the highest we can hope for? Why not aim for the "the right decision"? There is a fact that becomes very evident whenever one is faced with an ethical problem and multiple parties have a stake in the outcome: We live in a pluralistic society. *Ethical pluralism* holds that it is just a fact that people don't always agree on what is the right action to take in a given situation, or even on how to arrive at the right answer. Of course, a right answer may or may not actually exist. If the question is a matter of taste, such as "Which indie rock band is the best?" or "Who makes the best barbecue?" or "Which theory of nursing is best for teaching nurses?," there may not be a single right answer. However, the mere fact that just about everyone disagrees about the best course of action does not mean there is not a right answer. A jury in a trial may not ever agree at all whether the defendant is guilty or not guilty, and no one may ever really know except the defendant, the plaintiff, and (if the defendant is not guilty) the actual guilty party. Regardless, there is a fact of the matter. The defendant is either guilty or not even though no one can agree.

It would be foolish to think that, in our politically charged society, there would be a consensus about how to ensure a fair distribution of wealth. However, that does not mean there is not a fair way to divide wealth in a given economy. The most we can hope for is that the laws passed are not arbitrary or self-serving. Likewise, medical staff may never agree on whether to honor a patient's request to turn off a pacemaker, but that does not mean there is no right answer about honoring that request. The most we can hope for is that whatever decision is made is one that can be explained to the patient and the family such that anyone would say, "I may not agree, but I understand why the decision was made."

This kind of pluralism should be contrasted with *ethical relativism* and *ethical monism*. In ethical relativism, all moral values are viewed as relative to something; nothing is good or bad, right or wrong, in itself. For instance, cultural relativists argue that moral values (right/wrong/good/bad) are dependent on the culture one is operating in. This means that nothing can be said to be right or wrong outside the culture in question. If you want to do right, then follow the old maxim "When in Rome, do as the Romans do," because literally that is what is right. Protagoras, an ancient Greek philosopher, is said to have argued that "whatever things seem to each city to be fine and just are so for that city, so long as it maintains them." In other words, what is ethically just is relative to a particular city. I guess you could call that municipal relativism. But instead of "city" substitute "region," "state," or "country" and you get the bigger picture.

Ethical monists say that some actions are right or wrong, good or bad, independently of a culture or a person. More importantly, they say that all morality is reducible to one single value. For instance, if you believed that all morality was a question of acting on what produced the least amount of pain for everyone, then you would be an ethical monist. Ethical monists believe that all moral dilemmas can be resolved by asking which action produces the one value the most. That choice then becomes the best resolution morally. For instance, philosopher Jeremy Bentham (1748–1832) was an ethical monist. He thought that you could figure out every ethical dilemma based on which action would produce the most amount of good, where good was measured in terms of pleasure, and bad in terms of pain, for the greatest number. He called this value *utility* and his theory *utilitarianism*. Later utilitarians like J.S. Mill (1806–73) would modify Bentham's proposal, but the core idea remained. The right thing to do was always whatever action would create the most amount of pleasure and the least amount of pain for everyone.

Ethical pluralists sit in between ethical monists and ethical relativists. Ethical pluralists say that there is not just one value that matters, like pleasure. An ethical pluralist might say there are several equally important ethical values, such as reducing pain and honoring patient requests, and there is no reason these values will not conflict. In the opening gambit, the choice about switching surgical procedures is a dilemma precisely because there may be more than one value at stake. On the one hand, we value medical progress, not the least because it results in less pain overall for everyone. The development of the smallpox vaccine involved some unpleasant suffering, but it resulted in a lot fewer people dead in the long run.

We also value our obligation to protect individuals from risk of harm or death. The question we asked about how much we should tell the patient about our lack of expertise in doing this procedure pits our value of what is best for everyone in the long run (surgeons getting good at the procedure through practice) against the value of patients' ability to decide what's best for them with adequate information. In Chapter 2 we will give names to those values, but for now it is important for us to see that an ethical dilemma is so difficult because we tend to think that values are plural, not monistic or relative.

If moral values were singular (ethical monism), resolving the "damned if you do, damned if you don't" moment might be simple. Figure out the single value and choose which option produces that single value the best. If the absence of pain for everyone is the single value, then we should most likely choose to implement the new procedure as much as possible, since surgeons who are good at the procedure will produce a better quality of life for everyone they operate on once they become experts.

If values were relative, ethical dilemmas would not be as problematic. If our prevailing culture thinks the right of the individual is more important than the good of the community, as is often the case in the United States for example, then the hospital has an obligation to warn patients about how inexperienced surgeons are even if this means surgeons never really get good at the new procedure. On the other hand, if the culture values the collective good of the community over the individual, then it may be permissible to inform but not warn. The point is that dilemmas are not as difficult or as vital if we are either ethical monists or ethical relativists.

Let's review: An ethical dilemma is one where there are at least two options about what is the right thing to do. Choosing any option will cause us to sacrifice some value. We are damned if we do this and we are damned if we don't. The reason we feel this clash of values is that ethical values seem inescapably plural. There seems to be more than one value and no good way to say that one value is more important than any other. We should respect patients, but we should also make their lives better. What happens when respecting patients' decisions actually leads to things being worse off for them (and everyone else)? Which value wins so we can have a resolution that is clear, coherent, and justified?

Answering that question is the heart of what we call *ethical decision making* or *moral reasoning*. Throughout this text, we will be referring to cases where an ethical decision has to be made. These are usually real-life stories of patients and providers who faced a dilemma. The goal of looking at these cases is to figure out how to resolve the dilemma in a way that is clear, coherent, and justifiable.

This sort of analysis goes on all the time in health care. A patient's family asks the doctor to shut off a defibrillator that keeps the patient's heart beating at the correct rhythm. This is not some machine to unplug; it is a device implanted in the patient's chest. A code must be transmitted to stop the tiny electric shocks that keep the patient's heart beating properly. The family wants this device deactivated because the patient is in the end stages of the dying process. The family feels that the device is prolonging the patient's life unnecessarily. However, we also find out that the patient is awake, eats with some help, and can communicate, though they aren't capable of making their own decisions. Some nursing staff worry that shutting off the defibrillator will hasten the patient's death.

Since the patient is not capable of making their own decisions, standard policy is to defer to the patient's designated surrogate as if their wishes were the patient's themselves. We value a patient's right to make their own decisions, what we often refer to as their *autonomy*. Families request that staff remove breathing tubes every day, and all things considered, we should treat their request as if it came from the patient. This is referred to as *substituted judgment*. However, we also value *non-maleficence*, the duty not to harm someone without a compelling reason.

We know this is an ethical dilemma because if we agree to the family's request we may violate the principle of non-maleficence, but if we don't agree then we violate the family's autonomy. Now, we value autonomy in bioethics, but not at the expense of causing harm. Medical staff have to make the call that a patient could harm themself or others every time they restrain a patient.

So now that we can recognize a dilemma, what do we do with it?

There are several ways to analyze an ethical dilemma. The most frequently used method in bioethics and medicine today is usually called *principlism* because it focuses on principles like autonomy and non-maleficence and tries to balance them in a way that is clear, coherent, and justified.

We can think of ethical dilemmas as being like a diagnosis and treatment, whereby we break our process down into problem, data (including facts, medical goals, patient goals, and context), ethical assessment, dialogue, and best course of action.* It turns out that more or less every professional, ethical-decision-making model has the same sorts of elements even if they are not labeled the same. For instance, The American Accounting Association categorizes its ethical decision making as follows:

1. Determine the facts
2. Define the ethical issue
3. Identify the major principles, rules, and values
4. List the courses of action
5. Compare values and alternatives (see if a clear decision is evident)
6. Assess the consequences
7. Make a decision.†

The one thing missing, however, is the place of identifying the ethical dilemma. Can you find the dilemma in the accounting model? It is in step 5. But we've seen that what makes ethical reasoning difficult is when major principles, rules, and values clash in a "damned if we do, damned if we don't" moment. It certainly is true that lots of ethical issues have clear and evident decisions. If you have a choice between lying to a client and not lying to a client, all things being equal, you shouldn't lie to clients mainly because, all things being equal, we shouldn't lie. Accountants, nurses, and administrators should do likewise. But what everyone needs is a way to resolve those thorny ethical issues that represent a dilemma. Let's combine these similar models into one that emphasizes the dilemmas in bioethics.

The first step to any treatment is to examine the patient and sort out what things are relevant and what things are not. Let's call this step the "describe" phase. Here we want to pay close attention to the facts of the case and the stake-holders—all the people who have an interest in the outcome of the dilemma. Stakeholders typically include the medical staff, the hospital administration, the patient, and the family members. Scientific researchers might also be involved. In a public health department, the public at large would be included.

What does each of the stakeholders want? It may not be readily apparent that during the describe phase we need to isolate those facts that are ethically important. A patient's temperature is medically relevant, but is it ethically relevant? Only if it contributes to what makes our case a dilemma. Some facts should not even be considered in case analysis. Suppose we are part of an organ

---

* For a discussion of this method, see Lauris C. Kaldjian, Robert F. Weir, and Thomas P. Duffy, "A Clinician's Approach to Clinical Ethical Reasoning," *Journal of General Internal Medicine* 20, no. 3 (2005): 306–11.

† See https://www.accaglobal.com/gb/en/student/exam-support-resources/professional-exams-study-resources/strategic-business-leader/technical-articles/ethical-decision-making.html.

transplant network and have two equally sick people in need of a kidney: Does it matter that one is a woman and one is a man? How about if one is single and the other is married with three children? These factors should be considered only if they contribute to a better chance of long-term survival because we already want the organ to go to the person who will benefit the most from it.

Now let's examine another case study concerning the use of a ventilator. After going through the *describe* phase, we will move on to the other elements of our bioethics dilemma model: *dilemma*, *discern*, *decide*, and *defend*.

> A 48-year-old man with no immediate family suffers from a rare paralysis of the diaphragm. He has been on a ventilator (breathing machine) for the last ten years. He is dependent on the ventilator and cannot breathe unaided. He arrives at the ER because his home ventilator was malfunctioning and not giving him enough air. After the staff hook him up to a hospital ventilator, his breathing returns to normal. Nonetheless, he is admitted for observation. After he regains consciousness, he requests that his ventilator be removed and that he be allowed to die. He says he is tired of having this machine breathing for him. In another age he would have died a long time ago. When the medical staff express to him that other than the ventilator he is fairly healthy and can expect to live into his 70s, he remarks that this is precisely the problem. The staff is reluctant to remove the ventilator because the patient is not terminally ill. The patient insists that the right to refuse treatment is one of the strongest rights he has.

Describe

In the describe phase, we are interested only in which details of the story are relevant ethically:

1. The patient can't breathe unaided.
2. He's been on a vent for 10 years.
3. He is otherwise healthy.
4. His vent was blocked, and he almost died.
5. Now he wants the vent permanently removed.
6. The medical staff are reluctant to comply.
7. He has no immediate family.

Now let's get philosophical. Why is the fact that the patient can't breathe unaided *ethically* relevant? If we comply with his request, he will die fairly soon. What about the fact that he's been on a ventilator for ten years? Does it matter that he is otherwise healthy? Should we include that in our ethical analysis? Of course: The fact that he is otherwise healthy is what is giving the staff ethical fits.* Does it matter that he has no immediate family? Well, yes and no. Even if he did have immediate family, that wouldn't mean we could ignore his autonomy, but it would mean that there would be people he should ethically consider in his decision.

See how this works? Every fact that we allow into our analysis has to be ethically relevant. Does it matter that he is 48 as opposed to 70? If so, why?

> Notice that this scenario is relevant not only if you are interested in medicine. The person asking for the breathing tube to be removed is making an ethical decision as well. This person is choosing to refuse treatment, and that refusal is likely to end up killing him. Patients and their family members will often face ethical dilemmas. People with a family history of genetic abnormalities face a dilemma involving testing for that disease. If they test for the genetic marker and find they have it, the symptoms could take years to materialize and be very mild. On the other hand, if they do not test, they could risk passing on the trait to others. Consider that the patient in this case is requesting that medical staff do something many of them find unethical.

Dilemma

If we look at the case above, there is a very clear dilemma, which we can articulate as follows: If the staff comply with the request, they may harm someone unnecessarily. But if the staff refuse to honor the request, they violate the patient's freedom to refuse treatment. Of course, if there were more than two options, we could articulate the trilemma using all three options, etc. If it helps, think of dilemmas in terms of the following formula:

> *If we do (action), we violate (value), but if we don't do (action), we violate (other value).*

---

* I deal with this in more detail in the chapter on end-of-life issues (Chapter 5), but we have strong intuitions about how people should die, and it usually means they are terminal.

Once we isolate the dilemma, we can check to see if it is a true dilemma. Is there any way to compromise? Is there a way to honor the patient's desires even if we don't obey his request? Is there a way to minimize harm to the patient while allowing him the freedom to do wrong?

Discern

So now we've gone below the average intuitions about harm and freedom to discern two very real principles of bioethics: non-maleficence and autonomy. I say more about principles in the next chapter, but for now let's assume that no laws will be broken regardless of whether we remove the ventilator. We make this assumption because we want to zero in on the ethical issues of the case. We have to decide, as medical providers (in this scenario), whether we will remove the breathing tube as the patient requests.

The discern phase of the ethical analysis does not easily admit of hard and fast rules. If it did, there would be no need for case analyses. We would just subject our dilemma to a foolproof test and get a resolution. Unfortunately, ethics is not that precise. Remember, we want a decision that is clear, coherent, and justified. There is no clear consensus in ethics about which principle should take precedence: autonomy or non-maleficence. There are some rules of thumb, however, some of which are provided by Beauchamp and Childress:

1. There are good reasons for choosing one principle over the other
2. There's a realistic chance that choosing the option can be achieved
3. No morally preferable options are available
4. The best option is one that violates a principle the least
5. All negative effects of the violated principle are minimized
6. All stakeholders have been treated impartially.[*]

Decide

It would be a lot easier if we could just do all this analysis in the discern phase and then say something like "There are good arguments on all sides and I'm not sure which I prefer." Unfortunately, the nature of dilemmas is that if we refuse to take a side, it is like opting for the status quo, resulting in one of the options happening

---

[*] Tom L. Beauchamp and James F. Childress, *Principles of Biomedical Ethics*, 8th ed. (Oxford University Press, 2019), p. 23.

regardless. So we have to make a decision. We can't stay on the fence. (In real life, hospital ethics committees almost never "decide"; however, they recommend a resolution, but ultimately it is up to the provider to take the advice or not.)

Defend

The last step is to defend the conclusion. This involves justifying the choice that was made by the individual or the committee. In this stage, various objections to the decision that is reached are considered. Suppose your conclusion is that the medical providers should honor the man's request and remove the breathing tube. In that case, they would be honoring his autonomy at the expense of beneficence. What sort of objections might you hear from those who disagree, and what would you say in reply? Throughout this book, you will be asked to settle in your mind your position on a controversial issue. Part of that settling process is considering objections to your position. Are there any long-range implications of your decision? If everyone were to adopt your decision, would it lead to consequences with which you are uncomfortable? The key idea in this step is having a clear, consistent, and justified position.

WHAT'S THE DEBATE?

Now that we have some idea about how moral dilemmas work, let's look at how some other authors wrestle with ethical dilemmas. The first reading is from Sir David Ross (1877–1971). Ross was an ethical pluralist, and he writes about how to handle conflicts of duties in "What Makes Right Actions Right?" The second reading is from another Englishman, John Stuart Mill. Mill was an ethical monist who thought that all ethical dilemmas can be resolved by appeal to one value: utility. The last reading is from British philosopher Stephen Toulmin (1922–2009) about the ways in which we look at cases.

Reading 1.1: W.D. Ross, "What Makes Right Actions Right?"*

Ross's argument is relevant to bioethics because he attempts to find a way to resolve ethical dilemmas by identifying several prima facie duties. "Prima facie" (pronounced prime-a face-yah) literally means "on the face of it." The idea is that prima facie duties are duties we have unless there are very good reasons not to fulfill them. For example, all things being equal, we ought not to lie. But we can all think of exceptions to this prima facie duty. What if someone's life is at stake? What if lying will spare someone's feelings and won't hurt anyone (a white lie)? Ross tries to answer these questions.

The real point at issue between hedonism and utilitarianism on the one hand and their opponents on the other is not whether "right" means "productive of so and so"; for it cannot with any plausibility be maintained that it does. The point at issue is that to which we now pass, viz. whether there is any general character which makes right acts right, and if so, what it is. Among the main historical attempts to state a single characteristic of all right actions which is the foundation of their rightness are those made by egoism and utilitarianism. But I do not propose to discuss these, not because the subject is unimportant, but because it has been dealt with so often and so well already, and because there has come to be so much agreement among moral philosophers that neither of these theories is satisfactory.

> Philosophers often start off by differentiating their argument from others. Ross begins by distinguishing himself from some other theories. These theories will be discussed in a later chapter. He also states his driving concern: "... whether there is any general character which makes right acts right, and if so, what it is."

A much more attractive theory has been put forward by Professor Moore: that what makes actions right is that they are productive of more *good* than could have been produced by any other action open to the agent.[1]

---

* Ross, W.D. Chapter 2: "What Makes Right Acts Right?" from *The Right and the Good*, ed. Philip Stratton-Lake, Clarendon Press. Copyright © Oxford University Press 1930, 2002. pp. 16–47 [excerpted] Reproduced with permission of Oxford Publishing Limited (Academic) through PLSclear.

This theory is in fact the culmination of all the attempts to base rightness on productivity of some sort of result. The first form this attempt takes is the attempt to base rightness on conduciveness to the advantage or pleasure of the agent. This theory comes to grief over the fact, which stares us in the face, that a great part of duty consists in an observance of the rights and a furtherance of the interests of others, whatever the cost to ourselves may be. Plato and others may be right in holding that a regard for the rights of others never in the long run involves a loss of happiness for the agent, that "the just life profits a man." But this, even if true, is irrelevant to the rightness of the act. As soon as a man does an action *because* he thinks he will promote his own interests thereby, he is acting not from a sense of its rightness but from self-interest.

Ross considers a new attempt by one his contemporaries, G.E. Moore (1873–1958), who said that the right thing to do when faced with a choice between two actions is to choose the one that produces more *good*. Ross says that Moore's modest proposal is the last in a long line of theories that say the right thing to do is determined by the outcomes it produces, or the "results." One sort of good result is what is good for the person making the decision. This self-interest is sometimes called "egoism," which Ross mentioned in his opening. The really important thing to note is that Ross absolutely rejects self-interest as a moral reason to do something. It might be useful or pragmatic, but it isn't acting "from a sense of rightness."

To the egoistic theory hedonistic utilitarianism supplies a much-needed amendment. It points out correctly that the fact that a certain pleasure will be enjoyed by the agent is no reason why he ought to bring it into being rather than an equal or greater pleasure to be enjoyed by another, though, human nature being what it is, it makes it not unlikely that he will try to bring it into being. But hedonistic utilitarianism in its turn needs a correction. On reflection it seems clear that pleasure is not the only thing in life that we think good in itself, that, for instance we think the possession of a good character, or an intelligent understanding of the world, as good or better. A great advance is made by the substitution of "productive of the greatest good" for "productive of the greatest pleasure."

Not only is this theory more attractive than hedonistic utilitarianism, but its logical relation to that theory is such that the latter could not be true unless it were true, while it might be true though hedonistic utilitarianism were not. It is in fact one of the logical bases of hedonistic utilitarianism. For the view that what produces the maximum pleasure is right has for its bases the views

- that what produces the maximum good is right, and
- that pleasure is the only thing good in itself.

If they were not assuming that what produces the maximum *good* is right, the utilitarians' attempt to show that pleasure is the only thing good in itself, which is in fact the point they take most pains to establish, would have been quite irrelevant to their attempt to prove that only what produces the maximum *pleasure* is right. If, therefore, it can be shown that productivity of the maximum good is not what makes all right actions right, we shall *a fortiori* have refuted hedonistic utilitarianism.

> Ross then rejects utilitarianism, which says what matters is not maximizing self-interest but the most pleasure for the greatest number of people. Each individual's pleasure matters, of course, but only as one tiny part of the overall pleasure of the greatest number of people. Why does Ross think utilitarianism is no better than egoism?

When a plain man fulfils a promise because he thinks he ought to do so, it seems clear that he does so with no thought of its total consequences, still less with any opinion that these are likely to be the best possible. He thinks in fact much more of the past than of the future. What makes him think it right to act in a certain way is the fact that he has promised to do so—that and, usually, nothing more. That his act will produce the best possible consequences is not his reason for calling it right. What lends color to the theory we are examining, then, is not the actions (which form probably a great majority of our actions) in which some such reflection as "I have promised" is the only reason we give ourselves for thinking a certain action right, but the exceptional cases in which the consequences of fulfilling a promise (for instance) would be so disastrous to others that we judge it right not to do so. It must of course be admitted that such cases exist. If I have promised to meet a friend at a particular time for some trivial purpose, I should certainly think myself justified in breaking my engagement if by doing so I could prevent a serious accident or bring relief to the victims of one. And the supporters of the view we are examining hold that my thinking so is due to my thinking that I shall bring more good into existence by the one action than by the other.

> Ross thinks promises are the best example of why right actions are not about consequences, results, or outcomes. Keeping a promise is a right action because we have a duty to fulfill our promises. What happens when breaking our promise will save someone's life? Ross addresses this sort of objection below.

A different account may, however, be given of the matter, an account which will, I believe, show itself to be the true one. It may be said that besides the duty of fulfilling promises I have and recognize a duty of relieving distress,[2] and that when I think it right to do the latter at the cost of not doing the former, it is not because I think I shall produce more good thereby but because I think it the duty which is in the circumstances more of a duty. This account surely corresponds much more closely with what we really think in such a situation. If, so far as I can see, I could bring equal amounts of good into being by fulfilling my promise and by helping someone to whom I had made no promise, I should not hesitate to regard the former as my duty. Yet on the view that what is right is right because it is productive of the most good I should not so regard it.

There are two theories, each in its way simple, that offer a solution of such cases of conscience. One is the view of [Immanuel] Kant [1724-1804], that there are certain duties of perfect obligation, such as those of fulfilling promises, of paying debts, of telling the truth, which admit of no exception whatever in favour of duties of imperfect obligation, such as that of relieving distress. The other is the view of, for instance, Professor Moore and Dr. [Hastings] Rashdall [1858-1924], that there is only the duty of producing good, and that all "conflicts of duties" should be resolved by asking "by which action will most good be produced?" But it is more important that our theory fit the facts than that it be simple, and the account we have given above corresponds (it seems to me) better than either of the simpler theories with what we really think, viz. that normally promise-keeping, for example, should come before benevolence, but that when and only when the good to be produced by the benevolent act is very great and the promise comparatively trivial, the act of benevolence becomes our duty.

In fact the theory of "ideal utilitarianism," if I may for brevity refer so to the theory of Professor Moore, seems to simplify unduly our relations to our fellows. It says, in effect, that the only morally significant relation in which my neighbours stand to me is that of being possible beneficiaries by my action.[3] They do stand in this relation to me, and this relation is morally significant. But they may also stand to me in the relation of promisee to promiser, of creditor to debtor, of wife to husband, of child to parent, of friend to friend, of fellow countryman to fellow countryman, and the like; and each of these relations is the foundation of a *prima facie* duty, which is more or less incumbent on me according to the circumstances of the case.

> The problem, Ross says, with theories that center on results or conse-
> quences is that they make our relationships with others one-dimension-
> al. Everyone is a potential beneficiary of my actions, and that's it. If we
> accept the idea of prima facie duties, however, we have a much richer,
> more varied set of relationships. This is why Ross thinks we should buy
> into his theory.

When I am in a situation, as perhaps I always am, in which more than one of these *prima facie* duties is incumbent on me, what I have to do is to study the situation as fully as I can until I form the considered opinion (it is never more) that in the circumstances one of them is more incumbent than any other; then I am bound to think that to do this *prima facie* duty is my duty *sans phrase* [i.e., simply put] in the situation.

I suggest *"prima facie* duty" or "conditional duty" as a brief way of referring to the characteristic (quite distinct from that of being a duty proper) which an act has, in virtue of being of a certain kind (e.g., the keeping of a promise), of being an act which would be a duty proper if it were not at the same time of another kind which is morally significant. Whether an act is a duty proper or actual duty depends on *all* the morally significant kinds it is an instance of....

There is nothing arbitrary about these *prima facie* duties. Each rests on a definite circumstance which cannot seriously be held to be without moral signif-icance. Of *prima facie* duties I suggest, without claiming completeness or finality for it, the following division.[4]

1. Some duties rest on previous acts of my own. These duties seem to include two kinds,

    a. those resting on a promise or what may fairly be called an implicit promise, such as the implicit undertaking not to tell lies which seems to be implied in the act of entering into conversation (at any rate by civilized men), or of writing books that purport to be history and not fiction. These may be called the duties of fidelity.

    b. Those resting on a previous wrongful act. These may be called the duties of reparation.

2. Some rest on previous acts of other men, i.e., services done by them to me. These may be loosely described as the duties of gratitude.[5]

3. Some rest on the fact or possibility of a distribution of pleasure or happiness (or of the means thereto) which is not in accordance with the merit of the persons concerned; in such cases there arises a duty to upset or prevent such a distribution. These are the duties of justice.

4. Some rest on the mere fact that there are beings in the world whose condition we can make better in respect of virtue, or of intelligence, or of pleasure. These are the duties of beneficence.

5. Some rest on the fact that we can improve our own condition in respect of virtue or of intelligence. These are the duties of self-improvement.

6. I think that we should distinguish from (4) the duties that may be summed up under the title of "not injuring others." No doubt to injure others is incidentally to fail to do them good; but it seems to me clear that non-maleficence is apprehended as a duty distinct from that of beneficence, and as a duty of a more stringent character.

To see how relevant Ross's list is to bioethics, notice that we can find almost every ethical duty between providers and patients in his list: (1) medical providers have a duty to keep their promises to patients, and vice versa; (2) if a physician has a duty to repair things when they do something wrong like make a mistake in surgery, they have a duty to disclose their error; (3) providers have a duty to treat patients fairly ("not in accordance with the merit of the persons"); (4) providers have a duty to make patients better if they can; (5) a patient may have a duty to comply with a doctor's recommendations because doing so will make the patient improve their situation; and (6) the duty to "do no harm to patients" is different from and stronger than the duty to "do patients good."

It will be noticed that this alone among the types duty [*sic*] has been stated in a negative way. An attempt might no doubt be made to state this duty, like the others, in a positive way. It might be said that it is really the duty to prevent ourselves from acting either from an inclination to harm others or from an inclination to seek our own pleasure, in doing which we should incidentally harm them. But on reflection it seems clear that the primary duty here is the duty not to harm others, this being a duty whether or not we have an inclination that if followed would lead to our harming them; and that when we have such an inclination the primary duty not to harm others gives rise to a consequential duty to resist the inclination. The recognition of this duty of non-maleficence is the first step on the way to the recognition of the duty of beneficence; and that accounts for the prominence of the commands

"thou shalt not kill,"
"thou shalt not commit adultery,"
"thou shalt not steal,"
"thou shalt not bear false witness,"

in so early a code as the Decalogue. But even when we have come to recognize the duty of beneficence, it appears to me that the duty of non-maleficence is recognized as a distinct one, and as *prima facie* more binding. We should not in general consider it justifiable to kill one person in order to keep another alive, or to steal from one in order to give alms to another.

The essential defect of the "ideal utilitarian" theory is that it ignores, or at least does not do full justice to, the highly personal character of duty. If the only duty is to produce the maximum of good, the question who is to have the good—whether it is myself, or my benefactor, or a person to whom I have made a promise to confer that good on him, or a mere fellow man to whom I stand in no such special relation—should make no difference to my having a duty to produce that good. But we are all in fact sure that it makes a vast difference.

> Ross really emphasizes the importance of "First, do no harm." He thinks it is important to see this duty as separate from the duty to do good. Why does he think this? Which duty does he see as more important: "do no harm" or "do good"? Do you agree?

One or two other comments must be made on this provisional list of the divisions of duty....

It may, again, be objected that our theory that there are these various and often conflicting types of *prima facie* duty leaves us with no principle upon which to discern what is our actual duty in particular circumstances. But this objection is not one which the rival theory is in a position to bring forward. For when we have to choose between the production of two heterogeneous goods, say knowledge and pleasure, the "ideal utilitarian" theory can only fall back on an opinion, for which no logical basis can be offered, that one of the goods is the greater; and this is no better than a similar opinion that one of two duties is the more urgent. And again, when we consider the infinite variety of the effects of our actions in the way of pleasure, it must surely be admitted that the claim which *hedonism* sometimes makes, that it offers a readily applicable criterion of right conduct, is quite illusory.

I am unwilling, however, to content myself with an **argumentum ad hominem**, and I would contend that in principle there is no reason to anticipate that every act that is our duty is so for one and the same reason. Why should two sets of circumstances, or one set of circumstances, not possess different characteristics, any one of which makes a certain act our *prima facie* duty? When I ask what it is that makes me in certain cases sure that I have a *prima facie* duty to do so and so, I find that it lies in the fact that I have made a promise; when I ask the same question in another case, I find the answer lies in the fact that I have done a wrong. And if on reflection I find (as I think I do) that neither of these reasons is reducible to the other, I must not on any *a priori* ground assume that such a reduction is possible....

It is necessary to say something by way of clearing up the relation between *prima facie* duties and the actual or absolute duty to do one particular act in particular circumstances. If, as almost all moralists except Kant are agreed, and as most plain men think, it is sometimes right to tell a lie or to break a promise, it must be maintained that there is a difference between *prima facie* duty and actual or absolute duty. When we think ourselves justified in breaking, and indeed morally obliged to break, a promise in order to relieve someone's distress, we do not for a moment cease to recognize a *prima facie* duty to keep our promise, and this leads us to feel, not indeed shame or repentance, but certainly compunction, for behaving as we do; we recognize, further, that it is our duty to make up somehow to the promisee for the breaking of the promise. We have to distinguish from the characteristic of being our duty that of tending to be our duty. Any act that we do contains various elements in virtue of which it falls under various categories. In virtue of being the breaking of a promise, for instance, it tends to be wrong; in virtue of being an instance of relieving distress it tends to be right....

Our judgements about our actual duty in concrete situations have none of the certainty that attaches to our recognition of the general principles of duty. A statement is certain, i.e., is an expression of knowledge, only in one or other of two cases: when it is either self-evident, or a valid conclusion from self-evident premises. And our judgements about our particular duties have neither of these characters. (1) They are not self-evident. Where a possible act is seen to have two characteristics, in virtue of one of which it is *prima facie* right, and in virtue of the other *prima-facie* wrong, we are (I think) well aware that we are not certain whether we ought or ought not to do it; that whether we do it or not, we are taking a moral risk. We come in the long run, after consideration, to think one duty more pressing than the other, but we do not feel certain that it is so. And though we do not always recognize that a possible act has two such characteristics, and though there may be cases in which it has not, we are never certain that any particular possible act has not, and therefore never certain that it is right, nor certain that it is wrong. For, to go no further in the analysis, it is enough to point out that any particular act will in all probability in the course of time contribute to the bringing about of good or of evil for many human beings, and thus have a *prima facie* rightness or wrongness of which we know nothing. (2) Again, our judgements about our particular duties are not logical conclusions from self-evident premises. The only possible premisses [sic] would be the general principles stating their *prima facie* rightness or wrongness *qua* having the different characteristics they do have; and even if we could (as we cannot) apprehend the extent to which an act will tend on the one hand, for example, to bring about advantages for our benefactors, and on the other hand to bring about disadvantages for fellow men who are not our benefactors, there is no principle by which we can draw the conclusion that it is on the whole right or on the whole wrong. In this respect the judgement as to the rightness of a particular act is just like the judgement as to the beauty of a particular natural object or work of art. A poem is, for instance, in respect of certain qualities beautiful and in respect of certain others not beautiful; and our judgement as to the degree of beauty it possesses on the whole is never reached by logical reasoning from the apprehension of its particular beauties or particular defects. Both in this and in the moral case we have more or less probable opinions which are not logically justified conclusions from the general principles that are recognized as self-evident.

There is therefore much truth in the description of the right act as a fortunate act. If we cannot be certain that it is right, it is our good fortune if the act we do is the right act. This consideration does not, however, make the doing of our duty a mere matter of chance. There is a parallel here between the doing of duty and the doing of what will be to our personal advantage. We never *know* what act will in the long run be to our advantage. Yet it is certain that we are more likely in general to secure our advantage if we estimate to the best of our ability the probable tendencies of our actions in this respect, than if we act on caprice. And similarly we are more likely to do our duty if we reflect to the best of our ability on the *prima facie* rightness or wrongness of various possible acts in virtue of the characteristics we perceive them to have, than if we act without reflection. With this greater likelihood we must be content.

Many people would be inclined to say that the right act for me is not that whose general nature I have been describing, viz. that which if I were omniscient I should see to be my duty, but that which on all the evidence available to me I should think to be my duty. But suppose that from the state of partial knowledge in which I think act A to be my duty, I could pass to a state of perfect knowledge in which I saw act B to be my duty, should I not say "act B was the right act for me to do"? I should no doubt add "though I am not to be blamed for doing act A." But in adding this, am I not passing from the question "what is right" to the question "what is morally good"? At the same time I am not making the *full* passage from the one notion to the other; for in order that the act should be morally good, or an act I am not to be blamed for doing, it must not merely be the act which it is reasonable for me to think my duty; it must also be done for that reason, or from some other morally good motive. Thus the conception of the right act as the act which it is reasonable for me to think my duty is an unsatisfactory compromise between the true notion of the right act and the notion of the morally good action.

The general principles of duty are obviously not self-evident from the beginning of our lives. How do they come to be so? The answer is, that they come to be self-evident to us just as mathematical axioms do. We find by experience that this couple of matches and that couple make four matches, that this couple of balls on a wire and that couple make four balls: and by reflection on these and similar discoveries we come to see that it is of the nature of two and two to make four. In a precisely similar way, we see the *prima facie* rightness of an act which would be the fulfilment of a particular promise, and of another which would be the fulfilment of another promise, and when we have reached sufficient maturity to think in general terms, we apprehend *prima facie* rightness to belong to the nature of any fulfilment of promise. What comes first in time is the apprehension of the self-evident *prima facie* rightness of an individual act of a particular type. From this we come by reflection to apprehend the self-evident general principle of *prima facie* duty. From this, too, perhaps along with the apprehension of the self-evident *prima facie* rightness of the same act in virtue of its having another characteristic as well, and perhaps in spite of the apprehension of its *prima facie* wrongness in virtue of its having some third characteristic, we come to believe something not self-evident at all, but an object of probable opinion, viz. that this particular act is (not *prima facie* but) actually right....

Notes

1.   I take the theory which, as I have tried to show, seems to be put forward in *Ethics* rather than the earlier and less plausible theory put forward in *Principia Ethica*....

2.   These are not strictly speaking duties, but things that tend to be our duty, or *prima facie* duties....

3.   Some will think it, apart from other considerations, a sufficient refutation of this view to point out that I also stand in that relation to myself, so that for this view the distinction of oneself from others is morally insignificant.

4.   I should make it plain at this stage that I am *assuming* the correctness of some of our main convictions as to *prima facie* duties, or, more strictly, am claiming that we know them to be true. To me it seems as self-evident as anything could be, that to make a promise, for instance, is to create a moral claim on us in someone else. Many readers will perhaps say that they do not know this to be true. If so, I certainly cannot prove it to them; I can only ask them to reflect again, in the hope that they will ultimately agree that they also know it to be true. The main moral conviction of the plain man seem [*sic*] to me to be, not opinions which it is for philosophy to prove or disprove, but knowledge from the start; and in my own case I seem to find little difficulty in distinguishing these essential convictions from other moral convictions which I also have, which are merely fallible opinions based on an imperfect study of the working for good or evil of certain institutions or types of action.

5.   For a needed correction of this statement, cf. pp. 22–23 [of *The Right and the Good*, the 1930 book by Ross from which this extract is taken].

Reading 1.2: John Stuart Mill, from *Utilitarianism*

One of the biggest criticisms of Ross's prima facie duties is that they do not give us any way to decide when duties conflict. Ross does say that some of these duties will trump others, but he does not actually give us a system for deciding when one prima facie duty trumps another. Does Ross's pluralistic ethics really help us resolve dilemmas? We turn now to a monist response to this problem. Monists like J.S. Mill argue that their way is better because all dilemmas are resolvable in terms of one value. If all goodness is reducible to one value, then all dilemmas are resolvable.

There must be some standard by which to determine the goodness or badness, absolute and comparative, of ends, or objects of desire. And whatever that standard is, there can be but one; for if there were several ultimate principles of conduct, the same conduct might be approved by one of those principles and condemned by another; and there would be needed some more general principle, as umpire between them.

Accordingly, writers on Moral Philosophy have mostly felt the necessity not only of referring all rules of conduct, and all judgments of praise and blame, to principles, but of referring them to some one principle; some rule, or standard, with which all other rules of conduct were required to be consistent, and from which by ultimate consequence they could all be deduced. Those who have dispensed with the assumption of such a universal standard, have only been enabled to do so by supposing that a moral sense, or instinct, inherent in our constitution, informs us, both what principles of conduct we are bound to observe, and also in what order these should be subordinated to one another.

In the next section, notice that Mill doesn't argue for what he calls the greatest happiness principle (we should do whatever action produces the most amount of happiness for the most number of people, embraced by utilitarians). He does that elsewhere. Rather, he argues that this principle is the one value to which all other values can be reduced. He admits that virtue is a worthy goal, but what makes it worthy is that it produces utility.

Without attempting in this place to justify my opinion, or even to define the kind of justification which it admits of, I merely declare my conviction, that the general principle to which all rules of practice ought to conform, and the test by which they should be tried, is that of conduciveness to the happiness of mankind, or rather, of all sentient beings; in other words, that the promotion of happiness is the ultimate principle of Teleology.

I do not mean to assert that the promotion of happiness should be itself the end of all actions, or even of all rules of action. It is the justification, and ought to be the controller, of all ends, but it is not itself the sole end. There are many virtuous actions, and even virtuous modes of action (though the cases are, I think, less frequent than is often supposed), by which happiness in the particular instance is sacrificed, more pain being produced than pleasure. But conduct of which this can be truly asserted, admits of justification only because it can be shown that, on the whole, more happiness will exist in the world, if feelings are cultivated which will make people, in certain cases, regardless of happiness. I fully admit that this is true; that the cultivation of an ideal nobleness of will and conduct should be to individual human beings an end, to which the specific pursuit either of their own happiness or of that of others (except so far as included in that idea) should, in any case of conflict, give way. But I hold that the very question, what constitutes this elevation of character, is itself to be decided by a reference to happiness as the standard. The character itself should be, to the individual, a paramount end, simply because the existence of this ideal nobleness of character, or of a near approach to it, in any abundance, would go farther than all things else toward making human life happy, both in the comparatively humble sense of pleasure and freedom from pain, and in the higher meaning, of rendering life, not what it now is almost universally, puerile and insignificant, but such as human beings with highly developed faculties can care to have.

In the next section, Mill addresses the sort of moral laws Ross mentioned in the previous reading. Why does Mill think his one moral law (utility) is better than relying on several moral laws "all claiming independent authority"?

There exists no moral system under which there do not arise unequivocal cases of conflicting obligation. These are the real difficulties, the knotty points both in the theory of ethics, and in the conscientious guidance of personal conduct. They are overcome practically, with greater or with less success, according to the intellect and virtue of the individual; but it can hardly be pretended that any one will be the less qualified for dealing with them, from possessing an ultimate standard to which conflicting rights and duties can be referred. If utility is the ultimate source of moral obligations, utility may be invoked to decide between them when their demands are incompatible. Though the application of the standard may be difficult, it is better than none at all: while in other systems, the moral laws all claiming independent authority, there is no common umpire entitled to interfere between them; their claims to precedence one over another rest on little better than sophistry, and unless determined, as they generally are, by the unacknowledged influence of considerations of utility, afford a free scope for the action of personal desires and partialities. We must remember that only in these cases of conflict between secondary principles is it requisite that first principles should be appealed to. There is no case of moral obligation in which some secondary principle is not involved; and if only one, there can seldom be any real doubt which one it is, in the mind of any person by whom the principle itself is recognised.

If the preceding analysis, or something resembling it, be not the correct account of the notion of justice; if justice be totally independent of utility, and be a standard per se, which the mind can recognise by simple introspection of itself; it is hard to understand why that internal oracle is so ambiguous, and why so many things appear either just or unjust, according to the light in which they are regarded.

We are continually informed that Utility is an uncertain standard, which every different person interprets differently, and that there is no safety but in the immutable, ineffaceable, and unmistakable dictates of justice, which carry their evidence in themselves, and are independent of the fluctuations of opinion. One would suppose from this that on questions of justice there could be no controversy; that if we take that for our rule, its application to any given case could leave us in as little doubt as a mathematical demonstration. So far is this from being the fact, that there is as much difference of opinion, and as much discussion, about what is just, as about what is useful to society. Not only have different nations and individuals different notions of justice, but in the mind of one and the same individual, justice is not some one rule, principle, or maxim, but many, which do not always coincide in their dictates, and in choosing between which, he is guided either by some extraneous standard, or by his own personal predilections....

Who shall decide between these appeals to conflicting principles of justice? Justice has in this case two sides to it, which it is impossible to bring into harmony, and the two disputants have chosen opposite sides; the one looks to what it is just that the individual should receive, the other to what it is just that the community should give. Each, from his own point of view, is unanswerable; and any choice between them, on grounds of justice, must be perfectly arbitrary. Social utility alone can decide the preference ...

> Mill now turns to one of the strongest "moral laws," that of justice (people should get what they deserve), and shows that even that principle needs an ultimate grounding in utility. Why does he say that justice as a moral requirement has a "more absolute obligation" than other moral rules? How does this square with Mill's utilitarianism?

While I dispute the pretensions of any theory which sets up an imaginary standard of justice not grounded on utility, I account the justice which is grounded on utility to be the chief part, and incomparably the most sacred and binding part, of all morality. Justice is a name for certain classes of moral rules, which concern the essentials of human well-being more nearly, and are therefore of more absolute obligation, than any other rules for the guidance of life; and the notion which we have found to be of the essence of the idea of justice, that of a right residing in an individual implies and testifies to this more binding obligation. The moral rules which forbid mankind to hurt one another (in which we must never forget to include wrongful interference with each other's freedom) are more vital to human well-being than any maxims, however important, which only point out the best mode of managing some department of human affairs. They have also the peculiarity, that they are the main element in determining the whole of the social feelings of mankind. It is their observance which alone preserves peace among human beings: if obedience to them were not the rule, and disobedience the exception, every one would see in every one else an enemy, against whom he must be perpetually guarding himself. What is hardly less important, these are the precepts which mankind have the strongest and the most direct inducements for impressing upon one another. By merely giving to each other prudential instruction or exhortation, they may gain, or think they gain, nothing: in inculcating on each other the duty of positive beneficence they have an unmistakable interest, but far less in degree: a person may possibly not need the benefits of others; but he always needs that they should not do him hurt. Thus the moralities which protect every individual from being harmed by others, either directly or by being hindered in his freedom of pursuing his own good, are at once those which he himself has most at heart, and those which he has the strongest interest in publishing and enforcing by word and deed. It is by a person's observance of these that his fitness to exist as one of the fellowship of human beings is tested and decided; for on that depends his being a nuisance or not to those with whom he is in contact. Now it is these moralities primarily which compose the obligations of justice. The most marked cases of injustice, and those which give the tone to the feeling of repugnance which characterises the sentiment, are acts of wrongful aggression, or wrongful exercise of power over someone; the next are those which consist in wrongfully withholding from him something which is his due; in both cases, inflicting on him a positive hurt, either in the form of direct suffering, or of the privation of some good which he had reasonable ground, either of a physical or of a social kind, for counting upon....

It appears from what has been said, that justice is a name for certain moral requirements, which, regarded collectively, stand higher in the scale of social utility, and are therefore of more paramount obligation, than any others; though particular cases may occur in which some other social duty is so important, as to overrule any one of the general maxims of justice. Thus, to save a life, it may not only be allowable, but a duty, to steal, or take by force, the necessary food or medicine, or to kidnap, and compel to officiate, the only qualified medical practitioner. In such cases, as we do not call anything justice which is not a virtue, we usually say, not that justice must give way to some other moral principle, but that what is just in ordinary cases is, by reason of that other principle, not just in the particular case. By this useful accommodation of language, the character of indefeasibility attributed to justice is kept up, and we are saved from the necessity of maintaining that there can be laudable injustice.

Justice remains the appropriate name for certain social utilities which are vastly more important, and therefore more absolute and imperative, than any others are as a class (though not more so than others may be in particular cases); and which, therefore, ought to be, as well as naturally are, guarded by a sentiment not only different in degree, but also in kind; distinguished from the milder feeling which attaches to the mere idea of promoting human pleasure or convenience, at once by the more definite nature of its commands, and by the sterner character of its sanctions.

Reading 1.3: Stephen Toulmin, "How Medicine Saved the Life of Ethics"

Philosopher Stephen Toulmin argues that bioethics changed the trends in moral philosophy for the better. As you read, ask yourself what the strengths and faults of bioethics are as moral reasoning, according to Toulmin. (Numbers in brackets are keyed to the list of references at the end of the reading.)

... The new attention to applied ethics (particularly medical ethics) has done much to dispel the miasma of subjectivity that was cast around ethics as a result of its association with anthropology and psychology. At least within broad limits, an ethics of "needs" and "interests" is objective and generalizable in a way that an ethics of "wishes" and "attitudes" cannot be. Stated crudely, the question of whether one person's actions put another person's health at risk is normally a question of ascertainable fact, to which there is a straightforward "yes" or "no" answer, not a question of fashion, custom, or taste, about which (as the saying goes) "there is no arguing." This being so, the objections to that person's actions can be presented and discussed in "objective" terms. So, proper attention to the example of medicine has helped to pave the way for a reintroduction of "objective" standards of good and harm and for a return to methods of practical reasoning about moral issues that are not available to either the dogmatists or the relativists.

Before you move on to the next paragraph, can you summarize Toulmin's thesis?

... Let me here mention one of these, which comes out of my own personal experience. From 1975 to 1978 I worked as a consultant and staff member with the National Commission for the Protection of Human Subjects of Biomedical and Behavioral Research, based in Washington, DC; I was struck by the extent to which the commissioners were able to reach agreement in making recommendations about ethical issues of great complexity and delicacy.[1] If the earlier theorists had been right, and ethical considerations really depended on variable cultural attitudes or labile personal feelings, one would have expected 11 people of such different backgrounds as the members of the commission to be far more divided over such moral questions than they ever proved to be in actual fact. Even on such thorny subjects as research involving prisoners, mental patients, and human fetuses, it did not take the commissioners long to identify the crucial issues that they needed to address, and, after patient analysis of these issues, any residual differences of opinion were rarely more than marginal, with different commissioners inclined to be somewhat more conservative, or somewhat more liberal, in their recommendations. Never, as I recall, did their deliberations end in deadlock, with supporters of rival principles locking horns and refusing to budge. The problems that had to be argued through at length arose, not on the level of the principles themselves, but at the point of applying them: when difficult moral balances had to be struck between, for example, the general claims of medical discovery and its future beneficiaries and the present welfare or autonomy of individual research subjects.

How was the commission's consensus possible? It rested precisely on this last feature of their agenda: namely, its close concentration on specific types of problematic cases. Faced with "hard cases," they inquired what particular conflicts of claim or interest were exemplified in them, and they usually ended by balancing off those claims in very similar ways. Only when the individual members of the commission went on to explain their own particular "reasons" for supporting the general consensus did they begin to go seriously different ways. For, then, commissioners from different backgrounds and faiths "justified" their votes by appealing to general views and abstract principles which differed far more deeply than their opinions about particular substantive questions. Instead of "deducing" their opinions about particular cases from general principles that could lend strength and conviction to those specific opinions, they showed a far greater certitude about particular cases than they ever achieved about general matters.

This outcome of the commission's work should not come as any great surprise to physicians who have reflected deeply about the nature of clinical judgment in medicine. In traditional case morality, as in medical practice, the first indispensable step is to assemble a rich enough "case history." Until that has been done, the wise physician will suspend judgment. If he is too quick to let theoretical considerations influence his clinical analysis, they may prejudice the collection of a full and accurate case record and so distract him from what later turn out to have been crucial clues. Nor would this outcome have been any surprise to Aristotle, either. Ethics and clinical medicine are both prime examples of the concrete fields of thought and reasoning in which (as he insisted) the theoretical rigor of geometrical argument is unattainable: fields in which we should above all strive to be *reasonable* rather than insisting on a kind of exactness that "the nature of the case" does not allow [5, 1.3.1094b12–27].

In this next section, Toulmin is worried about the reputation casuistry has acquired as a check on priniciplism. Does his defense of taking each ethical dilemma on a case-by-case basis sound compelling to you? Why or why not?

This same understanding of the differences between practical and theoretical reasoning was taken over by [thirteenth-century philosopher Thomas] Aquinas, who built it into his own account of "natural law" and "case morality," and so it became part of the established teaching of Catholic moral theologians. As such, it was in harmony with the pastoral practices of the confessional [12, D.3, Q.5, A.2, Solutio]. Thus, Aquinas's own version of the fundamental maxim was framed as an injunction to the confessor—"like a prudent physician"—to take into account *peccatoris circumstantiae atque peccati*, that is, "the circumstances both of the sinner and of the sin." Later, however, the alleged readiness of confessors to soften their judgments in the light of irrelevant "circumstances" exposed them to criticism. In particular, the seventeenth-century French Jesuits were attacked by their Jansenist coreligionists on the ground that they "made allowances" in favor of rich and high-born penitents that they denied to those who were less well favored. And, when the Jansenist [Antoine] Arnauld [1612–94] was brought before an ecclesiastical court on a charge of heterodoxy, his friend [Blaise] Pascal [1623–62] launched a vigorous counterattack on the Jesuit casuists of his time by publishing the series of anonymous *Lettres provinciales* which from that time on gave "casuistry" its unsavory reputation.[2]

Looking back, however, we may wonder how far this reputation was really justified. No doubt, a venal priest could corrupt the confessional by showing undue favor to penitents of wealth or power: for example, by fabricating specious "extenuating circumstances" to excuse conduct that was basically inexcusable. But we have no reliable way of knowing how often this really happened, and the mere possibility of such corruption does nothing to change the original point—namely, that practical decisions in ethics can never be made by appeal to "self-evident principles" alone and rest rather on a clinical appreciation of the significant details characteristic of particular cases. No doubt, we are free to use the word "casuistry"—like the parallel words "wizardry" and "sophistry"—to refer to "the *dishonest* use of the casuist's (or the clinician's) arts,"[3] but that does no more to discredit the honest use of "case morality" than it does the honest use of case methods in clinical medicine.

By taking one step further, indeed, we may view the problems of clinical medicine and the problems of applied ethics as two varieties of a common species. Defined in purely general terms, such ethical categories as "cruelty" and "kindness," "laziness" and "conscientiousness," have a certain abstract, truistical quality: before they can acquire any specific relevance, we have to identify some *actual* person, or piece of conduct, as "kind" or "cruel," "conscientious" or "lazy," and there is often disagreement even about that preliminary step. Similarly, in medicine: if described in general terms alone, diseases too are "abstract entities," and they acquire a practical relevance only for those who have learned the diagnostic art of identifying real-life cases as being cases of one disease rather than another.

In its form (if not entirely in its point) the *art* of practical judgment in ethics thus resembles the art of clinical diagnosis and prescription. In both fields, theoretical generalities are helpful to us only up to a point, and their actual application to particular cases demands, also, a human capacity to recognize the slight but significant features that mark off, say, a "case" of minor muscular strain from a life-threatening disease or a "case" of decent reticence from one of cowardly silence. Once brought to the bedside, so to say, applied ethics and clinical medicine use just the same Aristotelean kinds of "practical reasoning," and a correct choice of therapeutic procedure in medicine is the *right* treatment to pursue, not just as a matter of medical technique but for ethical reasons also.

> Toulmin thinks that ethical reasoning about bioethics is very much like the way in which doctors diagnose and treat illnesses. This was a point made in the introduction. This time it's not a doctor but a philosopher who makes this claim. Do you agree that deciding the right thing to do in a dilemma is similar to how a doctor decides the right way to treat an illness? Are there places where the analogy breaks down?

"My Station and Its Duties"

In the last decades of the nineteenth century, F.H. Bradley of Oxford University expounded an ethical position that placed "duties" in the center of the philosophical picture, and the recent concern of moral philosophers with applied ethics (most specifically, medical ethics) has given them a new insight into his arguments also.... [D]ifferent people are subject to different moral claims, depending on where they "stand" toward the other people with whom they have to deal, for example, their families, colleagues, and fellow citizens [13].

> Toulmin "name drops" F.H. Bradley's (1846–1924) concept of duties to make his point. Do you agree with the statement "Different people are subject to different moral claims depending on where they stand toward the other people they have to deal"?

For Bradley, that is to say, the central consideration in practical ethics was the agent's standing, status, or station.... As the modern discussion of medical ethics has taught us, professional affiliations and concerns play a significant part in shaping a physician's obligations and commitments, and this insight has stimulated detailed discussions both about professionalism in general and, more specifically, about the relevance of "the physician/patient relationship" to the medical practitioner's duties and obligations.[4]

Once embarked on, the subject of professionalism has proved to be rich and fruitful. It has led, for instance, to a renewed interest in Max Weber's [1864–1920] sociological analysis of vocation (*Beruf*) and bureaucracy, and this in turn has had implications of two kinds for the ethics of the professions. For, on the one hand, the manner in which professionals perceive their position as providers of services influences both their sense of calling and also the obligations which they acknowledge on that account. And, on the other hand, the professionalization of medicine, law, and similar activities has exposed practitioners to new conflicts of interest between, for example, the individual physician's duties to a patient and his loyalty to the profession, as when his conduct is criticized as "unprofessional" for harming, not his clients, but rather his colleagues.

In recent years, as a result, moral philosophers have begun to look specifically and in greater detail at the situations within which ethical problems typically arise and to pay closer attention to the human relationships that are embodied in those situations. In ethics, as elsewhere, the tradition of radical

individualism for too long encouraged people to overlook the "mediating structures" and "intermediate institutions" (family, profession, voluntary associations, etc.) which stand between the individual agent and the larger scale
context of his actions....

"Intermediate institutions" (i.e., neither the government nor the individual): hospitals, research facilities, and international organizations like the
World Health Organization would count as these sorts of institutions.

On this alternative view, the only just—even, properly speaking, the only
moral—obligations are those that apply to us all equally, regardless of our standing. By undertaking the tasks of a profession, an agent will no doubt accept certain special duties, but so it will be for us all. The obligation to perform those
duties is "just" or "moral" only because it exemplifies more general and univer-
salizable obligations of trust, which require us to do what we have undertaken
to do. So, any exclusive emphasis on the universal aspects of morality can end
by distracting attention from just those things which the student of applied
ethics finds most absorbing—namely, the specific tasks and obligations that any
proession lays on its practitioners.

Think about your own profession (or future profession). There are certainly ethical codes in any profession. What about the ethics of implementing technology like stem cell or abortion? What happens when our
professional duties clash with our universal moral demands? Which ones
win out?

Most recently, Alasdair MacIntyre [b. 1929] has pursued these considerations further in his new book, *After Virtue* [16]. MacIntyre argues that the public
discussion of ethical issues has fallen into a kind of Babel, which largely springs
from our losing any sense of the ways in which *community* creates obligations
for us. One thing that can help restore that lost sense of community is the recognition that, at the present time, our professional commitments have taken on
many of the roles that our communal commitments used to play. Even people
who find moral philosophy generally unintelligible usually acknowledge and
respect the specific ethical demands associated with their own professions or

jobs, and this offers us some kind of a foundation on which to begin reconstructing our view of ethics. For it reminds us that we are in no position to fashion individual lives for ourselves, purely as *individuals*. Rather, we find ourselves born into communities in which the available ways of acting are largely laid out in advance: in which human activity takes on different *Lebensformen*, or "forms of life" (of which the professions are one special case), and our obligations are shaped by the requirements of those forms.

In this respect, the lives and obligations of professionals are no different from those of their lay brethren. Professional obligations arise out of the enterprises of the professions in just the same kinds of way that other general moral obligations arise out of our shared forms of life; if we are at odds about the *theory* of ethics, that is because we have misunderstood the basis which ethics has in our actual *practice*. Once again, in other words, it was medicine—as the first profession to which philosophers paid close attention during the new phase of "applied ethics" that opened during the 1960s—that set the example which was required in order to revive some important, and neglected, lines of argument within moral philosophy itself.

Equity and Intimacy

Two final themes have also attracted special attention as a result of the new interaction between medicine and philosophy. Both themes were presented in clear enough terms by Aristotle in the *Nicomachean Ethics*. But, as so often happens, the full force of Aristotle's concepts and arguments was overlooked by subsequent generations of philosophers, who came to ethics with very different preoccupations. Aristotle's own Greek terms for these notions are *epieikeia* and *philia*, which are commonly translated as "reasonableness" and "friendship," but I shall argue here that they correspond more closely to the modern terms, "equity" and "personal relationship" [5].

Modern readers sometimes have difficulty with the style of Aristotle's *Ethics* and lose patience with the book, because they suspect the author of evading philosophical questions that they have their own reasons for regarding as central. Suppose, for instance, that we go to Aristotle's text in the hope of finding some account of the things that mark off "right" from "wrong": if we attempt to press this question, Aristotle will always slip out of our grasp. What makes one course of action better than another? We can answer that question, he replies, only if we first consider what kind of a person the agent is and what relationships he stands in toward the other people who are involved in his actions; he sets about explaining why the kinds of relationship, and the kinds of conduct, that are possible as between "large-spirited human beings" who share the same social standing are simply not possible as between, say, master and servant, or parent and child [5].

The bond of *philia* between free and equal friends is of one kind, that between father and son of another kind, that between master and slave of a third, and there is no common scale in which we can measure the corresponding kinds of conduct. By emphasizing this point, Aristotle draws attention to an important point about the manner in which "actions" are classified, even before we say anything ethical about them. Within two different relationships the very same deeds, or the very same words, may—from the ethical point of view—represent quite different *acts* or *actions*....

... For, surely, the very deed or utterance by Dr. A toward Mrs. B which would be a routine inquiry or examination within a strictly professional "physician–patient relationship"—for example, during a gynecological consultation—might be grounds for a claim of assault if performed outside that protected context.

> Removing a breathing tube is moral and legal if you are a doctor and someone authorized gives consent, but it is considered assisted suicide if not done by a medical professional. Can you think of other acts that would be immoral outside of a particular profession?

The *philia* (or relationship) between them will be quite different in the two situations, and, on this account, the "circumstances" do indeed "alter cases" in ways that are directly reflected in the demands of professional ethics.

With this as background, we can turn to Aristotle's ideas about *epieikeia* ("reasonableness" or "equity"). As to this notion, Aristotle pioneered the general doctrine that principles never settle ethical issues by themselves: that is, that we can grasp the moral force of principles only by studying the ways in which they are applied to, and within, particular situations. The need for such a practical approach is most obvious, in judicial practice, in the exercise of "equitable jurisdiction," where the courts are required to decide cases by appeal, not to specific, well-defined laws or statutes, but to general considerations of fairness, of "maxims of equity." In these situations, the courts do not have the benefit of carefully drawn rules, which have been formulated with the specific aim that they should be precise and self-explanatory: rather, they are guided by rough proverbial mottoes—phrases about "clean hands" and the like. The questions at issue in such cases are, in other words, very broad questions—for example, about what would be *just* or *reasonable* as between two or more individuals when all the available facts about their respective situations have been taken into account [17–19]. Similar patterns of situations and arguments are, of course, to be found in everyday ethics also, and the Aristotelean idea of *epieikeia* is a direct intellectual ancestor of a central notion (still referred to as "epikeia") in the Roman Catholic traditions of moral theology and pastoral care [11].

... [The] demand for intelligent discussion of the ethical problems of medical practice and research obliged them to pay fresh attention to applied ethics, however philosophers found their subject "coming alive again" under their hands. But, now it was no longer a field for academic, theoretical, even mandarin investigation alone. Instead, it had to be debated in practical, concrete, even political terms, and before long moral philosophers (or, as they barbarously began to be called, "ethicists")5 found that they were as liable as the economists to be called on to write "op ed" pieces for the *New York Times*, or to testify before congressional committees.

Have philosophers wholly risen to this new occasion? Have they done enough to modify their previous methods of analysis to meet these new practical needs? About those questions there can still be several opinions. Certainly, it would be foolhardy to claim that the discussion of "bioethics" has reached a definitive form, or to rule out the possibility that novel methods will earn a place in the field in the years ahead. At this very moment, indeed, the style of current discussion appears to be shifting away from attempts to relate problematic cases to general theories—whether those of Kant, [John] Rawls [1921–2002], or the utilitarians—to a more direct analysis of the practical cases themselves, using methods more like those of traditional "case morality." (See, e.g., the discussion in a recent issue of the *Hastings Center Report* of the moral issues that are liable to arise in cases of sex-change surgery [23, pp. 8–13].)

Whatever the future may bring, however, these 20 years of interaction with medicine, law, and the other professions have had spectacular and irreversible effects on the methods and content of philosophical ethics. By reintroducing into ethical debate the vexed topics raised by *particular* cases, they have obliged philosophers to address once again the Aristotelean problems of *practical reasoning*, which had been on the sidelines for too long. In this sense, we may indeed say that, during the last 20 years, medicine has "saved the life of ethics," and that it has given back to ethics a seriousness and human relevance which it had seemed—at least, in the writings of the interwar years—to have lost for good.

References [to this extract]

5. ARISTOTLE. *Nicomachean Ethics*.
11. JONSEN, A. R. Can an ethicist be a consultant? In *Frontiers in Medical Ethics*, edited by A. ABERNATHY. Cambridge: Bollingen, 1980.
12. AQUINAS, THOMAS. *Commentarium Libro Tertio Sententiarum*.
13. BRADLEY, F. *Ethical Studies*. London, 1876.
14. BLEDSTEIN, B. *The Culture of Professionalism*. New York: Norton, 1976.
16. MACINTYRE, A. *After Virtue*. South Bend, Ind.: Notre Dame Univ. Press, 1981.
17. DAVIS, K. *Discretionary justice*. Urbana: Univ. Illinois Press, 1969.
18. NEWMAN, R. *Equity and Law*. Dobbs Ferry, N.Y.: Oceana, 1961.
19. HAMBURGER, M. *Morals and Law: The Growth of Aristotle's Legal Theory*. New Haven, Conn.: Yale Univ. Press, 1951.
23. Marriage, morality and sex change surgery: four traditions in case ethics. *Hastings Cent. Rep.*, August 1981.

Notes

1. The work of the national commission generated a whole series of government publications—mainly reports and recommendations on the ethical aspects of research involving research subjects from specially "vulnerable" groups having diminished autonomy, such as young children and prisoners. I have written a fuller discussion of the commission's work for a forthcoming Hastings Center book on the "closure" of disputes about matters of technical policy. As a member of the commission, A.R. Jonsen was also struck by the casuistical character of its work, and this led to the research project of which this paper is one product.

2. The *Lettres provinciales* were published periodically, and anonymously, in 1656–57, but it did not take long for their authorship to be discovered, and they have remained perhaps the best-known documents on the subject of "case reasoning" in ethics. The intellectual relationship between the vigorous attack on the laxity of the Jesuits' case morality contained in the *Lettres* and the larger program of seventeenth-century philosophy deserves closer study than it has yet received.

3. For the word "casuistry," see the entry in the complete *Oxford English Dictionary*, which revealingly points out how many English nouns ending in "ry" (e.g., "sophistry," "wizardry," and "Popery") are dyslogistic. It seems to be no accident that the earliest use of the word "casuistry" cited in the OED dates only from 1725—i.e., after Pascal's attack on the Jesuit casuists. This helps to explain, and confirm, the current derogatory tone of the word.

4. See Bledstein's discussion [14, p. 107] of the nineteenth-century confusion between codes of ethics and codes of etiquette within such professional societies as the American Medical Association.

5. Once again, the *Oxford English Dictionary* has a point to make. It includes the word "ethicist" but leaves it without the dignity of a definition, beyond the bare etymology, "ethics + ist."

<hr>

ETHICS COMMITTEE

A Minor in a Research Trial

Suppose that you sit on the ethics committee of a hospital or you are a family member. Your job is to recommend a course of action. Review the following case.

> Timmy is a bright 14-year-old boy with a rare lung cancer. He is currently ventilator dependent and has undergone both chemotherapy and a bone-marrow transplant but to no avail. He has less than six months to live. He has discussed end-of-life care with his doctor and

his parents. His parents want his ventilator removed so that Timmy can die with dignity. Timmy agrees. However, two days later, Timmy and his parents are approached to participate in a clinical trial for lung cancer. This would require Timmy to stay on the ventilator and receive IV infusions of an experimental drug researchers are hoping will help lung-cancer patients. Timmy wants to enroll in the trial. He is aware that there is little hope that the treatment will do anything for his condition. He tells his parents: "I want to help other kids before I die." Timmy even writes an essay for his school newspaper arguing that terminal patients have an obligation to help others in research.

The medications do have potential for some very nasty side-effects. Animal testing showed that vomiting, diarrhea, and night sweats are common. One rare side-effect found in 20% of animal subjects is a fatal heart condition. Timmy, however, tells his parents that "this is no worse than all that chemotherapy I did and so what if it quickens my death? I'm going to die anyway." His parents are very reluctant to give their consent. They worry about the suffering Timmy might experience and insist that Timmy previously agreed to palliative (comfort care) only. Timmy is adamant that he wants to help others. He has appealed to the hospital to let him make his own decisions. His doctor does not want him to participate because of the possibility of fatal side-effects. The legal department has expressed that Timmy could go to court against his parents in order to enter the clinical trial; however, it would likely take months to sort it out— months Timmy does not have. The hospital staff are willing to declare Timmy a mature minor and allow him to make his own decision, but they ask for a recommendation from the ethics committee.

As a group or individually, work through the steps of ethical reasoning and then vote on the best course of action. What is the "damned if you do and damned if you don't" aspect of this case? What facts do you wish you knew but do not? How could you honor the patient and the duty not to put him at risk? What ethical reasons can your committee agree on in order to make a recommendation?

CHAPTER 2

Ethical Principles for Resolving Dilemmas

Sophie's Choice without the Nazis

Sophie's Choice, William Styron's 1979 novel about a mother forced to choose which of her children lives and which dies in the ovens of Auschwitz, fills every parent with dread. The Nazis give Sophie a choice: choose one of her children to die, or they both die. Thankfully, this sort of tragic choice rarely happens. Except when it does. Consider the choice Michelangelo and Rina Attard had to make.

Rina's ultrasound revealed conjoined twins. The smaller of the twins was not expected to survive. The parents, devout Catholics, declined the option to terminate the pregnancy. At birth, the babies were dubbed "Mary and Jodie" in the interest of privacy. Jodie was relatively healthy: She had a normal brain, heart, lungs, and liver. Mary, however, had many difficulties: Her brain was underdeveloped; her heart was poorly functioning. The bottom line was that Mary could not survive without Jodie. Jodie, however, likely could not survive *with* Mary. The girls shared a bladder and an aorta. This meant Jodie's heart was doing double duty and could not sustain the life of both girls. Three options were available:

A. Keep both girls conjoined until the certain death of both twins, probably within three to six months or at best in a few years.
B. Separate the twins. This would give Jodie the opportunity to live. The surgery carried a five-per cent risk of death. Jodie would need several

61

operations for her bladder and genitals; however, her future would be good. According to her doctors, she would be able "to participate in normal life activities appropriate for her age and development." Mary would not survive the separation, however.

C. Perform an emergency separation after Mary dies. This option greatly increased Jodie's risk. The chance of surviving surgery would be about 40 per cent, with a significantly worse long-term prognosis than in option B.

What is the most moral option?

WHAT'S AT STAKE?

In the last chapter, we learned about dilemmas. These are "damned if we do, damned if we don't" situations we all face sometimes. Physicians face them. Nurses face them daily. Patients who have to decide which treatment has the fewest side effects face them. Family members who have to decide the fate of their loved one face them. Such is the case here. The Attards did not want to sacrifice one child to save the other. However, if they did nothing they would have lost both children. It is *Sophie's Choice* without the Nazis.

The parents were devout Catholics, and even though Catholic teaching does allow for the removal of extraordinary measures, the parents were "quite happy for God to decide what happened" rather than decide between their children.*

From the point of view of the hospital, there was a patient they could save—Jodie. Mary wasn't likely to survive no matter what happened. She couldn't live without Jodie and she was killing her sister. The hospital wanted to try option B. One child saved was better than no child saved.

For our purposes, this tragic choice can provide some insight into the principles that often form our moral reasoning. Consider the parents' refusal to choose between their children. One of the principles in moral reasoning is the principle of non-maleficence. This principle has a long history in medicine: *Primum non nocere*—"First, do no harm" (you won't find the term in the Hippocratic oath, but the sentiment is there). From Jodie and Mary's parents' point of view, saving Jodie by separation meant sacrificing Mary—a clear case of doing harm. However, if the parents did nothing, and both girls died, it would

---

* John Paris and A.C. Elias Jones, "'Do We Murder Mary to Save Jodie?': An Ethical Analysis of the Separation of the Manchester Conjoined Twins," *Postgraduate Medical Journal* 77, no. 911 (2001): 593–98.

be tragic but the parents would not have harmed Mary; the disease (conjoined twins) would have harmed them, not the parents.

An equally strong intuitive principle is that it is better to save one rather than lose two. The better outcome is one where one life is preserved rather than both lives being lost. This principle might look familiar: in the last chapter we examined the idea that we ought to maximize utility. That is, the right thing to do is to do those actions that lead to the best overall outcomes in terms of pleasure and pain for everyone. It seems intuitive that saving Jodie rather than losing both Jodie and Mary would represent more pleasure and less pain for everyone.

Of course, you might be thinking, "Who cares what the hospital wants? What matters is the wishes of the patients, or in this case, the parents of the minor children." In other words, the principle that should matter here is the autonomy of the parents to make decisions about their children. There is something very wrong with doing surgery on the girls against the wishes of the parents.

Because these principles (utility, autonomy, and non-maleficence) clashed so violently, a legal solution was sought. The British court sided with the hospital, and Mary and Jodie were separated. Jodie is alive and well. Mary died soon after surgery.

In this chapter we are going to talk about resolving dilemmas using principles and ethical theories. We are also going to learn the weaknesses of the principle approach and a few alternative ways of resolving ethical dilemmas.

From Intuitions to Principles

The first thing to notice is that principles are different from our intuitions. When I mentioned the parents' point of view, most of us can feel the sense of unease at having to choose between one's children. That visceral feeling is a sort of intuition. Let's call moral intuitions untested moral opinions. They are automatic; they don't involve a lot of reflective thinking. To get an idea of what I mean, take a look at this simple math problem:

A bat and ball cost $1.10. The bat costs one dollar more than the ball. How much does the ball cost?

This simple problem has been posed to thousands of people. Some of them are very smart. Fifty per cent of Harvard undergraduates get the answer wrong. Did you?

The answer is not ten cents. If you are like most people however, your first (dare we say automatic?) intuition was that the ball costs ten cents. This is a very strong intuition. If you think about it carefully, however, you will see it is wrong.

This is not a moral intuition like our untested feeling that if a parent decides which child dies they have harmed one of their children. Yet moral intuitions are the same in many respects. Just as we feel silly that we got the bat-and-ball problem wrong because a few moments of reflection would have served us to get the problem right, we also do not want to make the same mistake with moral intuitions. We want to reflect on those intuitions—test them to see if they hold up and if they can be applied in many situations. Those intuitions that stand the test of time and are useful over many situations we call *principles*. Now, principles are not absolute. For instance, we can't always "do no harm"; otherwise, doctors would never be able to do surgery (a definite harm). Principles are more like qualified intuitions.

Our intuitions can be mistaken. When you look at the math problem did you have an immediate thought that the bat should cost a dollar? Did you really test that thought? What you had was an intuition: The ball must cost ten cents. The intuition would be wrong, since the correct answer is five cents. (Google "bat and ball problem" if you have not already.)

Intuitions can be correct or they can be mistaken. Ethical principles, on the other hand, are time-tested ideas about what is right or wrong over a wide number of cases. Jonathan Haidt identifies five foundational ethical values found in every culture. Each foundational value has its opposing value:

Care: cherishing and protecting others; opposite of harm.

Fairness or proportionality: rendering justice according to shared rules; opposite of cheating.

Loyalty or ingroup: standing with your group, family, nation; opposite of betrayal.

Authority or respect: submitting to tradition and legitimate authority; opposite of subversion.

Sanctity or purity: abhorrence for disgusting things, foods, actions; opposite of degradation.

A sixth foundation, Liberty, was theorized by another author as the opposite of Oppression.*

Haidt calls these the moral foundations that are hard-wired into each of us. They represent settled intuitions—intuitions that have been tested over many cultures, eras, and situations.

When we apply these principles to ethical dilemmas in medicine, we get a set of tested intuitions that have come to be called *cardinal principles* in medical ethics. There are four that are common:

1. Autonomy (we should respect the self-determination of the patient)
2. Non-maleficence (we should never cause unnecessary harm to the patient)
3. Beneficence (any intervention should be for the patient's benefit)
4. Justice (we should treat everyone fairly)

You can see some of Haidt's moral foundations within these principles. Justice is commonly associated with fairness, beneficence with care, and non-maleficence with the Hippocratic oath to "do no harm."

Let's look at each of these principles more carefully.

Autonomy

The word autonomy literally means "self-rule" and refers to the conditions under which people should be free from interference in their actions. The principle of autonomy says that there is a presumption in favor of people being free to make their own decisions. People need two things to be able to make their own decisions: non-interference (or liberty) and an ability to make decisions (or agency). Let's look at both of these in terms of patients making decisions about their care.

The reference to non-interference or liberty means that patients have a presumption in favor of letting them make their own decisions, and any interference with those decisions needs a compelling reason. The court in our opening gambit thought it had a compelling reason for interfering in the parents' decision to forgo the separation, so they interfered.

The reference to decisional capacity or agency is also important. It is not enough that patients are allowed to make their own decisions; they must have

---

* Jesse Graham et al., "Moral Foundations Theory: The Pragmatic Validity of Moral Pluralism," *Advances in Experimental Social Psychology* 47 (2013): 55–130, https://doi.org/10.1016/B978-0-12-407236-7.00002-4.

the means to do so. A patient who is in and out of consciousness may not be able to go through the process of making a decision even though they are not hindered from doing so. It would be wrong to consider a four-year-old's decision to avoid surgery as autonomous because they do not have the requisite capacity to make these sorts of decisions.

One very important element regarding the means of making a decision is whether the patient has the information necessary to make an informed decision. That is, does the patient know enough about what they are agreeing to freely? Not having enough information because it has not been provided by a medical provider limits personal autonomy.

Alan the Pebble Splitter

The political philosopher Stanley Benn (1920–86) gives a story that illustrates our intuitions about autonomy and interference.* There's this guy Alan sitting on a public beach and he's got rocks in his hand and he is very calmly breaking those rocks into pebbles and then splitting those pebbles into smaller ones. Suppose you come up to Alan and ask him, "Why are you doing that?" It is a reasonable question but Benn reminds us that Alan is not bound, beyond politeness, to give reasons for his actions. He is not obligated to account to you for his actions. If you handcuffed him or removed the pebbles, you had better have a good reason.

Benn's point is that, morally, justification falls on the interferer to justify why they are interfering. A person exercising their autonomy in a way that does not harm others is not obligated to give a reason for their actions. How does this apply to medicine? Patients have a presumption against interference in their lives without some moral justification like consent to treatment or to prevent harm to others. This gives us a reason to think autonomy may not be inviolable. If Benn is correct, autonomy is the default, any interference by medical providers requires justification, and patients who refuse treatment do not owe a justification for their decision because it does not harm others.

We might say that the conditions for a patient's decision to be autonomous means at least that they are free to make the decision. No one is actively interfering with their decision by ignoring it or restraining them in some way. It also

---

* Stanley I. Benn, *A Theory of Freedom* (Cambridge: Cambridge UP, 1988).

means that they have sufficient agency. They have the means to make a decision, and this includes enough information and understanding of that information. If these minimal requirements are met, then we are honoring the principle of autonomy.

Autonomy is, minimally, a presumption in favor of people having both the means and the opportunity to make their own decisions. There are two common principles that provide exceptions to this non-interference: the harm principle and paternalism. The harm principle says we can interfere with autonomy to prevent harm to others, while paternalism says we can do the same but to prevent someone from harming themselves or to make them better people. Because paternalism, as an exception to autonomy, has a special history in health care, and because it is far, far more controversial than the harm principle, we will cover it in Chapter 3.

THE HARM PRINCIPLE AS AN EXCEPTION TO AUTONOMY

The harm principle can be traced back to John Stuart Mill and is one of the most important ideas in modern liberalism. It is called the harm principle because Mill says that the only justification for interference with someone's liberty is that their actions will harm others. This is a powerful intuition. The judge in the conjoined twins case justified interfering with the parents' refusal to separate the twins because their autonomous decision threatened Jodie's life (and Mary's life was already "marked for death").

Mill does say there are conditions on this simple principle. He does not think we should honor the autonomous decisions of children, even if their choices do not harm others. They lack the agency to make autonomous decisions. He also makes exceptions for those people who would do themselves *permanent* harm, such as selling themselves into slavery. He also thinks the harms that trigger the exception to autonomy must be those actions that violate a "clear and assignable duty" in society. In other words, not every form of emotional distress or hurt feelings constitutes a harm in Mill's sense of the word. Only violating those obligations that can be specifically applied to an individual, such as their right to consent to treatment, counts as harming them.

In bioethics, the harm principle exception would apply only when a patient violates a clear and assignable duty to someone else. You might think that Mary and Jodie's parents had a clear and assignable duty to save both children, if possible, and failing that, to save at least one. It seems the court in the case thought so too.

Non-maleficence

Discussion of the harm principle is a fitting segue into the principle of non-maleficence. Never confuse the principle of non-maleficence with the harm principle: The harm principle provides an exception to a patient's autonomy, while non-maleficence is the general moral principle that says we should avoid intentionally doing harm; it is the "do no harm" principle. Just as the principle of autonomy requires a justification for interfering with someone's decision, the principle of non-maleficence requires a justification for hurting someone. We should have a good reason for intentionally hurting someone.

This raises the question, what do we mean by harm? Just as with the principle of autonomy, this is tricky because if we narrowly define harm as involving only physical pain, then we leave out mental suffering, which is surely important. On the other hand, if we expand the definition of harm to include mental states, we run the risk of any sort of "hurt feelings" becoming a kind of harm. Just what the middle ground is between those two is a very big debate in moral and political philosophy, and I'm afraid we won't resolve that debate here. We can say, however, that minimally, to harm is to make someone worse off than they were before. That definition has its problems, but it will do for now.

Beneficence

It is important that we distinguish between non-maleficence (the moral obligation to refrain from doing unnecessary harm to others) and beneficence (the moral obligation to do good or benefit others). Often we distinguish these obligations in terms of positive and negative obligations. A negative obligation is one that requires us only *not* to do something. A positive obligation, on the other hand, requires us to do something substantive. The hospital staff in the conjoined twins case considered it not only their duty not to harm but also their duty to help those who could be helped. In that case, Mary seemed beyond help, but Jodie could be saved and the staff thought they had a duty to save Jodie if they could, rather than lose both infants.

We could say that beneficence as a bioethical principle means that any action a provider takes should make the patient better off. If a physician orders a test that the patient's insurance will pay for but ultimately is not necessary, the physician may not have harmed the patient (she did not violate her duty to non-maleficence), but she has failed to make the patient better off (a violation of the principle of beneficence). So-called "futile treatment," where continued medical intervention will not help the patient, may not technically harm the patient, but most medical staff are distressed when some intervention is futile such that it will not improve the patient's health.

If this is true, the principle of beneficence, as a bioethical principle, is role dependent: The patient may not have a duty to beneficence nearly as much as the provider does—especially a doctor. Patients who come for diagnosis or treatment expect that their provider will have their best interest in mind. This is what it means for medicine to be a profession and not merely a trade.

COVID-19 and Beneficence

During the height of the pandemic, several drugs were rumored to help with COVID symptoms, hydroxychloroquine for example. This drug was prescribed by some doctors under an emergency use authorization. The FDA issues such authorizations when there is no clinical evidence and the possible benefits outweigh the risks of harm. A clinical trial determined that the drug had no benefit, however, and some risk to those with heart conditions. Some might argue that since the risks are low, people should have the right to try hydroxychloroquine. This is up for debate. However, doctors who prescribe the drug would arguably violate beneficence. It is not enough that providers do not harm others with their prescribing; they must also reasonably believe that their treatments will benefit the patient.

Justice

Justice is a lofty concept, much admired but rarely examined. The term *fairness*, however, is a more readily understood concept. Plato defines justice provisionally as "getting what one deserves." Aristotle later laid out the form for any just action, namely that it treat equals equally and unequals unequally. This is not just a platitude. Do not confuse equality and fairness: There are times when treating someone equally might be unjust and treating someone unequally would be consistent with justice. For instance, it would be unjust to give everyone in a class the median class grade regardless of their test scores, though it would be treating everyone equally. It would be just, but certainly not equal, to give priority in distributing vaccines to the people most at risk for exposure to a virus.

In our opening gambit, the Attards did not wish to choose between their daughters because that would be to treat one child better than the other, violating the principle of equality. They would rather let God decide. However, the court did not find it just to allow Jodie to die even though Mary was likely to die.

The philosopher John Rawls famously defined justice as fairness. What counts as fairness are those standards of who gets what that reasonable people would agree to if (and only if) those same people could not tell if their decision of who gets what would benefit them individually or not. Rawls thinks we would all agree to fair conditions in this state of "ignorance." The upshot of Rawls's theory was that behind this veil of ignorance reasonable people would give priority to the least advantaged (since those deciding might actually turn out to be the least advantaged once the veil is lifted).

The idea that justice is about who gets what (distributive justice) can be filled out in a number of ways, all of which are pertinent to patients and providers. For instance, we must start with the assumption that almost all medical resources are scarce resources. Medical staff are limited. Medications are limited. Beds in the Intensive Care Unit are scarce. This means inevitably there will be rationing of these resources. The question for ethics is what is the just way to do so? Following are some principles for distributing scarce resources justly.

UTILITY AS JUSTICE

"Utility" is a fancy word for "the most pleasure and least amount of pain for the greatest number." There is a strong moral intuition that, all things being equal, we ought to do those actions that result in the greatest amount of good for everyone involved. This intuition is tied to the idea of non-maleficence and beneficence. The principle of utility, however, says that while we have an obligation to do good and avoid harm, we have this obligation for the greatest number of beings.

Utility is a very egalitarian principle. Everyone's individual well-being counts morally, but no one's well-being counts more than anyone else's. This means that if we have a conflict between one person's good and the good of the many, the good of the many should win. In the words of *Star Trek*'s Commander Spock, "The good of the many outweighs the good of the few or the one." Spock would make an excellent utilitarian. Also, it is important to mention that the utility principle states that we should maximize utility for everyone. "Everyone" might just refer to people, but animals can also suffer and feel pleasure. Indeed, many utilitarians would include animal well-being in the utility calculation.

NEED/ACUTENESS AS JUSTICE

One of the most important principles of distributive justice is that priority should be given to those who are the most in need. This principle governs the norms of triage in the emergency department: Those in the greatest need deserve the greatest distribution of medical staff attention. Even this gets more complicated the more closely we examine it. "Greatest need" could mean greatest *immediate* need: When doctors have one patient with a blocked airway and the other with failing kidneys, both have great need but one patient's need is immediate.

The choking patient is more "acute" because she will die first without intervention, but without restored kidney function, the other patient will be just as dead in a day or two at the most. Furthermore, someone might have the greatest need but also the worst prospects of surviving, whereas another might have less need but a much better prognosis. If providers have limited resources and personnel, who is the priority? It is standard that in conditions of great scarcity, like a disaster, the most acute patients with the worst prognosis are less of a priority than patients who have a better chance of surviving. The standard is grounded in utility, maximizing the best consequences overall.

FIRST-COME-FIRST-SERVED AS JUSTICE

The least complicated way to distribute scarce resources is by using a line, where the first in line gets the goods first. We use this to distribute tickets for concerts, for example. Doctors' offices see people by appointment, and if today is full, patients have to wait until someone cancels or wait "in line" for another appointment. Even most vaccines are distributed on a first-come-first-served basis.

From Principles to Principlism

It is one thing to recognize that there are ethical principles. It is another to advocate that these principles are the primary way to resolve ethical dilemmas. This latter claim is what is known as *principlism* in bioethics. It is by far the dominant theory for resolving ethical dilemmas in health care, and it is easy to see why it is so popular. It is relatively easy to employ four principles already hardwired into our moral foundations. This sort of principlism is not without controversy, however. There are those who think it rash and detrimental to focus on principles to the exclusion of other models.

We already saw in the last chapter that W.D. Ross gave us a list of prima facie duties but that there was no satisfactory way of ranking them. What do we do when our duty to benefit the patient (beneficence) conflicts with our duty to let the patient make their own decisions (autonomy)? What do we do when the duty not to harm conflicts with the duty to do what is just and fair? Critics of principlism point out that having a set of four or more principles does not preclude having to weigh them against each other in order to reach a prudent decision.

Casuistry

We can best think of principlism and its critics as traditions within bioethics. Principlism is the dominant tradition, but this was not always the case. Long before Beauchamp and Childress articulated principlism, there was a tradition that emphasized the need for prudence in weighing options in ethical dilemmas—*casuistry*.

Casuistry emphasizes practical wisdom—wisdom about what to do—and gets its name from the Latin word for an event or a circumstance. Casuistry emphasizes comparison of like cases in order to form a moral judgment. You are already doing some rudimentary casuistry as you think through the cases in this book, if you start asking yourself, "If the right answer in that case was x, then how does that relate to this case before me?" Stephen Toulmin's reading in the last chapter also champions casuistry.

Care Ethics

Care ethics, sometimes called "ethics of care," refers to a strand of ethics that criticizes principlism as primarily a male-driven ethic. In 1982, Carol Gilligan (b. 1936) wrote, "Yet in the different voice of women lies the truth of an ethic of care, the tie between relationship and responsibility."* Caring as a moral concept is certainly contained in the concept of beneficence mentioned earlier, but it is not necessary. Doing good toward others is certainly easier if we care for them in some way, but the concept of care is not prominent in principlism. Nor is the concept that I might have special obligations to those I care about that I do not have toward others. This suggests that an ethic based on care as a moral concept is far different from the principle of beneficence.

Still, care is one of the moral foundations mentioned earlier, and it also seems to be a very important intuition. Consider the following case inspired by moral philosopher Michael Slote (b. 1941). Suppose you are about to undergo a very risky surgery that will require a great deal of aftercare. Suppose also that you do not have anyone close to you who can be there for you during this trying time. Now suppose I fly across the country at great personal expense and, when I arrive at your side, I tell you that I am going to stay with you throughout this ordeal. You might rightly ask, "Why would you do that?" Now, think of the kinds of answers that would seem fitting for me: "I calculated the utility (the overall happiness minus the overall suffering for everyone) and so I am here" or "I

---

* Carol Gilligan, *In a Different Voice* (Cambridge, MA: Harvard UP, 1982).

have a duty to beneficence and so I do good for others when I can. I can so I am here." Even "I want to be the kind of person who does this sort of thing" rings hollow. None of these really captures that the only fitting reason for making this trip is that "I care about you. We are friends." In other words, the relationship gives moral reasons that the principles cannot. This is the intuition behind care ethics. Care ethics has a strong following in nursing.

From Principles to Theories

Andrew Stimpson, 25, was diagnosed HIV-positive in 2002. He despaired and even contemplated suicide. When he returned to a clinic fourteen months later, he was pronounced HIV free. Andrew was elated but felt he had been a victim of a bad first test. He sued the clinic that tested him. After a thorough investigation including several more tests, the court ruled that Andrew had no standing because both the positive and subsequent negative tests were all accurate.

A spokesman for the National Health Service (NHS) in the United Kingdom, where Andrew lives, said, "This is a rare and complex case. When we became aware of Mr. Stimpson's HIV negative test results we offered him further tests to help us investigate and find an explanation for the different results." Andrew has not stepped forward to do this. A trust spokeswoman added, "We urge him, for the sake of himself and the HIV community, to come in and get tested." While there have been anecdotes of a handful of other people seemingly cured of HIV, Andrew represents a very small and valuable group of potential research subjects. But he isn't interested in being tested further. He said, "There are 34.9 million people with HIV globally and I am just one person who managed to control it, to survive from it and to get rid of it from my body." One researcher expressed the stakes involved: "Inside [Andrew's] immune system is perhaps a key that could allow us to develop some kind of vaccine."[*]

In this chapter so far, we have learned about ethical principles that help us evaluate our moral intuitions. But what happens when those ethical principles clash? Which principles take precedence? In the story of Andrew Stimpson we find several principles clashing. Andrew may very well have the key to curing the plague of the twenty-first century running around in his body. Many people would say he has, at the very least, a prima facie duty to help the research for a cure or a vaccine for HIV. Yet he has thus far refused.

---

* Hugh Muir and James Meikle, "Mysterious case of the man who claims to have beaten HIV by taking vitamins," *Guardian*, Nov. 14, 2005, https://www.theguardian.com/uk/2005/nov/14/health.aids.

The principle of utility mentioned above would indicate that in order to maximize the amount of good for the most people, it would be morally permissible to compel Andrew to give some blood or even some bone marrow (a painful procedure) to help find a vaccine. Indeed, if one is concerned only with utility, researchers might be justified in sacrificing Andrew's life if it would make the lives of thousands of HIV sufferers better. You probably had that intuition when you read the case. You probably also felt a twinge of conscience that we should not compel people to do things with their body without their consent—evoking the principle of autonomy. Indeed, it is Andrew's life after all, and he has a right to live it as he pleases even if we would like him to cooperate with researchers.

We have three ethical principles all clashing here. How do we decide which principle (or principles) has priority? In this section, we are going to learn about ethical theories and how they provide guidance on what to do when ethical principles clash.

It is likely that if you were asked which ethical theory you subscribe to, you might not have an answer. We don't go through life consciously doing moral reasoning according to some ethical theory. If you are like most people, you do not consciously think about exactly how you resolve any ethical choice—you just do it. Maybe, just maybe, you recognize a principle like "don't harm people" or "this is best for everyone," but most people do not go deeper than that.

But we want to go deeper here. We want to look at ethical theories that will help us figure out what is the right thing to do when principles like "do no harm" clash with others like "maximize the good." It would be best for everyone if Andrew cooperated with researchers, but if he didn't, it might be best for everyone if we forced him to cooperate. This would harm him egregiously because we would do something to him without his consent. Normally that would be very wrong, but what if harming Andrew would actually be the best thing we could do for thousands of people who are suffering from HIV? Which principle wins? Each of the ethical theories we will consider have something to say about that.

A good way to distinguish between moral theories is to remember the Cs

Moral theories prioritize either **c**onsequences, moral **c**odes, or **c**haracter. If consequences are prioritized, the theory is consequentialist. Utilitarianism is the go-to example. If the priority is on moral codes apart from consequences, we call it deontological. Ross's theory from Chapter 1 is deontological. If it is based on character, then it best associated with virtue. Virtue ethics is an example, as is Care Ethics.

Utilitarianism holds that the right thing to do is always whatever produces the most amount of utility for the greatest number. Recall the principle of utility: "produce the most amount of pleasure and the least amount of pain for the greatest number of people." Utilitarianism as a theory says that when any two principles clash, utility always wins. It is a very simple and elegant theory. However, it seems to condone some pretty awful things. If thousands of HIV positive people could be cured by hurting—even killing—one person, utilitarianism might say that would not only be permissible but actually the right thing to do. For some people, though, that is just counter-intuitive; it runs against their intuitions about right and wrong. Many people would say that sometimes there are duties we have not to harm people that must be honored no matter how many people would be helped if we ignored those duties.

When rights and duties come first, we call those theories *deontological*. There are moral codes that everyone must follow, even if breaking them every now and then would make more people better off. When consequences like maximizing utility are what matters, we call those theories *consequentialist*. For consequentialist theories like utilitarianism, the only factor that determines what is the right thing to do is the likely consequences of the action.

Punishment for not Vaccinating?

Under New York City's policy, people in four Brooklyn zip codes who resist vaccination could face fines of up to $1,000, but it is not clear whether they could actually be compelled to get vaccinated if they continue to refuse. Health Commissioner Dr. Oxiris Barbot said those who refuse vaccination would be dealt with on a "case-by-case basis."[*]

How would a consequentialist decide the morality of punishing those who don't vaccinate?

The third branch of ethical theory has to do with character, not consequences or moral codes. *Virtue theories* start not with the question "What is the right

---

[*] Mark Osborne, "New York City issues fines of $1,000 to 3 people who refused to be vaccinated against measles," *ABC News*, April 19, 2019.

thing to do?" but rather with "What sort of persons should we be?" In a way, this is both consequentialist and rule-based, and in a way it is neither. It is kind of consequentialist because what matters morally is the right sort of outcome—the cultivation of a set of virtues. Forcing Andrew Stimpson to comply with our research on HIV against his will violates many character traits such as kindness, fairness, and integrity. It would also violate a common moral code in medicine that says we do not do things to people medically without their consent. Our reasons for this are not just consequentialist or even based on a slavish adherence to some sort of rule. Instead, we follow these rules and seek good resolutions because of the kind of people—indeed the kind of society—we want to be.

Virtue ethics as a theory is older than either consequentialist theory or deontological theory; the Greeks elucidated the concept as far back as 400 BCE. It is a theory that in many ways is hard to implement because it does not give us clear action-guiding principles. Adopting a virtue ethics method doesn't tell you definitively what is the right thing to do. Instead, it relies on our understanding about what a good person would do in the situation, and then we are to emulate it.

How do we use ethical theories like the ones above to aid in moral reasoning? One way is that they provide a way to prioritize those ethical principles we mentioned earlier. In a clash between autonomy and beneficence, a duty-based theory like Ross's from Chapter 1 would tell you that the duty to not interfere with a person's autonomy is stronger than the duty to do good to someone.

All of these theories have their problems, though. Nothing in philosophy (especially ethics) is easy. You might be asking yourself whether you have to commit to one of these theories, since they all seem to have their pros and cons. The short answer is you do not have to commit. Just try them out—a bit like speed dating or taking a test drive. This is not to say that picking an ethical theory is like choosing which car to buy. Ethical analysis does not require you to operate only from one particular theory. You should choose your ethical theory based on which one seems the most clear, consistent, and justified, just like the way you seek to resolve ethical dilemmas. This may take a long time; in fact, you may not settle on a theory until long after this course.

There is a value to having an ethical theory to work from, however. What does an ethical theory do for you when it comes to ethical reasoning? It sets boundaries. If you are committed to the framework of deontology, then you are not going to be okay with sacrificing the life of one person to save thousands, hundreds, or even a couple of people. As one character from the movie *Avengers: Infinity War* says, "We don't trade lives."

On the other hand, if you are committed to a consequentialist theory, you commit yourself to doing what produces the greatest number of good consequences and the fewest bad consequences, even if sacrifices have to be made. In the sequel to *Infinity War*, Tony Stark (Iron Man) trades his own life for the lives of billions of people. He would be an excellent consequentialist.

Having an ethical theory also helps to solve a problem from Chapter 1. If you remember the W.D. Ross reading, Ross lists several prima facie duties that we ought to strive to honor. However, what happens when these duties conflict? What happens when telling a lie will save a life? What happens when telling the truth will destroy someone's life? What should we do when experimenting on Andrew Stimpson against his will could yield results that could save thousands, maybe millions of lives? Ross does not give us much guidance. Ethical theories, however, give us ways to prioritize some principles over others.

Deontology and rule-based systems won't ignore utility altogether, but in a clash between respect for a person's right to bodily integrity (we can't do experiments on Andrew) and the utility of advancing research on HIV, "respect for persons" or the autonomy of the individual will always win out over consequences.

To illustrate this, take the concept of a "right." This is one of the most used and most misunderstood concepts in public discourse. A right, as we use it in legal terminology, is a claim on other people's behavior. If I say I have a right to practice my religion freely, then this is a claim on everyone else's behavior. No one must interfere with my practice of my religion. Likewise, if I have a right to a fair trial or an attorney without having to pay for one, then it is up to society to provide me one free of charge. That is the claim I make on others when I invoke my right.

Now take a quote from a consequentialist, the "father" of utilitarianism, Jeremy Bentham: "Rights are nonsense on stilts." Bentham does not think much of the concept of a right, does he? To a utilitarian, consequences are all that matter. And the only consequences that matter are the ones that bring the most pleasure into the world. An individual right flies in the face of that sort of calculus, doesn't it?

Suppose that interfering with my religious practice would actually produce more goodness in the world. Maybe my religion is toxic, violent, or degrading. Interfering would make fewer and fewer people believe my awful religion. What if not only society but even practitioners like me would be better off if society interfered? A rights-based theory would say, "Sorry, but even if society would be better off, we don't get to sacrifice rights for well-being. My rights ought to be protected even if fewer people are happy." Do you see now why a utilitarian like Bentham would think rights were nonsense? If we elevate those rights the way we do in documents like the United Nations Declaration of Human Rights or the US Bill of Rights, if we are prepared to endure a great deal of societal unhappiness to protect those rights even if the people invoking them are despicable, hateful, and degrading, Bentham might think we are putting that nonsense up on stilts.

Who is correct—Bentham or the rights theorists? Does it surprise you that no one agrees definitively? Remember back in Chapter 1 when we discussed how we may not always come to a consensus about resolving an ethical dilemma? The same applies to picking an ethical theory. Bentham wrote about utilitarianism in the first half of the nineteenth century, and rights theorists have been around since before then. Nobody has conceded defeat.

Do not feel that you have to choose between being a utilitarian championing the greater good and a rights advocate championing respect for persons. There are many shades in between. Take the case of J.S. Mill. Mill was the son of one of Jeremy Bentham's closest friends. He was raised to carry on the utilitarian legacy of his father, and he did—sort of. Mill wrote an essay on Bentham, in which it was expected that he would praise his father's friend. Instead, Mill used the occasion to critique Bentham's brand of utilitarianism and begin a different sort of consequentialist theory. Today we call it *rule utilitarianism*.

We have already read a bit of Mill's new utilitarian theory in Chapter 1. Bentham's utilitarianism says that the right action in any dilemma is to do what will produce the most amount of good (pleasure) and the least amount of bad (pain) overall. We do this for each moral action we take. So let's call that *act utilitarianism*. Mill agreed with his father's friend about the value of utility, saying that he regarded utility as the ultimate appeal on all ethical questions. Then he inserts a "but": "But utility as it is expressed in man as a progressive being." What in the world did Mill mean by this? Simply put, morality does ultimately reduce to utility, but how we make ethical decisions does not. In Mill's words, "Don't confuse moral evaluation with a decision procedure."

Mill thinks we make decisions about the right thing to do in general by following rules or principles, not by calculating utility in every single act. In fact, if we were to calculate utility for every single act, we might end up not maximizing utility for everyone. Humans, it turns out, are really bad at calculating utility in the moment of making ethical decisions—just as bad as they are at recognizing they are operating on bad intuitions. Remember the bat and ball problem? A whole bunch of data from social psychology backs this up. In one book, Nobel Prize-winning economist Daniel Kahneman lists around thirty biases that humans have both as individuals and especially when in large groups.[*] Think about how these might sabotage maximizing utility.

---

[*] Daniel Kahneman, *Thinking Fast and Slow* (New York, NY: Farrar, Straus, and Giroux, 2011).

Some Common Cognitive Biases

- confirmation bias (we tend to believe data that confirm our prior beliefs)
- hindsight bias (we tend to believe we could have predicted outcomes in hindsight)
- anchoring bias (we tend to focus strongly on the first piece of data we encounter and evaluate other data based on it)
- availability bias (we tend to overestimate the value of data we can recall quickly and easily)
- sunk-cost fallacy (we don't want to abandon projects we have heavily invested in, even if they are a losing proposition)
- the framing effect (we can draw different conclusions for the data depending on the order in which it is presented)

Mill knew about some of these biases, but not nearly as much as we know now. Given the human proclivity for biases in calculation, it makes sense that humans would not be good at predicting which decisions will maximize utility for everyone. We could even end up causing more suffering in the end.

Instead, Mill advised that we set up some rules of thumb, such as "don't lie," "don't cheat," "don't steal," "keep your promises," and so on. In this he sounds like a deontologist: rules, obligations, codes. However, Mill still claims the mantle of his mentor Bentham because he says we chose those rules or codes based on what has produced the most utility in the past. In other words, we do an inventory of moral rules from the past (the Ten Commandments, rules of etiquette, etc.) and then we hypothesize which rules in general lead to more happiness for the greatest number of people: "net happiness." If there are significant enough changes in society (e.g., we go from a tribal society to a democracy), then those rules are apt to change. But they do not change very often, and they do not change from day to day.

If experimenting on Andrew Stimpson might save thousands, even millions of lives in the end, we might miss many of the unintended consequences of our actions. If we make an exception to the general rule against violating patient autonomy to advance HIV research, people might start to think the rule itself does not mean a lot. That sort of fear and distrust could lead to a lot of suffering, especially in medicine.

We could overestimate the bad consequences, however. Consider another case. There was a time before 1975 when psychiatrists had strict confidentiality rules in place to prevent disclosing anything that was said in a therapy session to anyone, including the police. There were several incidents of patients threatening to kill or injure someone they knew. In such cases, don't medical professionals have a duty to warn the potential victim or the police? Many psychiatric professionals believed that violating this rule of confidentiality would cause a lot of negative consequences. "Patients won't trust us anymore," they claimed. "We can't give good care if we can't talk about everything without fear of some therapist blabbing about what a patient says." The therapist's office is like the seal of confession in the Catholic Church, they argued.

When a very high-profile case (*Tarasoff v. Regents of the University of California*) resulted in the California Supreme Court ruling that psychiatrists do have a duty to warn potential victims or the police, the psychiatric community was outraged. Don't change this rule, they claimed, or it will lead to bad consequences. Patients will be afraid to open up to their therapist and as a result won't get well.

Except they were wrong. Today, it is standard practice for therapists to warn patients that they cannot keep threats to others confidential. Psychiatrists and therapists have a duty to warn the police if a patient makes credible threats. And there has been no evidence that this has hampered therapy all that much. Changing the rule did not lead to more suffering. I use this example to show that sometimes our concerns about what is called a "slippery slope" have proven overblown, and uncertainty in expected consequences should make us wary of making exceptions to rules, especially in a medical setting.

Why study ethical theories if I don't have to hold to one?

Think of ethical theories as a record of people thinking through multiple ethical dilemmas and trying to find consistency among them. One value of studying them is that you get the benefit of looking at how a whole body of people have anticipated some very uncommon ethical dilemmas.

Think of it like an engineering problem. Some engineering principles are confirmed by a great deal of theoretical physics. Is it important for engineers to be familiar with how bodies operate in motion? Definitely. Studying theoretical physics makes engineers sensitive to the implications of their engineering because they are, in a sense, thinking the thoughts after the physicists. It is the same with ethics.

WHAT'S THE DEBATE?

Reading 2.1: Ruth Macklin, "Applying the Four Principles"

In this reading, Ruth Macklin (b. 1938) takes the four cardinal principles and applies them to some cases. She is in a dialogue with another author named Raanan Gillon (b. 1941). It is not necessary to read Gillon's article because Macklin reproduces his argument enough for us. (Numbers in brackets are keyed to the list of references at the end of the reading.)

As one who endorses the approach using the four principles, I maintain that they are always in need of interpretation and further analysis. Moreover, problems may lurk when applying them to specific cases. I shall comment on each of the four scenarios in turn.

The "Standard" Jehovah's Witness Case

A traditional approach to the four principles might view the "standard" Jehovah's Witness case as a prominent example of a conflict of ethical principles [1]. A competent adult patient is refusing a treatment that has the best chance of saving his life, according to well-documented studies published in medical journals. Nevertheless, the respect for persons principle mandates that physicians should comply with the expressed wishes of a competent adult patient even if the predicted consequences are unfavorable or grave.

Arguably, two ethical principles could support the opposite judgment: that the physician may—or must—seek to override the patient's refusal of a blood transfusion. The principle of non-maleficence requires physicians to avoid harm, whenever possible, so withholding a proven, beneficial treatment is likely to have the consequence of producing harm. Although withholding a treatment is an omission rather than an action, it represents a deliberate decision taken by a physician and therefore, constitutes a course of action. The related principle of beneficence, which calls for maximizing benefits and minimizing harms, could also be used in support of the physician's duty to administer a blood transfusion in contravention of a patient's refusal.

If this is all that can be said about an analysis that relies on the four principles, this methodology could yield no clear resolution of the physician's dilemma. One reason no resolution is forthcoming is, as Gillon has pointed out, that "the four principles approach does not provide a method for choosing" [2].

Notice that the author has set up the "damned if you do, damned if you don't" characteristic of a dilemma: the clash between the principles of autonomy (respect the patient's right to refuse) and beneficence/non-maleficence (do what is in the patient's best interest). In this next section, Macklin entertains some objections to using the principles at all. Can you spot the two objections to principlism?

The principles are not a set of ordered rules with instructions for making inferences and arriving at deductive conclusions. One of the common (and misguided) criticisms of the four principles is that they constitute a deductive system and therefore, presumably, a rigid method for arriving at solutions to complex ethical dilemmas. A quite different criticism of the method makes the opposite point, finding it deficient because it does not yield clear answers to troubling moral quandaries. As Gillon notes, moral agents have to come to their own answers, using their preferred moral theories, and at the same time consider the set of common moral commitments provided by the four principles [2]. Since I am in substantial agreement with Gillon on the soundness and utility of the four principles, I reject both criticisms: that the method is unacceptable because it is inflexible, and that the principles are useless because they fail to provide a unique solution to moral dilemmas.

Gillon's resolution of this dilemma brings the allegedly conflicting principles of respect for persons and beneficence into congruence. It is clear (at least prima facie) that respect for persons requires the physician to accede to the patient's refusal of a blood transfusion.

So Macklin agrees with Gillon on this case. Autonomy is more important than non-maleficence/beneficence. But why? She argues that the Jehovah's Witness doctrine on blood transfusions is internally rational. If one believes the doctrine, the refusal of a blood transfusion is rational.

What about the balance of benefits and harms? According to the patient's calculus of values, the harm resulting from receiving a transfusion (denial of eternal salvation) is greater than the harm caused by refusing the transfusion (the end of mortal life on earth). Arguably, this is a rational calculation for anyone who believes in the metaphysical scheme of the Jehovah's Witness faith. If one has to choose between eternal salvation and a few more years of mortal life in which one is merely "passing through," the choice of eternal salvation appears rational. From the perspective of the Jehovah's Witness, refusal of a blood transfusion has a favorable balance of benefits over harms.

Gillon argues, further, that the expense of a non-blood alternative treatment is not so great as to warrant overriding the patient's wishes based on a financial cost benefit assessment [1]. Finally, rights based justice and legal justice are on the side of honoring the patient's wishes, so all three principles line up in favor of the conclusion that the ethical solution to the dilemma is to honor the Jehovah's Witness's refusal of blood transfusions.

> Now Macklin is going to "up the ante" by suggesting that a change in some of the facts could alter how the balance of principles turns out. Do you think Macklin's change to the case really changes the moral dilemma? To which principle does Macklin appeal to change the calculation?

While I find this solution compelling, based on the underlying moral presuppositions and empirical assumptions, we can imagine an alternative analysis—also using the four principles—that could arrive at a different conclusion. At least implicitly, Gillon's analysis gives great weight to the patient's stated wishes and, as a result, the respect for persons principle. Physicians who believe that their primary obligation is to save lives, when possible, will, however, almost always subordinate respect for persons to beneficence. More importantly, if the empirical facts are considerably different from what Gillon has hypothesised, it is at least plausible to think that accepting a patient's refusal of blood could cause more harm than good.

Consider the following scenario. The Jehovah's Witness patient is a married man with four children. His wife is not employed, as she is occupied rearing the children. The family lives in the US, not the UK, and they would have no health insurance for the family if the breadwinner dies. The wife has no occupational skills, and could therefore obtain only a low paying job if she were forced to go to work upon her husband's death. The husband has only a small life insurance policy that could support his family for a year or two after he dies. In addition, the closely-knit Jehovah's Witness community becomes incensed when physicians override patients' refusal of blood. Elders of the church have urged Witnesses not to seek medical attention for conditions that might result in a recommendation of a blood transfusion. If that were to become a reality, there would be a likely increase in morbidity and mortality among Jehovah's Witnesses even in situations where they do not need blood transfusions. The net result would be a significant balance of harms over benefits, thereby contravening the principle of beneficence. On this scenario, the principles of respect for persons and beneficence are not congruent, but are in conflict.

Whether or not this scenario is plausible should not concern us. What is relevant to an analysis of this case is the scope of the principle of beneficence, that is, to whom the physician owes a moral obligation. In considering a patient's refusal of life saving treatment, is it appropriate to include harms that may come to others besides the patient—the patient's family or the Jehovah's Witness community? I am uncertain what Gillon would answer, since he notes that "the controversial issue of who falls within the scope of beneficence is answered unambiguously for at least one category of people": patients and clients of health care workers [2]. Gillon does not discuss family members of patients or clients in his discussion of the scope of beneficence, although he poses the difficult question: "whom or what do we have a moral duty to help and how much should we help them?" In addition to the problem of scope, there is the classic methodological difficulty with utilitarian calculations: the difficulty of predicting which of several possible future scenarios will actually come about, and determining the likelihood of an array of potential good and bad consequences.

Macklin appeals to consequences. A patient's refusal could have wider harms, not just their loss of life. Harm to families and communities count if we are talking about utility. So why shouldn't these social harms factor into the discussion?

Let us consider one final possibility. There is anecdotal evidence that at least some Jehovah's Witnesses waver in their decisions when confronted with life threatening situations. They firmly refuse recommended blood transfusions, according to the teachings of their religion. They assert their refusals in the presence of family members and often, an elder of the church. But when offered the option of speaking alone with a physician, they relent and accept blood. Alternatively, when hospital authorities seek judicial intervention, a Jehovah's Witness may utter the standard objection, "... against my will," yet in reality accept the transfusion. This possibility points to the difficulty in ascertaining whether a patient's stated wish is truly autonomous. Although it is generally true that people say what they mean and mean what they say, legitimate exceptions occur. The Jehovah's Witness who refuses blood in the presence of family members or an elder of the church may not be expressing an autonomous wish. In adhering to the respect for persons principle, physicians have an obligation to seek to determine whether their patients' refusals of recommended treatments are truly autonomous. If there is reason to suspect that a Jehovah's Witness patient's refusal of a blood transfusion is unduly influenced or lacking adequate understanding of the consequences, the physician should not accede immediately and unquestioningly to the patient's wish.

The foregoing considerations serve as a reminder that an ethical analysis using the four principles is complex. It requires an interpretation of the principles themselves in the context in which they are applied, as well as an accurate assessment of the factual circumstances of the situation. While I agree with Gillon's analysis of the "standard" Jehovah's Witness case, I have tried to show that a change in the background conditions could alter the conclusion that *respect for persons* and *beneficence* always line up in favor of accepting a competent adult patient's refusal of blood. Nevertheless, for the moral agent who is convinced that *respect for persons* always takes precedence over *beneficence*, any conflict between these two principles would still require the physician to adhere to the patient's refusal of blood. Moreover, because physicians owe stronger obligations to their patients than to other parties who may be affected (the patient's family or the community), it is ethically preferable to give priority to the patient's own assessment of the good and bad consequences of refusing of blood....

Why not take the Jehovah's Witness community as the relevant group in determining the existence of social agreement?

It is far from evident that what any society agrees upon is, therefore, morally right, even in that society and even if the majority of people in that society accept it. Slavery was accepted by a majority of people who lived in the American South before the civil war, but slavery is surely an unjust social arrangement when analyzed according to the four principles. It may still be true that a majority of the people in some African countries accept the traditional practice of female genital mutilation, despite ample medical evidence of the physical harm, often lifelong, that results from that cultural practice. The penalty of amputation of the hands of common thieves in countries that adhere to strict Islamic law appears unacceptably harsh to other societies that consider the practice to be cruel and unusual punishment. These few examples show that mere social agreement cannot be sufficient for determining what is in anybody's best interest, even within the relevant society or cultural group.

In the case of the child of Jehovah's Witnesses, how can the child's best interest be determined? According to the beliefs of parents and others in the Jehovah's Witness community, the individual who receives a blood transfusion—whether a child or adult—will be denied eternal salvation. Physicians in the UK and US, along with judges who are called upon to adjudicate such cases, do not subscribe to this metaphysical belief. Instead, physicians and judges compare two alternative states of affairs for a child in need of a blood transfusion: a high probability of death or serious, irreversible morbidity, on the one hand, versus continued mortal life, on the other. Modern medical science provides an objective, reasonably accurate way of determining which of these consequences is more likely in any given circumstance. In cases of decision making for those who are incapable of deciding for themselves, these admittedly narrow, scientific grounds should be the basis for deciding what is in a person's best interest. As Gillon notes, there are borderline cases and hard cases, but the case of a child who could easily be restored to full health with a blood transfusion and would almost certainly die without the transfusion is neither borderline nor hard [1].

A continued, healthy life and a premature death are not coequal values. Competent, adult patients should be permitted to decide for themselves whether other values override the usual wish they would normally have for a continued healthy life. Arguably (but still problematically), older adolescent children of adult Jehovah's Witnesses should be permitted to refuse blood if it can be ascertained that they are acting autonomously. But the two year old child has not yet developed a belief system or a value system on the basis of which to choose a hoped for eternal salvation over continued mortal life....

References

1. Gillon R. Four scenarios. J Med Ethics 2003;29:267–8.
2. Gillon R. Medical ethics: four principles plus attention to scope. BMJ 1994;309:184–8.

Reading 2.2: E. Arries, "Virtue Ethics: An Approach to Moral Dilemmas in Nursing"

Arries gives a survey of virtue ethics and applies it to moral dilemmas in nursing.

Introduction

The purpose of this essay is to discuss virtue ethics as an approach to moral dilemmas in nursing. Nurses, by virtue of their practice are the members of the health profession who have the most contact with patients. As a result, they are confronted with situations of intense potential moral conflict more often than any other member of the healthcare team. Most of the time, nurses find it difficult to respond in an appropriate way to such situations of moral conflict; as a consequence they can experience intense moral distress. The moral distress experienced by nurses often results from a conflict between a professional duty to care and personal convictions, such as values and beliefs. In this vein, the boundaries between professional obligations and personal convictions of what are right or wrong in the nurse-patient interaction become blurred, for example, the recent case of a theatre nurse who appealed against a demand by his/her employer to assist in surgery to terminate pregnancy.

> "Theatre nurse": i.e., a surgical nurse working in the operating room or "surgical theatre."

In this case, it is evident that tension exists between the nurse's personal moral convictions and his/her duty to care. It is in such situations that nursing ethics could play a role in providing nurses with guidance on how to behave and address conflicting issues.

We could consider nursing ethics as concerning itself with what is right (good) or wrong (bad) in the nurse-patient interaction. In this vein, nursing ethics revolves around three central concepts: nurse ("self"), patient ("other") and health ("the good") (Rossouw & Van Vuuren, 2004:3). It is the dynamic balance between these three dimensions that determines whether the response by the nurse to a situation of moral distress is ethical or not. At times, the dynamic balance in the nurse-patient interaction becomes so blurred that a choice between equally valid ethical outcomes or ideals, such as health, must be made. If this happens, we say that a moral dilemma has occurred. Generally, health care practitioners approach moral dilemmas based on two broad, divergent and opposing ethical perspectives.

> In this section, the author critiques principlism and consequentialism. What are the reasons Arries rejects these theories as insufficient for solving dilemmas particular to nurses?

For example, Botes (1997:3) indicates that doctors predominantly base their ethical decisions on a normative approach to ethics such as principilism with some consideration of consequentialism and utilitarianism. This approach uses the four principles of autonomy, justice, beneficence, and non-maleficence. However, at times when a moral dilemma ensues and these principles are in conflict, it is not always easy to decide which one should dominate. In addition, some consequences might not be that obvious in a moral situation or due to the lack of information and time, it is not always clear how to decide which consequences would be best within the context of the moral dilemma. Even applying the rule of the greatest good for the greatest number of people might pose problems in a healthcare situation where the rights of each and every individual patient are valued. Some nurses might find the aforementioned approaches very disturbing, because they do not accommodate the interpersonal element of nurse-patient interaction. To this effect, nurses often based their ethical decisions on their engagement with the holistic needs of the patient. This approach is associated with the ethics of care (Gilligan's, 1982 in Botes, 1997:3). Within an ethics of care approach to moral dilemmas, the involvement, harmonious relations between a nurse and a patient as well as the needs of other people within every unique ethical situation plays an important role in solving an ethical problem.

On the one hand, it appears that there is virtually no interaction between the two approaches. Differences in power and knowledge between nurses and doctors in the healthcare situation often lead to a situation where doctors play a dominant role in ethical decisions. This implies that ethical decision-making about moral dilemmas in particular, is based on a principilism approach with some consideration of consequentialism and utilitarianism. This gives rise to a situation where nurses feel they are marginalised and excluded from moral decisions that affect them equally. Nurses are often expected to carry out ethical decisions made by doctors, such as withdrawing life-support or following a do not resuscitate order. Most of the time, they have not been part of these decisions. This gives rise to conflict in the health team since nurses disagree with decisions made by doctors. This often leads to tension among members of the healthcare team, problems of job dissatisfaction and burn-out among nurses.

On the other hand, it seems that both approaches do not consider the dispositions or character of the nurse as a moral agent as an important factor during moral decision-making. In this vein, it seems that ethical decisions about moral dilemmas could be regarded as ineffective, because they give rise to unnecessary mental and physical suffering for patients and their families as well as conflict. Furthermore, the solution to moral dilemmas could be regarded as incomplete, because it does not accommodate the interpersonal nature of the nurse-patient relationship and the emotional elements of human experience.

As a possible solution to this ineffective and incomplete approach to solving moral dilemmas amongst members of the health team, I suggest a virtue ethics approach to moral dilemmas. The word "approach" is not intended to mean a set of rules that will guide a choice between alternatives, but rather a focus on the type of nurses that we ought to be. I think virtue ethics as an approach to moral dilemmas in nursing provide a more holistic analysis of moral dilemmas and facilitate more flexible and creative solutions when combined with a principalist, consequentialist, utilitarian or ethics of care approach to moral decision-making.

What does the author promise to argue for in this thesis statement? Why do you think Arries emphasizes that the approach is not a list of rules or principles that will tell us what is surely the right thing to do?

To advance this argument, I will present the reader with a rationale for a virtue ethics approach to moral decision-making in nursing. In addition, I will look at the nature of virtue ethics, and focus particularly on the central characteristics of virtue ethics, such as the concepts of virtue and virtuousness, the nature of human being and the telos or the good. To illuminate the aforementioned characteristics of virtue ethics and how they could be applied to moral dilemmas in nursing, I will relate it to the story of Martin. I wish to stress that it is not my intention with this article to provide a list of rules to be followed in order to solve a moral dilemma, because many such useful rules or ethical decision-making methods already exist. What is intended here, rather, is to provide the reader with an understanding of how virtues could be applied to illuminate and make moral decision-making so much more meaningful for the people involved.

Rationale for a Virtue Ethics Approach to Moral Dilemmas in Nursing

> In this section, the author gives four reasons for including virtue theory in our moral decision making. Which of these four do you think is the strongest/most compelling to you? Which is the weakest?

Firstly, ethical principles applied during moral decision-making insist on the use of reason only. Reason itself, as I shall indicate later, can be seen as a virtue. In this vein, they require from nurses as moral agents during moral decision-making to "bracket" their emotional experiences. In this vein, ethical principles only tell us what action to take and do not consider the holistic human nature of the nurse as a moral agent. People do not work very well without virtues. Virtues are beneficial to human interaction and communication, and to the functioning of human society (Scott, 1995:280). For example, acting only from a sense of duty is insufficient and likely to fail if one does not have personal virtues of dedication, perseverance and integrity to back it up.

Secondly, according to the Patient Rights Charter ([South Africa] Department of Health, 1999), patients and their significant others have a right to be involved in decision-making. Williams (1998:264) indicates that on the level of society, patients as consumers of health care demonstrate an increased demand for accessibility and interest in hospital processes, such as decision-making. In this vein, patients also become increasingly aware of their right to participate in health care decisions impacting on their health. This is especially true when it comes to moral decision-making. Worldwide and locally, patients and their family members are increasingly demanding to be involved in decisions about treatment, including the termination or withdrawal thereof (Biley, 1992:414; Avis, 1994; Sainio, Lauri & Eriksson, 2001:97–98). To this effect, moral decision-making based on a paternalistic, materialistic and deterministic way, especially in a pluralistic society does not hold water any longer. Today, patients and their families demand to be empowered in as far as decisions that affect their daily life is concerned. [To involve patients and their families in moral decision-making not only requires a paradigm shift; it also] demands certain kinds of dispositions and sensitivity. In other words, it demands certain virtues in order to tolerate differences in opinion that might arise during an ethical situation. Thus, an approach that demands the use of principles in an impartial way is not tolerated let alone fulfilling the expectations of consumers of health care.

Do you agree with the criticism of principles and ethical theories in the paragraph above as "impartial" and "paternalistic, materialistic, and deterministic"?

Thirdly, nurses who are in constant interaction with patients and their families are important stakeholders to moral decision-making in health care. As independent practitioners, they are accountable for their decisions, including moral decisions. Health care has become increasingly complex, and to this effect, the problems with which healthcare personnel are confronted are complex too. The complex nature of moral problems requires a collaborative approach. For this reason, it is no longer feasible for doctors as members of a complex and diverse team to assume a dominant position in solving moral dilemmas or making moral decisions and issuing prescriptions on behalf of other team members. A collaborative approach based on rational interaction through dialogue, discourse and moral sensitivity to moral decision-making in nursing is required. Becoming sensitive to different perspectives in moral decision-making in nursing requires certain dispositions of character. In this vein, it appears that virtue ethics as an approach that focuses on the moral character and disposition of the nurse as a moral agent is crucial to any approach to moral decision-making, whether based on principlism, consequentialism or deontology (Kristjansson, 2000:193–94).

Lastly, for nurses to participate in moral decision-making confidently, it is necessary for them to understand the language, theories and methods of analysis used in ethical discourse. As practitioners of nursing, nurses have a better understanding of nursing care than any other healthcare practitioner. However, they might sometimes find it problematic to consider ethical issues involved in such situations, let alone participate in decisions regarding what is good for everyone involved in a moral dilemma. In this vein, virtue ethics as an approach to moral dilemmas in nursing can provide important insights for them. Virtue ethics, in effect, proposes a very sophisticated theory of moral development. For this has crucial far-reaching implications for the teaching of ethics (Scott, 1995:284).

The Nature of Virtue Ethics (VE)

Virtue ethics refers to one of three major approaches in normative ethics (Rossouw & Van Vuuren, 2004:58). However, virtue ethics is not a problem-solving or decision-making tool. Virtue ethics can be defined as an approach that emphasises the character and disposition of a person, in contrast to an approach that emphasises duties, rules or principles (deontology), or one that emphasises the consequences of actions (consequentialism). In this vein, virtue ethics emphasises *being* rather than *doing* (Magee, 2001:32–33; Scott, 1995:283). Our being, in other words, who we truly are, influences our behaviour. Thus, virtue ethics in nursing can be viewed as an approach of ethical deliberation about the moral character and dispositions of nurses as moral agents that enables them, as virtuous human beings, to fulfil their purpose and function as professional people. In this vein, a description of a person's character and character traits portrays a way of being instead of acting. Character according to Drane (in Davis, Aroskar, Liaschenko & Drought, 1997:49) refers to the structure of one's personality with special attention to its ethical components. To this effect, one can argue that from one's way of being flows one's way of conducting the business of one's personal and professional life in ways that are identifiable and dependable over time (Davis, Aroskar, Liaschenko & Drought, 1997:49). A person's character is a source as well as the product of his/her value commitments and actions. Thus, if we consider ethics as a dynamic view between what can be regarded as right or wrong and revolving around three central concepts, namely "self," "other" and "the good," then virtues, from a virtue ethics perspective, can be seen as the golden thread that binds them together, and virtue ethics as a framework that can help us understand the virtues necessary for moral excellence.

Virtues

Virtues are some of the most central characteristics of virtue ethics. Virtue ethics as an approach to moral decision-making implies that moral conduct assumes good characteristics in a nurse as a moral agent. In this vein, for a nurse to act as a moral agent that advocates on behalf of a patient during moral decision-making in order to demonstrate excellence (*arete*) and behave well in a sustained manner, requires the development of good characteristics or virtues.

> The word in parentheses is the Greek term that Aristotle uses for "virtue" or "excellence."

In its purest form according to Trianosky (1990:336), virtue ethics holds that only judgements about virtue are basic in morality, and that the rightness of actions is always derivative from the virtuousness of traits.

> If this is true, is it accurate to say, as Arries does at the beginning of this section, "virtue ethics is not a problem-solving or decision-making tool"?

Virtues, from an Aristotelian perspective, can be defined as a characteristic habit of excellence of the soul (Arrington, 1998:71). From a nursing perspective, it implies a characteristic habit that allows the nurse to become a good practitioner who behaves well. The literature on virtue ethics (Arrington, 1998:71–72; MacIntyre, 1998:74–76) distinguishes between two kinds of virtues: those that relate to a person's character and those that relate to a person's intellect. The former is sometimes referred to as "moral virtue" and the latter as "intellectual virtue." Intellectual virtue as a disposition enables a nurse to reason well, while acting in accordance with right reason, requires moral virtue. However, the contrary is also true. For example, a nurse who applies the principle of benevolence, that is the wish to do good for his/her patient, decides to act in direct opposition to a doctor's do not resuscitate (DNR) prescription. Without apparent self-interest, the nurse might feel that the patient is being treated unfairly and thus decide to act on the patient's behalf. In this vein, the nurse demonstrates courage as a virtue. A courageous nurse is capable of free thought and undertakes responsible actions and carries them out, whatever their implications might be. However, in nursing practice, a courageous act cannot always be justified on the basis of being right or of its consequences. Nurses also need to assess the particular circumstances of a situation and demonstrate some common sense. In this vein, they have to find the "right balance" between extremes, which Aristotle refers to as vices (Arrington, 1998:76). Thus, Aristotle believed that a virtue lay in the middle of two contrary vices and is described as "choosing the mean between the vice of excess and the vice of deficiency" (Taylor, 2002:63). For example, a nurse demonstrating the virtue of courage chooses a mean state with fear on the one end and confidence on the other. Sometimes nurses are expected to act courageously and speak out or "blow the whistle" on actions, that are to the detriment of their patients, for example abusing of patients or making false recordings that could endanger the life of critically ill patients. In this vein, nurses ought to be confident and demonstrate a willingness and perseverance to stand up or speak out for those for whom they care. Failure to do so would indicate the morally deficient character of a cowardice nurse (Magee, 2001:38: Arrington, 1998:76).

On the contrary, it would also be inappropriate for nurses to act courageously if there was nothing worth acting courageously about, for example in situations where no facts are available or accusations that are purely based on hearsay. Acting on this basis would indicate the morally excessive character of a foolish or foolhardy nurse. Thus, in conclusion, the acts of a courageous nurse are appropriate and relevant to the particular circumstances of a case. Acting wisely in a particular situation of moral difficulty, requires, according to Aristotle (in Magee, 1987:48), the intellectual virtue of practical wisdom (*phronesis*). Practical wisdom as a virtue enables the nurse as a moral agent to know what action is correct in a specific situation. To this effect, virtues enable the nurse to discover the relevant moral aspects of a moral dilemma and to interpret, judge and evaluate them, and to apply rules, principles and moral theories wisely to a situation in order to resolve the dilemma. Therefore, both the intellectual virtues (practical wisdom) and the moral virtues (virtues of character) are necessary for the realisation of various types of moral obligations in nursing, including dealing with moral dilemmas.

> It should be noted that Aristotle mentions other intellectual virtues, not just "practical wisdom" (sometimes called "prudence").

Besides the cardinal virtues expounded by ancient Greek philosophers, such as the virtues of courage, temperance, prudence and justice, Botes and Rossouw (1995:26) described reflection, empathy, fairness, honesty, dedication, responsibility and respect for people as virtues for the nurse as a moral agent. In addition, Beauchamp and Childress (2001:32–38) consider the following five virtues as applicable to health professionals: trustworthiness, integrity, discernment, compassion and conscientiousness.

Decision-making about moral issues in health care demands that the health practitioner or the nurse exercise rational control over emotions. The virtues described in the preceding paragraphs are necessary for such rational control, because it takes a so-called mean position between the vices or excess and deficiency. Self-control in situations of moral difficulty is possible if the nurse possesses virtues. In this vein, a nurse who demonstrates these virtues in a balanced form can be seen as a virtuous nurse. Where virtues reflect the characteristic in itself, virtuousness refers to the quality of that virtue, especially when demonstrated in character. Virtuous nurses are ethical nurses, because they have a deep desire to behave well, irrespective of the circumstances.

> Arries now turns to the particular advantages of virtue ethics for decision
> making in nursing.

The Purpose of Moral Decision-Making in Nursing

One characteristic of nursing is its purposeful nature. This implies that with their action or interaction, nurses aim to achieve something. In this vein, the aim that nurses want to achieve must be worth the effort in other words, it must be good. As indicated elsewhere, ethics revolves around three central concepts: the "self," "other" and "good." The good can sometimes mean different things to different people.

In Aristotelian thought, there is a *telos* or ultimate goal at which all actions of human beings are directed. Aristotle regards this as *eudaemonia*, which is sometimes translated as "happiness" or "well-being" (Ashby, 1997:34; Hospers, 1997:254: Arrington, 1998:67). However, a particular state of happiness or well-being is intended by him. This state of *eudaemonia* or happiness involves inter-action between various facets of life in order to achieve the telos or the highest good. This state of *eudaemonia*, according to Aristotle, is found in the nature of human kind (Arrington, 1998:67). The nature of human beings for Aristotle is reflected in their function. Thus, for us to understand what *eudaemonia* is, we need to grasp what the function of human beings is. Our function as human beings is the one thing that distinguishes us from all other creatures in the universe, for example, our ability to reflect on our actions; in other words, to think rationally. Therefore, reason is our unique function, our *telos* in life (Washburn, 2003:77). The level of our reason is closely linked to our developmental state. This implies that as much as reason can vary across a continuum, so can our state of happiness. For example, a mentally impaired person might sometimes be happier than a person whose faculties are fully functional. A person living in the most physically and mentally appalling conditions can still be happy. Therefore, the state of *eudaemonia* or happiness that Aristotle had in mind is one that was deeply rooted in the joy a person gets from his/her ability to reason, a happiness that is lasting, and worth having, and that makes the person experiencing it flourish.

As stated previously, the purpose of nursing is to promote the health of the patient. Therefore, *eudaemonia* is sometimes translated as "health" in nursing (Botes & Rossouw, 1995:24). However, based on our understanding of what *eudaemonia* means, health in nursing could therefore mean different things for different people. Thus, health for a patient might not mean health for a nurse or any other health professional. This is a profound idea that nurses should consider. Health for a particular patient might be more transcendental rather than literal. Much as it can imply a state of well-being, happiness or feeling physically well, can also be seen from a spiritual point of view. Thus, a virtuous nurse who acts as a moral agent will have a deep understanding of the nature of human beings and grasp how this could affect a person's moral decisions or behaviour.

> What does Arries mean by health being "more transcendental rather than literal"? Is this another way of saying that "being healthy" might be more or less subjective (whatever the patient thinks it is)? If so, wouldn't this be, at the very least, in tension with Aristotle's idea of virtue being objective?

Virtues and the Role of Emotion and Motivation

The association between virtues, emotion and motivation as well as their relevance to moral decision-making are implicit in the following definition of emotion. Emotion is defined as "... *felt tendency toward anything intuitively appraised as good (beneficial), or away from anything intuitively appraised as bad (harmful). This attraction or aversion is accompanied by a pattern of physiological changes organized towards appropriate action. The patterns differ for the different emotions*" (http:// plato.stanford.edu). The aforementioned definition implies that virtues related to a person's emotions motivate him/her to do the right thing. According to Plato, Aristotle's teacher, virtues are related to both emotion and will (http:// aristotle'sethics.stanford.edu). In this vein, emotion and motivation are important characteristics of virtues (Kristjansson, 2000:193–95).

For the sake of so-called objectivity in moral decision-making, an ethical approach based on principlism demands that emotions be discarded or bracketed during moral decision-making (Edwards, 1996:123). However, as holistic human beings, nurses' emotions and feelings are fundamental to their nursing experience. Their emotions influence their perception of a moral situation of how and what they see as well as the quality or goodness of the circumstances. When challenged with a situation of moral difficulty, nurses are expected to assess and recognise the morally pertinent aspects of the situation, which requires the use of cognitive processes. However, perceiving the ethical nature of a situation does not only involve a cognitive process. Emotions of a balanced nature make us sensitive to particular circumstances and help to illuminate the perception we develop about a particular moral situation. In this vein, what we see shapes how and what we experience. Thus, perception and affect are closely related in informing our moral judgements. Therefore, it should not mean that nurses must not consider their emotions during moral decision making, but they should learn how to practice rational control over them. A virtuous nurse will understand the importance of this, because emotions that are over- or under-expressed could indicate a deficient character. Emotions should not be accepted as instinctive unmanageable reactions to moral dilemmas, but as sensitivities that inform our moral judgements (Kristjansson, 2000:194).

| The author now applies her understanding of virtue ethics to a case. |

Martin's Story

The following story of Martin demonstrates how virtue ethics could be applied to moral dilemmas in nursing.

Martin, a 58-year-old lawyer who is an atheist, is admitted to hospital with multiple musculo-skeletal and head injuries after a motor vehicle accident. After stabilisation in the resuscitation room, he is rushed to the operating theatre to drain a sub-dural hemorrhage and to reduce his fractures. Due to the extent of his injuries, Martin is admitted post-operatively to the critical care unit. Three days after admission to the unit, Martin regains consciousness and the doctors are able to assess the true extent of his injuries. It has been established that Martin is a known leukaemic sufferer who is currently in remission. He also has diabetes mellitus that is well controlled. As a result of his injuries, he has become a quadriplegic. Despite two occasions of being actively resuscitated in the critical care unit, Martin's cognition remained intact. After four weeks in hospital, Martin is miraculously discharged and sent home to the care of his family members as his primary care givers.

Two months after his discharge, Martin is readmitted to hospital with pneumonia. In a conversation with his family one month ago, Martin voiced his choice that should his condition deteriorate no more active resuscitation procedures should be carried out on him as he cannot bear the suffering any longer. His family was in agreement with him, as they were also deeply affected by his suffering. Despite his physical disabilities, the nurses described Martin as a "lovely patient to care for." Martin, being aware of his rights as a patient, voiced his choice of nor [sic] being actively resuscitated to the healthcare team.

From this story, it is evident that a moral dilemma has occurred. The dilemma involves the moral right of the patient to refuse treatment on the one hand and the nursing team's duty to care on the other hand. For both nurse and patient, the situation results in intense moral conflict, as it seems that a situation with equally right outcomes has arisen. The nurse has a moral duty to promote Martin's well-being or health. To do so, professionally, nurses are expected to balance their expert professional knowledge and understanding with the preference of their patients. In terms of their professional expectations, nurses ought to work collaboratively with patients, thus informing, guiding, advising and helping them, to make appropriate and responsible choices about their health. Factors that influence a person's health status, such as beliefs, cultural background and social circumstances must be taken into consideration. The nurse has to take into consideration the means by which the patient made decisions on the one hand, and ensure that he/she complies with the legal-ethical framework of his/her practice and own convictions on the other hand. In terms of their Professional Code of Conduct and regulations (Muller, 2001:3–8) guiding their practice and informing their decisions, nurses are professionally bound to do good by promoting the health of their patients. After all, they have pledged not only to uphold the legal-ethical and moral traditions of the profession, but also not to discriminate on the basis of race, colour, conviction or religion. In this vein, nurses have committed themselves to act virtuously. In Martin's situation, nurses are required to demonstrate virtues of honesty, caring, trustworthiness and respect.

> Is the above case really a dilemma with equally right outcomes? What is the "damned if we resuscitate and damned if we don't resuscitate" dilemma here?

Virtue ethics as an approach focuses on the moral character of the moral agent. In the next section, therefore, we shall focus on the patient and the nurse as moral agents in Martin's story.

In this next section, the author engages in moral reasoning about the case. See if you can find some of the steps of moral reasoning discussed in Chapter 1 (the 5 Ds).

The Patient as Moral Agent: Martin's Story

A patient's right to refuse health services, including treatment, is a legal reality in South Africa (Department of Health, 1999). In a long discourse on the issues of terminal care, McCartney and Trau (1990:443) indicate that any care that is painful or discomforting to a dying patient may be perceived as burdensome and the individual has an autonomous right to refuse such intervention. The ethical strength of this argument for autonomy is that it is based on moral thought. Furthermore, it has legal precedent in that many judicial decisions have been made in favour of an individual's right to refuse treatment or have treatment ceased. To accept an autonomous decision by a patient, Tschudin (1986:94) is of the opinion that there must be certainty that the individual has accurate information and that all the implications and outcomes of their decision are fully comprehended. From a virtue ethics approach, this implies that nurses need to establish what motivated Martin's decision.

It is important for the nurse as a moral agent to establish whether Martin's decision is motivated freely and sincerely by his faith and whether there is no element of coercion from his religious community or indeed his family. If it is proven beyond reasonable doubt that the patient is able to make an autonomous decision about his spiritual faith, then he is competent to make an autonomous decision about his health. In this instance, Martin's cognition has not been impaired by his illness and if all the concerned participants are satisfied that he has an accurate understanding of his situation, they should respect his choices. Martin for example could have chosen to prioritise what he believes is his eternal existence over what is his current quality of physical health. In this vein, recalling Aristotle's ideas on *eudaemonia*, health is more of a transcendental nature, for example, the patient might have come to terms with his situation and meaning of his life, based on his belief. This might include that he has come to terms with the existential condition about the inescapable nature of death. Thus, considering this, there is clearly an ethical duty on behalf of the nurse to accept his autonomous choice to refuse resuscitation. From a virtue ethics approach, it would be rather morally right of the nurse to respect the faith of their patients, including their choices based on their own free will, rather than to violate it. In these circumstances it is necessary for nurses to become aware of how this event has affected them, in other words, to become aware of their emotional responses and the virtues required in the situation....

> In the case presentation (p. 97) did you notice any discussion about Martin's faith? He is described as an atheist and then the author indicates that the nurse must decide if he is being unduly influenced by a religious community? It seems this is simply an assumption by the author as to why he would refuse resuscitation. Be careful that we do not make assumptions not presented as evidence when reasoning through a case. This is an example.

In the next paragraphs, the virtues inherent in Martin's case will be identified and discussed. Botes and Rossouw (1995:24–26) identified a list of virtues relevant to nursing. However, in my opinion, from a virtue ethics perspective, one virtue is not necessarily more important than another. It is rather the context of the moral dilemma in any opinion that dictates the virtues to be demonstrated by the nurse as a moral agent. The virtues necessary in Martin's story are care; respect and integrity; justice and courage; reason; and honesty and trust.

Care as a Virtue

There is general consensus among nurses that care is and should be a central characteristic of nursing. Therefore, care must be a virtue inherent in the character of a nurse. Noddings (in Botes, 1997:10) distinguishes between natural and ethical care. Natural care refers to situations where people act voluntarily in the interest of others. Ethical care on the other hand, arises from natural care. However, care as a virtue involves an inherent disposition or attitude and is based on a deep sense of responsibility and empathy.

Based on an analysis of acting from the virtue of caring, Van Hooft (1999:200) concludes that caring embraces both thinking right and feeling right, and having the right goal in the context of an ethical practice. It suffuses all aspects of healthcare workers and becomes a full and total orientation of their professional being. In this way both their feeling and their thinking will have the quality of caring. Acting from caring, or acting well or virtuously in the healthcare context, involves sensitive awareness, proper motivation, and rational and evaluative judgement. Accordingly, being a caring nurse is enough to ensure that one will act well (Van Hooft, 1999:200). In this vein, when nurses act from the virtue of care, they will be doing what anyone could judge to be right. By demonstrating sensitivity and empathy in Martin's case regarding his decision from his perspective and understanding one's own emotions and those of others would enable nurses to develop an unbiased view of Martin's decision and communicate an understanding thereof (Wiseman, 1996:1165; Barker, 2000:332). Thus, a virtuous nurse who approaches Martin's situation from a virtue of care will view his decision with empathy and a deep sense of responsibility. In so doing, the nurse as a virtuous moral agent realises the courage Martin demonstrates, which might in turn provoke feelings of respect and admiration.

Respect and Integrity as Virtues

In his [second] Categorical Imperative, Kant stipulates that one should never treat people as a means to achieve an end, but as ends in themselves (Arrington, 1998:104). This implies that we should treat people as human beings with respect. To demonstrate respect is to demonstrate a sensitivity to the differences in the views that people as human beings might hold and learn to understand them even if we disagree. As human beings, this also implies that we should respect the autonomy of others. The ethical strength of this argument for autonomy is that it is based on moral thought on the one hand and that it has legal precedent on the other, because many judicial decisions have been made in favour of people's right to express themselves freely, and to refuse treatment or have treatment ceased (National Health Act, 2004). In Martin's case it would be the morally right thing for the nurse to respect the faith of the patient and his choices, which he has made based on his own free will, rather than to violate them. Violating the faith of the patient might jeopardise the inherent trust relationship between nurse and patient, which might have detrimental effects for both as moral agents.

Integrity means being faithful to one's commitments; it focuses on nurses as people and their dedication to their patients (Gaul, 1995:133). Thus the focus of integrity is on the nurse-patient relationship. Nurses with integrity take the quality of patient care seriously, not only because they owe it them, but also because they judge themselves in meeting this standard. Integrity also demands that they speak up on behalf of the patient when issues of incompetence or immoral actions against patients by fellow healthcare workers arise. Acting based on integrity in Martin's case requires the nurses to support his decision or, if they do not, to ensure that patient care is transferred to another qualified caregiver. Integrity does not require nurses who are ethically opposed to, for example, the patient's "right to die" decision to participate in planning or carrying out a treatment plan. However, it does require that continuity of care be ensured (Gaul, 1995:134).

Justice and Courage as Virtues

Justice can be seen as a principle and as a virtue. Justice as a principle implies fairness and equality. Justice as a virtue enables the nurse to have an awareness of, and a special concern for, the vulnerability of a patient. Therefore, justice can be expressed in concrete actions, i.e., when the nurses in Martin's situations understand his vulnerability and then develop the need to act in his best interests. From this perspective, justice is not only a matter of fairness in the distribution of nursing care and health resources, but also what Pellegrino and Thomasma (1993) call "loving justice" (Lutzen & Da Silva, 1996:208). The virtue of "loving" justice can also be related to the virtue of benevolence, which implies a wish to do good for other (Edwards, 1996:68–69).

Considering the case of Martin, if the nurse wishes to demonstrate the virtue of a "loving justice" he/she will feel the need to act on behalf of the patient, if he/she perceives the latter to be unfairly treated. In other words, what motivates nurses is the intention to do good or what they as virtuous moral agents perceive to be in the best interests of the patient. For example, after a consideration of all the facts and the consequences, nurses might be convinced that not resuscitating the patient might be in the patient's best interest, and in response to this they voice their thoughts to the rest of the ethical decision-making team. In this way, the nurse demonstrates some courage in advocating on behalf of the patient, even if it sometimes means upsetting other team members who might feel that the responsibility is solely that of the doctors. To this end, the nurse demonstrates courage by speaking out and questioning existing practice.

A courageous nurse is someone who is capable of free thought, undertakes responsible actions and carries them out. However, acting courageously cannot always be justified as right on the basis of its consequences, for example when driven by compassion. Other normative aspects need to be considered (Lutzen & Da Silva, 1996:209). In this regard, it is not the consequence of the action that is the guiding principle, but the virtuous conscience and the trust the patient has in the nurse to advocate on his behalf that should motivate the nurse (MacIntyre, 1998:57). To demonstrate justice as a virtue implies exercising practical wisdom (intellectual virtue), which is motivated by the virtues of character (moral virtues) to decide how to act in order to make the best possible decision. Thus, the nurses' virtues enable them not only to do what is right, as in the case of applying rules and law, but also to do the right thing right. Thus, justice as a virtue also implies respect for the patient's integrity or dignity, which is not only a matter of being fair or just (Lutzen & Da Silva, 1996:209).

Reason as a Virtue

Nurses are often accused of responding to ethical situations in an emotional and irrational way. This is claimed by Botes (1997:13) to be the main reason why doctors are intolerant of including them in moral clinical decision-making. Thus, the intolerance is not aimed at the approach, e.g., virtue ethics or the ethics of care, but at the way in which it is operationalised by nurses. This intolerance will probably continue until nurses apply virtue ethics in a rational way. However, reason does not only imply the use of abstract rules and principles to make decisions or solve problems, but also certain dispositions. Reason must be supported by virtues, but virtues alone are not sufficient to make a moral choice. Therefore, nurses as moral agents also need a certain disposition to use their reason. Reason as a virtue in Aristotelian terms implies a certain kind of excellence (*arete*) of the soul. Like Plato, Aristotle is of the opinion that the excellence of reason is wisdom (Arrington, 1998:54). This implies that wisdom is the virtue of reason. MacIntyre (1984:150) also states that "... *the exercise of the virtues requires ... a capacity to judge and to do the right thing in the right place at the right time in the right way. The exercise of such judgement is not a routinizable application of rules.*" Therefore, nurses as moral agents in Martin's case must demonstrate practical wisdom to decide how to respond to a situation. In other words to do what is right in this case, and that is to respect the choices Martin has made.

...

Honesty and Trust as Virtues

Honesty is one of the cornerstones of the nurse-patient relationship. Honesty refers to the quality of not lying, cheating, stealing or being insincere, but qualities of truth, sincerity and reliability (Botes & Rossouw, 1995:25). Every patient has the right to honest information about the nature of their health status. Honesty is a pre-condition for a trust relation. Patients often reveal their deepest and most personal concerns and problems with nurses. This means that patients trust nurses, thus confiding their private vulnerabilities. For example, Martin's vulnerable state leaves him with almost no option but to trust the nurses to honour and respect his choices. However, a virtuous nurse will realise this profound dependence of the patient and knows not to exploit them so as not to cause them harm. Trust can be lost if the nurses decide to violate the faith of the patient. Trust must be earned, because if there is distrust on the part of the patient, it could be because the nurses fail to perform what is necessary for the patient. Patients rely on the nurses' moral character and competence and trust that nurses will behave well. The least that nurses as moral agents acting in the situation can do is not to violate this trust (Lutzen & Da Silva, 1996:207).

References [to this extract]

ARRINGTON, RL 1998: Western ethics: An historical introduction. Massachusetts: Blackwell Publishers.

AVIS, M 1994: Choice cuts: An exploratory study of patients' view about participation in decision-making in a day surgery unit. *International Journal of Nursing Studies.* 31:289–98.

BARKER, P 2000: Reflections on caring as a virtue ethic within an evidence-based culture. *International Journal of Nursing Studies.* 37:329–36.

BEAUCHAMP, T & CHILDRESS, J 2001: Principles of bio-medical ethics. Fifth edition. Oxford: Oxford University Press.

BILEY, F 1992: Some determinants that affect patient participation in decisionmaking about nursing care. *Journal of Advanced Nursing.* 17:414–21.

BOTES, AC & ROSSOUW, G 1995: The reconstruction of virtue based ethics in nursing. *RAUCUR.* 1(2), Nov. 1995: 19–26.

BOTES, AC: The ethics of care and of justice in ethical decision-making in the health team: Inaugural address presented on 27 August 1997. Johannesburg: Rand Afrikaans University.

DAVIS, AJ; AROSKAR, MA; LIASCHENKO, J & DROUGHT, TS 1997: Ethical dilemmas in nursing practice. Fourth Edition. New Jersey: Prentice-Hall, Inc.

DEPARTMENT OF HEALTH (SOUTH AFRICA) 1999: A Patients' Rights Charter. Pretoria: Department of Health.

DRANE, JF: Character and the moral life (In: Davis, AJ; Aroskar, MA; Llaschenko, J & Drought, TS 1997: Ethical dilemmas in nursing practice. Fourth Edition. New Jersey: Prentice-Hall. Inc).

EDWARDS, SD 1996: Nursing ethics: A principle-based approach. London: MacMillan

GAUL, AL 1995: Care: An ethical foundation for critical care nursing. *Critical Care Nurse.* June 1995: 131–35.

GILLIGAN, C 1982: In a different voice: Psychological theory and women's development. Cambridge: Harvard University Press.

HOSPERS, J 1997: An introduction to philosophical analysis. Fourth edition. London: Routledge.

KRISTJÁNSSON, K 2000: Virtue ethics and emotional conflict. *American Philosophical Quarterly.* 37(3), July 2000: 193–207.

LUTZEN, K & DA SILVA, AB 1996: The role of virtue ethics in psychiatric nursing. *Nursing Ethics.* 3(3): 202–11.

MACINTYRE, A 1984: After virtue. Second edition. Notre Dame, IN: University of Notre Dame Press.

MACINTYRE, A 1998: A short history of ethics. London: Routledge.

MAGEE, B 2001: The story of philosophy. London: Dorling Kindersley Limited.

MCCARTNEY, JJ & TRAU, JM 1990: Cessation of the artificial delivery of foods and fluids: Defining terminal illness and care. *Death Studies.* 14: 443–47.

MULLER, ME 2001: Nursing Dynamics. Third edition. Sandown: Heinemann.

PELLEGRINO, ED & THOMASMA, DC 1993: The virtues in medical practice. New York: Oxford University Press.

ROSSOUW, D & VAN VUUREN, L 2004: Business ethics. Third edition. Cape Town: Oxford University Press for Southern Africa.

SAINIO, C; LAURI, S & ERIKSSON, E 2001: Cancer patients' views and experiences of participation in care and decision-making. *Nursing Ethics.* 8(2):97–113.

SCOTT, PA 1995: Aristotle, nursing and health care ethics. *Nursing Ethics.* 2(4):279–85.

SOUTH AFRICA (REPUBLIC). National Health Act (Act 61 of 2003). Pretoria: Government Printer.

TAYLOR, R 2002: An introduction: Virtue ethics. New York: Prometheus Books.

TRIANOSKY, G 1990: What is virtue ethics all about? *American Philosophical Quarterly*. 27(4), October 1990:335–44.

TSCHUDIN, V 1986: Ethics in nursing: The caring relationship. Oxford: Butterworth Heinemann.

VAN HOOFT, S 1999: Acting from the virtue of caring in nursing. *Nursing Ethics*. 6(3): 189–201.

WASHBURN, P (ED) 2003: The many faces of wisdom: Great philosophers' visions of philosophy. New Jersey: Upper Saddle River.

WISEMAN, T 1996: A concept analysis of empathy. *Journal of Advanced Nursing*. 23: 1162–67.

Internet Sources

Aristotle's ethics. Stanford Encyclopedia of Philosophy. (https://plato.stanford.edu/entries/aristotle-ethics/) Accessed on 04 April 2004.

Plato's ethics: An overview. Stanford Encyclopedia of Philosophy. (http://plato.stanford.edu) Accessed on 04 April 2004.

ETHICS COMMITTEE

Billy Likes to Eat Mud

Billy is a 30-year-old developmentally disabled individual who has an oral fixation. Billy has an IQ of 68 and is nonverbal, occasionally making a groaning or yelping noise. He currently lives in an eight-bed group home. Over the years Billy's oral fixation has led to macroglossia (enlarged tongue) and dysphasia.

A normal day for Billy includes:

- Slapping his tongue with anything he can. This has caused chronic parasitic infections and occasional tongue lesions from trauma.

- Getting into the group home's kitchen, when staff are not watching, and stuffing large quantities of bread into his mouth. This has led to incidents of choking.

Billy's room is comfortable and stimulating. He has a swing in his room and a larger swing in a gated area right outside the group home's door. He likes to use a "sit and spin" toy to spin on the floor for hours.

Billy's care aid, Damian, noticed that Billy was outside swinging and decided to interact with him. To Damian's dismay, he found Billy sitting next to his swing slapping mud on his tongue. Damian immediately said to Billy, "NO BILLY, that's ucky, let's go get cleaned up." Damian washed Billy's mouth out with mouthwash and a toothbrush, pulling clumps of mud out of his mouth. Afterwards, Damian redirected Billy to something besides slapping his tongue with mud. Later, Damian found Billy slapping his tongue with mud when delivering his oral medication. Damian repeated the process of washing his mouth out and gave him his medication. When Damian found Billy slapping mud on his tongue a third time that week, he made the decision to restrict Billy from going outside to his swing for the rest of the day and documented what had happened. It is not unusual for staff to make these restrictions.

A few days later, Damian received a letter from management reprimanding him for restricting Billy. The letter stated it was "not in their mission to restrict individuals from achieving their potential" and "You are not qualified to make that decision." The letter demanded a justification for the restriction.

> Discuss the case using the 5 Ds in Chapter 1. Make an argument that defends or disagrees with Damian's decision.

CHAPTER 3

Dilemmas in the Patient–Provider Relationship

OPENING GAMBIT

∞∞∞∞∞∞∞∞∞∞∞∞∞∞∞∞∞∞∞∞∞∞∞∞∞∞∞∞∞∞∞

Prescribing Cebocap[*]

Mrs. Lightman, 74, had surgery four years ago to correct bowel obstruction, and the emotional and physical stress made it difficult for her to sleep. She was prescribed Seconal, a sleeping pill, following her surgery. Four years later, she just can't sleep without it. When Mrs. Lightman moved to a long-term care nursing facility, she came under the care of nurse Jeremy Cartman. Jeremy recognized that Mrs. Lightman was most likely addicted to sleeping pills, so he mentioned his concerns to her. She became agitated and worried that Jeremy would "take away her pills." Jeremy mentioned his concerns to the resident geriatric specialist, Dr. Kenny. Mrs. Lightman was experiencing symptoms like nausea, trouble concentrating, and constipation, which are the possible side-effects of long-term use of Seconal. Dr. Kenny promised to look into it. Jeremy was assigned to another wing of the facility.

A few months later, Jeremy was re-assigned to Mrs. Lightman's care and asked Dr. Kenny about Mrs. Lightman's sleeping issues. Dr. Kenny explained that he had the pharmacist gradually replace the dosage of Seconal with a placebo, and now she's receiving only the placebo and seems to be sleeping fine. "Don't worry, we aren't charging her for Seconal," Dr. Kenny explained. "I had

---

* This case study was adapted from "Placebos for Addiction Withdrawal," in Robert M. Veatch, Amy M. Haddad, and Dan C. English, eds., *Cases in Biomedical Ethics: Decision-Making, Principles, and Cases* (New York: Oxford, 2010), 137.

the pharmacist chart it as Cebocap." (Cebocap is the brand name of a placebo.) "I doubt she'll notice. If she does, just tell her I prescribed something different for her sleeping problems." It turns out that Mrs. Lightman did notice. The next time Jeremy checked on her, he asked how she was feeling. "The headaches and constipation are much better," she replied. "I bet it's the fiber and good sleep I'm getting. I noticed there's a medicine I don't recognize on my bill. It only costs 1.99, so it's no big deal, but have you heard of something called Cebocap?"

WHAT'S AT STAKE?

What could be the downside if Nurse Cartman told Mrs. Lightman that she'd had her Seconal replaced with a placebo? The alternative is to deceive her so that she keeps taking it. At the heart of the problem is the idea that Mrs. Lightman is getting a treatment that she did not consent to. Dr. Kenny took it upon himself to change her prescription without informing her of it first. This is a clear violation of autonomy. However, he did it because Mrs. Lightman didn't need the Seconal and because it was actually harming her—a clear example of the duty toward patient beneficence.

The problem of informed consent is a clash between the duty to autonomy and the duty to beneficence. Nurse Cartman can uphold autonomy and tell Mrs. Lightman that she is taking a placebo, honoring her autonomy at the risk of beneficence. The best case is that Mrs. Lightman accepts that she was being harmed by a drug that she had become dependent on and now will simply stop taking the placebo. Furthermore, she will understand and accept that Dr. Kenny did this for her good and not just to deceive her. The worry, however, is that she will feel betrayed and not trust either Dr. Kenny or Nurse Cartman in the future. The alternative is for Nurse Cartman to continue to keep Mrs. Lightman in the dark, upholding the benefit of Cebocap while violating her autonomy. He does not have to tell her an outright falsehood: He could claim that Cebocap is an alternative to Seconal as a sleep aid, which is true but is surely not the whole truth.

The established medical traditions for what constitutes informed consent do not help with this particular dilemma. Traditionally, there are five conditions for ethically permissible informed consent:

1. The patient has decisional capacity. The patient has the capacity to make their own decisions.

2. The patient has adequate information to make a decision. This presents a duty for the medical providers to disclose the information the patient needs to make a decision.
3. The patient understands the information. To be informed, the patient must be given the information in a manner and language they can comprehend.
4. The patient makes a voluntary choice. There is no unethical coercion or manipulation.
5. The patient authorizes the treatment. There is some procedure that says the patient agrees to undergo the treatment.

You can think of these conditions in the following way: The first three have to do with the patient being fully informed (or adequately informed), and the last two conditions have to do with the patient being free from coercion.

As you can imagine, there are some ethical problems with some of these terms. First, *decisional capacity* is a broad term. A patient can have decisional capacity for some medical decisions but not others. For example, an elderly patient may not have the capacity to decide to stop taking an antibiotic, but they may have the capacity to decide whether to refuse dialysis. Decisional capacity can also wax and wane; an Alzheimer's patient may have decisional capacity in the morning but not by the late afternoon.

Competence vs. Capacity

We often use the terms "competence" and "capacity" (short for "decision-making capacity") interchangeably. However, they are not exactly the same. Competence is a legal term. Competence is presumed unless a court has determined that an individual is incompetent. A judicial declaration of incompetence may be global, or it may be limited (e.g., to financial matters but not medical decisions). The person declared incompetent is considered incompetent until another court decision reverses the ruling.

Decision-making capacity, on the other hand, is a clinical term that is task-specific. A physician may determine that a patient does not have the capacity to make a decision for or against surgery for a hip fracture, but they may have the capacity to decide if they want a sleeping pill or a laxative.

What factors can affect capacity to give informed consent? Mental impairment, surely. Intoxication, surely, if only briefly. What about pain? Dax Cowart, a young pilot, was forcibly treated against his will for eighteen months. An exploding fuel tank had burned him severely. His treatment included very painful debriding processes and daily "tankings" in chemical solutions that also were very painful. Cowart repeatedly refused treatment, but because it was 1973 and paternalism was still very much a part of medicine, his requests to cease treatment were ignored.* One justification for ignoring his lack of consent was that the suffering was clouding his judgment; otherwise, he would have been able to see the value of the treatment.

There is a slippery slope here, and it shows up when we consider what to do when patients disagree with their providers. If fear, pain, or suffering in general can compromise decisional capacity, then to some degree or another all patients are compromised. If they are compromised, patient judgement can be overridden. But who decides this? The provider? If so, then doctors can override patients' wishes. Providers can engage in paternalism for the good of the patient; all they have to do is judge the patient's decisional capacity compromised.

Adequate information is an even bigger problem. The main debate concerns the standard we use to decide what is an adequate amount of information. Three standards have been applied in the history of bioethics. The "physician standard" was just what it sounds like: Adequate disclosure was whatever amount of information the physician thought was adequate. This was replaced by the "reasonable person standard": What was adequate disclosure of information was whatever a hypothetical reasonable person would need to consent to a treatment. However, it was a 1972 lawsuit that forced medical providers to adopt a "patient-centered" standard.

Jerry Canterbury suffered from excruciating pain in his back. Dr. William Spence recommended that he have surgery on his spine. Spence laid out the benefits and most of the risks; however, he left out one rare risk of paralysis, which is exactly what happened to Canterbury. Canterbury was paralyzed from the waist down after he fell in the hospital. Spence testified in his defense that he had left out this small risk because he thought the surgery was what his patient needed and was afraid that disclosing even the small risk of paralysis might cause Canterbury to refuse the surgery on his spine. The court found in favor of Canterbury, and while referencing a reasonable patient standard, it significantly broadened the scope of what must be disclosed to a patient. The standard must be "measured by the patient's need, and that need is the information material to the decision." The court went on to say that the test of whether a potential risk should be disclosed to the patient is whether the patient might need the

---

* Lonnie D. Kliever (ed.), *Dax's Case: Essays in Medical Ethics and Human Meaning* (Dallas, TX: Southern Methodist University Press, 1989).

information to make a decision. The court acknowledged that this would effectively mean that "all risks potentially affecting the decision must be unmasked."[*]

The easiest way for medical providers to meet the court's standard is to disclose all the risks, no matter how small. This has led to long disclosure forms, where every potential risk and alternative is spelled out and the patient is asked to sign acknowledging that they have read and understand the risks and alternatives of the procedure.

Can the disclosure of every promised benefit, no matter how unlikely, also undermine informed consent? Patients with no other options often volunteer themselves or in some cases their children for research trials, hoping for a miracle. Should medical providers even disclose the possible benefits, no matter how small, in these cases? The worry is that we will end up with something like the Charlie Gard case.[†] In 2017, Charlie Gard, a 10-month-old, was diagnosed with a rare disorder that caused him seizures, progressive brain damage, and muscle failure. There is no current treatment that is effective. One drug did hold some promise, but it wasn't even in research trials yet. The parents consented to the treatment in the hope that it might help Charlie. The medical staff opposed it, however, because they thought the treatment was prolonging Charlie's daily suffering. Charlie's case highlights an important point about disclosure of information. Normally the concern is disclosing enough information in the doctor-patient relationship so that consent can make a treatment permissible. But consent can also be an exercise of the patient's or family members' autonomy. Just because a patient will consent to a procedure does not mean it is morally permissible, let alone a moral obligation, for the medical providers to do the procedure.

What Counts as Informed Consent?

You might think there are two ways of saying what counts as valid moral consent. First, there is the *procedure of consent*. To say someone has consented to treatment is to say that the proper procedure was followed. They have read the form and have had their questions answered. This ensures that there was adequate disclosure of information because all the information was disclosed. However, the procedural conception of consent does not guarantee that the patient makes a choice based on the information. After all, patients may not know which

---

[*] *Canterbury v. Spence* (464 F.2d 772 (D.C. Cir. 1972), https://casetext.com/case/canterbury-v-spence.

[†] Debra Goldschmidt and Hilary Clarke, "Baby Charlie Gard dies after life support withdrawn," *CNN*, July 29, 2017, https://www.cnn.com/2017/07/28/health/charlie-gard-death.

questions to ask regarding treatment. In other words, a provider could give the patient the forms and ask if there are any questions, and the patient could decide whether to have surgery or therapy by flipping a coin; this would satisfy the conditions of adequate disclosure according to *Canterbury v. Spence*.

The other kind of consent is procedural in a way but we should call it *deliberative consent* since what counts as consent is that the patient has weighed the options and thought through the choices carefully. This sort of consent requires more of a relationship with the patient on the part of the provider because the patient may have to be guided through how to eliminate all but the most serious side-effects or risks for a routine procedure. The difficulty is that it is nearly impossible to measure this deliberative process and determine whether the patient has gone through it. It is not legally enforceable or quantifiable, so most providers will opt for the procedural model because of the legal risk.

Therapeutic Privilege as an Exception to Informed Consent

Notice that the court ruled that what was unacceptable was the *reason* that Dr. Spence withheld the information. He was concerned that disclosure would cause Jerry Canterbury to refuse the treatment Spence thought he needed. Could there be cases where a medical provider could ethically withhold information, not because it might sway the patient from treatment but because it might cause the patient undue distress? Some patients may have the capacity to consent, but emotional distress due to irrational fears or misunderstandings about medicine means they might overreact to information and give in to anxiety or depression. In some cases, this can affect treatment.

For example, multiple sclerosis (MS) is a debilitating neural disease that is incurable but treatable. Stress can exacerbate the symptoms of MS. There are several types of MS, and some have a worse prognosis than others. Neurologists surveyed have reported that sometimes if there is a concern that a diagnosis of MS will cause the patient undue distress and make their symptoms worse, the doctor will withhold saying "it's MS" until they can start the patient on a regimen of drugs to control the MS symptoms. A few weeks later, the neurologist will tell the patient they have MS. Such temporary withholding of information because it might cause distress is commonly called *therapeutic privilege*.

It is important to note that the physician's recommendation for treatment should be the same whether the diagnosis is disclosed immediately or later. It could be argued that the information being withheld in our example is of a different sort than what was withheld from Jerry Canterbury. Canterbury had to decide about the risks of surgery versus receiving no treatment. In the case of the MS patient, the information is not relevant for making a decision since the treatment would be the same and the risks are minimal. The doctor is concerned that the stress of being told they have an incurable, debilitating, but treatable disease would actually make the patient's symptoms worse.

The conditions of therapeutic privilege are as follows:

1. The information should be withheld, not altered as if lying to the patient.
2. The information must not be information that a patient would need to make a medical decision.
3. The information must be withheld for the patient's benefit, not in order to avoid negative patient interaction.
4. The information must be withheld only temporarily.

Let's consider each of these in turn. First, therapeutic privilege is not lying: In the case of Mrs. Lightman, above, or the MS patient, if the patient asked point-blank, "Do I have MS?" or "Is this a placebo?" both Nurse Cartman and the neurologist would have to answer "Yes."

Second, therapeutic privilege cannot run afoul of *Canterbury v. Spence*. Providers cannot withhold any information that any patient would need to make an informed decision about treatment. The treatment for MS is the same one already prescribed, and there is no alternative treatment medically approved. It seems reasonable, since MS is not a terminal illness and the treatment itself is not so burdensome, that any patient diagnosed with MS would want to be treated. Therefore, the MS patient in our scenario is not being deprived of information that they would need to exercise their autonomy. It is certainly a gray area, determining which information would be considered not relevant for medical decision making. However, it seems reasonable that counter-factual information—that is, information that would have given the patient a reason to choose otherwise—should be considered information that providers cannot withhold.

Third, therapeutic privilege is not a way of managing problem patients. It is considered unethical for providers to withhold information only to placate or pacify patients. If Dr. Kenny prescribed a placebo because he did not want to deal with a belligerent or annoying Mrs. Lightman, it would violate her autonomy. Likewise, if the neurologist withheld the MS diagnosis because he just could not take one more crying, hysterical patient today, that, too, would be a violation of patient autonomy.

Finally, therapeutic privilege is, ideally, temporary. At some point, the doctor should tell the patient what they did and why. It is to be hoped that the breach of trust is minimal and understandable. When Mrs. Lightman is completely off Seconal and sleeping well, her doctor should let her know that she is not receiving any treatment at all and that the weaning process was for her own good. This "temporary" requirement is one that is the most disputed because it is the most counter-intuitive. Isn't it better if the patient never knows? What does it hurt Mrs. Lightman to think she is getting a sleep aid when she is getting a sugar pill? The placebo is beneficial to her health and not very expensive. Or it might damage patient trust for the neurologist to admit he withheld diagnosis until the patient was on an MS drug. Word could also get around to other patients and the effect would be negated.

So what is the moral justification for the "temporary" part of therapeutic privilege? Essentially, it is because the patient is receiving treatment without their consent. In most cases, they are paying for treatment without knowing what is going on. It is a small but potentially exploitative violation of autonomy.

Consider the following scenarios. Which ones would you consider acceptable? questionable? unethical?

1. A primary-care physician knows that a patient suffers from severe anxiety and intrusive thoughts for which he has never received treatment. She needs to send the patient to an oncologist to have a biopsy to rule out cancer. The appointment is two weeks away, and she is concerned that if she tells the patient where she is sending him, he will suffer severe anxiety worrying about the upcoming biopsy. The physician tells him she's sending him to a "liver specialist" for a biopsy, knowing that as soon as the patient arrives, he will realize it is an oncologist.

2. A patient has an inoperable brain tumor and the neurologist is concerned about how the patient will take the news since there is no treatment indicated. The neurologist tells the patient that they have an incurable brain disorder and prescribes some medication to help with the symptoms. The patient dies in a few weeks.

3. A patient in the hospital has an irrational fear of antibiotics, concerned that she will become resistant to them. She refuses all antibiotics. Surgery is crucial for the patient's survival, and the surgeon has ordered pre-operative antibiotics. The nurse gives the antibiotic along with the patient's other daily meds but does not tell her she is getting an antibiotic, and the patient does not ask.

4. A patient is admitted to ER after taking an overdose of pain medication in a suicide attempt. He ends up in the ICU due to complications. Routine test results indicate that the patient may have pre-cancerous tumors in his stomach. The ICU staff do not tell him the results while he is in their care. He is informed of the results when he is moved to a regular room.

There are several factors affecting autonomous decision making in these cases. First, there is the duration of the violation. In three of the examples, information is withheld for a short period, and the patient is eventually given all the information. Second, there is the nature of the violation. Is information just omitted or is the patient told something that, while true, is not the whole truth? Third, there is the nature of the information itself. Is the information being withheld something the patient would need to make decisions that affect their life? This seems to be the ethical concern in case 2, where the patient needs this information to get their affairs in order and prepare for their death. Finally, there is the reason for the violation. Is it to prevent harm or merely to avoid a difficult patient?

In case 1, the information is withheld, but it is only for a short period. However, this case does seem to violate the standard definition since the psychological threat (the patient worrying about cancer for two weeks) doesn't seem to meet the threshold of being medically harmful.

According to a 2008 report, 62% of doctors think prescribing placebos is morally justified under certain conditions. In an anonymous survey, half of the doctors polled admitted to prescribing placebos.

- If a clinical trial showed a sugar pill was better than no treatment for fibromyalgia, would you recommend sugar pills to fibromyalgia patients? Yes, 58% of the doctors said.
- Do you ever actually recommend treatments primarily to enhance a patient's expectations? Yes, 80% of the doctors said.
- In the last year, did you recommend a placebo treatment to a patient? Yes, 55% of the doctors said.

Two-thirds of doctors polled told patients they were receiving "medicine not typically used for your condition but might benefit you."

Source: J.C. Tilburt et al., "Prescribing 'Placebo Treatments': Results of National Survey of US Internists and Rheumatologists," British Medical Journal 337 (2008), https://doi.org/10.1136/bmj.a1938.

Placebos and therapeutic privilege represent exceptions to informed consent. They are not to be considered rare, and both are controversial (placebos are controversial in treatment but less so in medical research; see Chapter 4). The foundation for informed consent is autonomy. The challenges to informed consent come from the provider's duties to beneficence and non-maleficence especially. Therapeutic privilege is withholding information the disclosure of which would be so contra-indicated as to violate non-maleficence.

The Duty to Warn

In the patient-provider relationship, there is often a conflict between the principles of autonomy and beneficence—between what the patient wants and what is best for the patient. Sometimes there is even a clash between what the patient wants and what is best for others. Take the dilemma inherent in the duty to warn. Valuing patient autonomy includes respecting a patient's privacy, but what happens when respecting privacy means harming others? This is a dilemma for medical providers who are asked by the patient to keep their HIV status from a partner who does not have HIV. Which is more important: the patient's privacy or their partner's health?

Paternalism

When we infringe on patient autonomy for their own good, it is called *paternalism*, from the Latin *pater*, meaning "father." In other words, we are treating them in much the same way we treat children. There are situations where paternalism is acceptable; for example, if someone does not have the ability to make their own decisions because they are temporarily impaired (intoxication or dementia, for instance), then medical providers may do what is in the patient's best interest until they are able to make their own decisions again. We can call this *weak* paternalism because the invasion is minimal. *Strong* paternalism, on the other hand, would involve violating a patient's autonomy when they do have decisional capacity, such as keeping a terminal diagnosis from a patient in order to spare their feelings. Strong paternalism is not very welcome in medicine.

The trend in medicine since the 1980s is to give patients more autonomy, not less. This is the result of several very public events that happened in the United States, where medical providers were seen to abuse their power in order to be paternalistic. We learned about Dax Cowart earlier. In 1973, Donald "Dax"

Cowart, a burn victim, was treated against his will for a year and a half. Cowart repeatedly refused painful treatments (e.g., bathing in a solution of bleach and other chemicals). Though he was an adult, both his requests to be discharged and his refusals of treatment were ignored.

The difficulty is, of course, determining when paternalism is weak or strong. It boils down to whether and when a patient has decisional capacity. The thing to remember is that ethically, decisional capacity is not an on/off switch in the way that the legal term "competent" is. If someone is declared incompetent by a court to make decisions, it usually takes another court hearing to declare them competent again. In contrast, decisional capacity can wax and wane. A person can have decisional capacity in the morning but not in the evening, as with Alzheimer's patients who have so-called "sundowner's syndrome." A person can also have partial decisional capacity. For instance, someone who cannot consent to surgery could still refuse treatment. It should not surprise you that the ethical concept of decisional capacity is a lot messier than the legal concepts of competent and incompetent.

WHAT'S THE DEBATE?

Reading 3.1: Gerald Dworkin, "Paternalism"

This article does not emphasize medical paternalism, but it is a clear exposition of paternalism. Dworkin's thesis is stated early: He argues that most paternalism is unethical, but there is a case to be made for interfering with someone's autonomy in order to prevent them from sabotaging their own future autonomy. From this simple exception, Dworkin (b. 1937) considers a host of cases.

... I take as my starting point the "one very simple principle" proclaimed by Mill in *On Liberty* ... "That principle is, that the sole end for which mankind are warranted, individually or collectively, in interfering with the liberty of action of any of their number, is self-protection. That the only purpose for which power can be rightfully exercised over any member of a civilized community, against his will, is to prevent harm to others. He cannot rightfully be compelled to do or forbear because it will be better for him to do so, because it will make him happier, because, in the opinion of others, to do so would be wise, or even right."[1]

This principle is neither "one" nor "very simple." It is at least two principles; one asserting that self-protection or the prevention of harm to others is sometimes a sufficient warrant and the other claiming that the individual's own good is never a sufficient warrant for the exercise of compulsion either by the society as a whole or by its individual members. I assume that no one with the possible exception of extreme pacifists or anarchists questions the correctness of the first half of the principle. This essay is an examination of the negative claim embodied in Mill's principle—the objection to paternalistic interferences with a man's liberty.

I

> In this section, Dworkin makes several distinctions. He points out that lots of laws might be proposed or passed for paternalistic reasons (for the good of some people) but those same laws could be justified for non-paternalistic reasons (for the good of society, etc.). Dworkin is not interested in these ulterior justifications. He then gives a list of the sort of paternalistic laws he's interested in.

By paternalism I shall understand roughly the interference with a person's liberty of action justified by reasons referring exclusively to the welfare, good, happiness, needs, interests or values of the person being coerced. One is always well-advised to illustrate one's definitions by examples but it is not easy to find "pure" examples of paternalistic interferences. For almost any piece of legislation is justified by several different kinds of reasons and even if historically a piece of legislation can be shown to have been introduced for, purely paternalistic motives, it may be that advocates of the legislation with an anti-paternalistic outlook can find sufficient reasons justifying the legislation without appealing to the reasons which were originally adduced to support it. Thus, for example, it may be that the original legislation requiring motorcyclists to wear safety helmets was introduced for purely paternalistic reasons. But the Rhode Island Supreme Court recently upheld such legislation on the grounds that it was "not persuaded that the legislature is powerless to prohibit individuals from pursuing a course of conduct which could conceivably result in their becoming public charges," thus clearly introducing reasons of a quite different kind. Now I regard this decision as being based on reasoning of a very dubious nature but it illustrates the kind of problem one has in finding examples. The following is a list of the kinds of interferences I have in mind as being paternalistic.

II

1. Laws requiring motorcyclists to wear safety helmets when operating their machines.
2. Laws forbidding persons from swimming at a public beach when lifeguards are not on duty.
3. Laws making suicide a criminal offense.
4. Laws making it illegal for women and children to work at certain types of jobs.
5. Laws regulating certain kinds of sexual conduct, e.g., homosexuality among consenting adults in private.
6. Laws regulating the use of certain drugs which may have harmful consequences to the user but do not lead to anti-social conduct.
7. Laws requiring a license to engage in certain professions with those not receiving a license subject to fine or jail sentence if they do engage in the practice.
8. Laws compelling people to spend a specified fraction of their income on the purchase of retirement annuities. (Social Security)
9. Laws forbidding various forms of gambling (often justified on the grounds that the poor are more likely to throw away their money on such activities than the rich who can afford to).
10. Laws regulating the maximum rates of interest for loans.
11. Laws against duelling.

In addition to laws which attach criminal or civil penalties to certain kinds of action there are laws, rules, regulations, decrees, which make it either difficult or impossible for people to carry out their plans and which are also justified on paternalistic grounds. Examples of this are:

1. Laws regulating the types of contracts which will be upheld as valid by the courts, e.g., (an example of Mill's to which I shall return) no man may make a valid contract for perpetual involuntary servitude.
2. Not allowing as a defense to a charge of murder or assault the consent of the victim.
3. Requiring members of certain religious sects to have compulsory blood transfusions. This is made possible by not allowing the patient to have recourse to civil suits for assault and battery and by means of injunctions.
4. Civil commitment procedures when these are specifically justified on the basis of preventing the person being committed from harming himself.

(The D.C. Hospitalization of the Mentally Ill Act provides for involuntary hospitalization of a person who "is mentally ill, and because of that illness, is likely to injure *himself* or others if allowed to remain at liberty." The term injure in this context applies to unintentional as well as intentional injuries.)

5. Putting fluorides in the community water supply.

To see how the five above might touch on medical decisions, consider that not allowing the consent of the victim as a defense for murder would apply to physician-assisted suicide (2 above). Of course, 3 above is referring to Jehovah's Witnesses and other groups refusing certain medical treatment for religious reasons. 4 above could apply not only to involuntary hospitalization but also to a physician deciding that a patient does not have decisional capacity and therefore doctors can make decisions for them.

All of my examples are of existing restrictions on the liberty of individuals. Obviously one can think of interferences which have not yet been imposed. Thus one might ban the sale of cigarettes, or require that people wear safety-belts in automobiles (as opposed to merely having them installed) enforcing this by not allowing motorists to sue for injuries even when caused by other drivers if the motorist was not wearing a seat-belt at the time of the accident.

I shall not be concerned with activities which though defended on paternalistic grounds are not interferences with the liberty of persons, e.g., the giving of subsidies in kind rather than in cash on the grounds that the recipients would not spend the money on the goods which they really need, or not including a $1000 deductible provision in a basic protection automobile insurance plan on the ground that the people who would elect it could least afford it. Nor shall I be concerned with measures such as "truth-in-advertising" acts and the Pure Food and Drug legislation which are often attacked as paternalistic but which should not be considered so. In these cases all that is provided—it is true by the use of compulsion—is information which it is presumed that rational persons are interested in having in order to make wise decisions. There is no interference with the liberty of the consumer unless one wants to stretch a point beyond good sense and say that his liberty to apply for a loan without knowing the true rate of interest is diminished. It is true that sometimes there is sentiment for going further than providing information, for example when laws against usurious interest are passed preventing those who might wish to contract loans at high rates of interest from doing so, and these measures may correctly be considered paternalistic.

III

Bearing these examples in mind let me return to a characterization of paternalism. I said earlier that I meant by the term, roughly, interference with a person's liberty for his own good. But as some of the examples show the class of persons whose good is involved is not always identical with the class of person's whose freedom is restricted. Thus in the case of professional licensing it is the practitioner who is directly interfered with and it is the would-be patient whose interests are presumably being served. Not allowing the consent of the victim to be a defense to certain types of crime primarily affects the would-be aggressor but it is the interests of the willing victim that we are trying to protect. Sometimes a person may fall into both classes as would be the case if we banned the manufacture and sale of cigarettes and a given manufacturer happened to be a smoker as well.

Thus we may first divide paternalistic interferences into "pure" and "impure" cases. In "pure" paternalism the class of persons whose freedom is restricted is identical with the class of persons whose benefit is intended to be promoted by such restrictions. Examples: the making of suicide a crime, requiring passengers in automobiles to wear seat-belts, requiring a Christian Scientist to receive a blood transfusion. In the case of "impure" paternalism in trying to protect the welfare of a class of persons we find that the only way to do so will involve restricting the freedom of other persons besides those who are benefitted. Now it might be thought that there are no cases of "impure" paternalism since any such case could always be justified on non-paternalistic grounds, i.e., in terms of preventing harms to others. Thus we might ban cigarette manufacturers from continuing to manufacture their product on the grounds that we are preventing them from causing illness to others in the same way that we prevent other manufacturers from releasing pollutants into the atmosphere, thereby causing danger to the members of the community. The difference is, however, that in the former but not the latter case the harm is of such a nature that it could be avoided by those individuals affected if they so chose. The incurring of the harm requires, so to speak, the active co-operation of the victim. It would be mistaken theoretically and hypocritical in practice to assert that our interference in such cases is just like our interference in standard cases of protecting others from harm. At the very least someone interfered with in this way can reply that no one is complaining about his activities. It may be that impure paternalism requires arguments or reasons of a stronger kind in order to be justified since there are persons who are losing a portion of their liberty and they do not even have the solace of having it be done "in their own interest." Of course in some sense, if paternalistic justifications are ever correct then we are protecting others, we are preventing some from injuring others, but it is important to see the differences between this and the standard case.

What Dworkin says here is subtle but important. A chart will be helpful. Paternalism is interfering with someone's autonomy (and only their autonomy) to prevent them from harming themself (Case 1). The harm principle, however, is interfering with Bob's autonomy to prevent harm *to someone else* like Adam (Case 2). What Dworkin means by "impure" paternalism is that sometimes our paternalism ends up interfering with others even though we didn't intend to (Cases 1 and 2). Sometimes our paternalism isn't to prevent harm but to benefit the person (Case 3), and sometimes we interfere with someone's autonomy only to benefit a third party (Case 4).

	Interfere with Bob's autonomy	Interfere with Adam's autonomy
To prevent harm to Bob	**1** CASE: Restraints for a dementia patient *Paternalism*	**2** CASE: Requiring vaccines *Harm principle*
To benefit Bob	**3** CASE: Mandatory exercise classes for workers *Paternalism*	**4** CASE: Taxing to pay for social services *Welfare principle*

Source: I am grateful to Dr. Arthur Ward for developing this diagram.

Paternalism then will always involve limitations on the liberty of some individuals in their own interest but it may also extend to interferences with the liberty of parties whose interests are not in question.

IV

Dworkin has one final exclusion from his class of paternalistic acts. He excludes from his discussion those laws or regulations that solve collective-action problems. A collective-action problem happens when individuals would be better off pursuing a collective good (e.g., better working hours). It is not rational for me to advocate as one person for an employee health-care subsidy even if I think it would be good for everyone. However, if enough people were to join me in my advocacy, then it would make sense for me to advocate for a subsidy. The regulation or legislation enforces what I would already agree to if there were enough people. This is not paternalism, Dworkin argues.

Finally, by way of some more preliminary analysis, I want to distinguish paternalistic interferences with liberty from a related type with which it is often confused. Consider, for example, legislation which forbids employees to work more than, say, 40 hours per week. It is sometimes argued that such legislation is paternalistic for if employees desired such a restriction on their hours of work they could agree among themselves to impose it voluntarily. But because they do not the society imposes its own conception of their best interests upon them by the use of coercion. Hence this is paternalism.

Now it may be that some legislation of this nature is, in fact, paternalistically motivated. I am not denying that. All I want to point out is that there is another possible way of justifying such measures which is not paternalistic in nature. It is not paternalistic because as Mill puts it in a similar context such measures are "required not to overrule the judgment of individuals respecting their own interest, but to give effect to that judgment: they being unable to give effect to it except by concert, which concert again cannot be effectual unless it receives validity and sanction from the law."[2]

The line of reasoning here is a familiar one first found in Hobbes and developed with great sophistication by contemporary economists in the last decade or so. There are restrictions which are in the interests of a class of persons taken collectively but are such that the immediate interest of each individual is furthered by his violating the rule when others adhere to it. In such cases the individuals involved may need the use of compulsion to give effect to their collective judgment of their own interest by guaranteeing each individual compliance by the others. In these cases compulsion is not used to achieve some benefit which is not recognized to be a benefit by those concerned, but rather because it is the only feasible means of achieving some benefit which is recognized as such by all concerned. This way of viewing matters provides us with another characterization of paternalism in general. Paternalism might be thought of as the use of coercion to achieve a good which is not recognized as such by those persons for whom the good is intended. Again while this formulation captures the heart of the matter—it is surely what Mill is objecting to in *On Liberty*—the matter is not always quite like that. For example when we force motorcyclists to wear helmets we are trying to promote a good—the protection of the person from injury—which is surely recognized by most of the individuals concerned. It is not that a cyclist doesn't value his bodily integrity; rather, as a supporter of such legislation would put it, he either places, perhaps irrationally, another value or good (freedom from wearing a helmet) above that of physical well-being or, perhaps, while recognizing the danger in the abstract, he either does not fully appreciate it or he underestimates the likelihood of its occurring. But now we are approaching the question of possible justifications of paternalistic measures and the rest of this essay will be devoted to that question....

> In this next section, Dworkin zeroes in on a tension in Mill's argument against paternalism. Mill is a committed utilitarian (see Chapter 1), and it doesn't seem that a committed utililitarian can advocate strongly against paternalism. Dworkin points out that there is a thread in Mill's argument that doesn't sound very utilitarian but advocates for the value of people living free of interference in their autonomy, with a few exceptions. Ask yourself whether Dworkin is fair to Mill and whether you think anyone committed to utilitarianism (not just the principle of utility) can be as anti-paternalistic as Dworkin thinks Mill should be.

Preventing a man from selling himself into slavery (a paternalistic measure which Mill himself accepts as legitimate), or from taking heroin, or from driving a car without wearing seat-belts may constitute a lesser evil than allowing him to do any of these things. A consistent Utilitarian can only argue against paternalism on the grounds that it (as a matter of fact) does not maximize the good. It is always a contingent question that may be refuted by the evidence. But there is also a non-contingent argument which runs through *On Liberty*. When Mill states that "there is a part of the life of every person who has come to years of discretion, within which the individuality of that person ought to reign uncontrolled either by any other person or by the public collectively" he is saying something about what it means to be a person, an autonomous agent. It is because coercing a person for his own good denies this status as an independent entity that Mill objects to it so strongly and in such absolute terms. To be able to choose is a good that is independent of the wisdom of what is chosen. A man's "mode of laying out his existence is the best, not because it is the best in itself, but because it is his own mode."[3]

> It is the privilege and proper condition of a human being, arrived at the maturity of his faculties, to use and interpret experience in his own way.[4]

As further evidence of this line of reasoning in Mill consider the one exception to his prohibition against paternalism.

> In this and most civilised countries, for example, an engagement by which a person should sell himself, or allow himself to be sold, as a slave, would be null and void; neither enforced by law nor by opinion. The ground for thus limiting his power of voluntarily disposing of his own lot in life, is apparent, and is very clearly seen in this extreme case. The reason for not interfering, unless for the sake of others, with a person's voluntary acts, is consideration for his liberty. His voluntary choice is evidence that what he so chooses is desirable, or at least endurable, to him, and his good is on the whole best provided for by allowing him to take his own means of pursuing it. But by selling himself for a slave, he abdicates his liberty; he foregoes any future use of it beyond that single act.
>
> He therefore defeats, in his own case, the very purpose which is the justification of allowing him to dispose of himself. He is no longer free; but is thenceforth in a position which has no longer the presumption in its favour, that would be afforded by his voluntarily remaining in it. The principle of freedom cannot require that he should be free not to be free. It is not freedom to be allowed to alienate his freedom.[5]

> Here we get to the heart of Dworkin's nuanced defense of paternalism. Mill, the anti-paternalist, says the state is justified in interfering with someone who wants to sell themself into perpetual servitude. Why does Mill make this exception? Dworkin attempts to tease out an answer. Can you find it in the paragraphs below?

Now leaving aside the fudging on the meaning of freedom in the last line it is clear that part of this argument is incorrect. While it is true that *future* choices of the slave are not reasons for thinking that what he chooses then is desirable for him, what is at issue is limiting his immediate choice; and since this choice is made freely, the individual may be correct in thinking that his interests are best provided for by entering such a contract. But the main consideration for not allowing such a contract is the need to preserve the liberty of the person to make future choices. This gives us a principle—a very narrow one—by which to justify some paternalistic interferences. Paternalism is justified only to preserve a wider range of freedom for the individual in question.

How far this principle could be extended, whether it can justify all the cases in which we are inclined upon reflection to think paternalistic measures justified remains to be discussed. What I have tried to show so far is that there are two strains of argument in Mill—one a straight-forward Utilitarian mode of reasoning and one which relies not on the goods which free choice leads to but on the absolute value of the choice itself. The first cannot establish any absolute prohibition but at most a presumption and indeed a fairly weak one given some fairly plausible assumptions about human psychology; the second while a stronger line of argument seems to me to allow on its own grounds a wider range of paternalism than might be suspected. I turn now to a consideration of these matters.

> There are two ways to look at autonomy. Autonomy is valuable as a free act. In this case, paternalism is always wrong because it interferes with a person's choice, full stop. Mill can't be arguing for this because it would flatly contradict with his utilitarianism, which says that actions are right solely because they produce the most good and the least harm for the greatest number. The other option is that what is valuable is not that each choice is without interference but rather that a person's life is filled

with autonomous choices. A life of autonomy is what is valuable, not each autonomous act. If this is your view, then some paternalism could be justified if it led to more future autonomy. It is the latter "autonomous lives" view that Dworkin says Mill has in mind, and the one Dworkin will go on to defend.

VI

We might begin looking for principles governing the acceptable use of paternalistic power in cases where it is generally agreed that it is legitimate. Even Mill intends his principles to be applicable only to mature individuals, not those in what he calls "non-age." What is it that justifies us in interfering with children? The fact that they lack some of the emotional and cognitive capacities required in order to make fully rational decisions. It is an empirical question to just what extent children have an adequate conception of their own present and future interests but there is not much doubt that there are many deficiencies. For example it is very difficult for a child to defer gratification for any considerable period of time. Given these deficiencies and given the very real and permanent dangers that may befall the child it becomes not only permissible but even a duty of the parent to restrict the child's freedom in various ways. There is however an important moral limitation on the exercise of such parental power which is provided by the notion of the child eventually coming to see the correctness of his parent's interventions. Parental paternalism may be thought of as a wager by the parent on the child's subsequent recognition of the wisdom of the restrictions. There is an emphasis on what could be called future-oriented consent— on what the child will come to welcome, rather than on what he does welcome.

So now Dworkin connects acceptable paternalism with consent. What principle could make paternalism permissible for children but not adults? Dworkin answers with a "you'll thank me later" principle. Parents make rational decisions that children do not have the ability to make but would consent to if they only had the rationality to do so. But doesn't this open up a possibility justifying paternalism against an adult who would consent to the interference in their autonomy if they could only see the big picture? Dworkin considers a few of these.

The essence of this idea has been incorporated by idealist philosophers into various types of "real-will" theory as applied to fully adult persons. Extensions of paternalism are argued for by claiming that in various respects, chronologically mature individuals share the same deficiencies in knowledge, capacity to think rationally, and the ability to carry out decisions that children possess. Hence in interfering with such people we are in effect doing what they would do if they were fully rational. Hence we are not really opposing their will, hence we are not really interfering with their freedom. The dangers of this move have been sufficiently exposed by [Isaiah] Berlin [1909–97] in his *Two Concepts of Liberty*. I see no gain in theoretical clarity nor in practical advantage in trying to pass over the real nature of the interferences with liberty that we impose on others. Still the basic notion of consent is important and seems to me the only acceptable way of trying to delimit an area of justified paternalism.

Let me start by considering a case where the consent is not hypothetical in nature. Under certain conditions it is rational for an individual to agree that others should force him to act in ways in which, at the time of action, the individual may not see as desirable. If, for example, a man knows that he is subject to breaking his resolves when temptation is present, he may ask a friend to refuse to entertain his requests at some later stage.

A classical example is given in the *Odyssey* [of Homer] when Odysseus commands his men to tie him to the mast and refuse all future orders to be set free, because he knows the power of the Sirens to enchant men with their songs. Here we are on relatively sound ground in later refusing Odysseus' request to be set free. He may even claim to have changed his mind but since it is just such changes that he wished to guard against we are entitled to ignore them.

> Medical examples might be 48-hour psychiatric holds, new medications with radio transmitters that digitally record when they are taken, or even suspension of Do Not Resuscitate orders during surgery.

A process analogous to this may take place on a social rather than individual basis. An electorate may mandate its representatives to pass legislation which when it comes time to "pay the price" may be unpalatable. I may believe that a tax increase is necessary to halt inflation though I may resent the lower pay check each month. However, in both this case and that of Odysseus the measure to be enforced is specifically requested by the party involved and at some point in time there is genuine consent and agreement on the part of those persons whose liberty is infringed. Such is not the case for the paternalistic measures we have been speaking about. What must be involved here is not consent to specific measures but rather consent to a system of government, run by elected representatives, with an understanding that they may act to safeguard our interests in certain limited ways.

I suggest that since we are all aware of our irrational propensities, deficiencies in cognitive and emotional capacities and avoidable and unavoidable ignorance it is rational and prudent for us to in effect take out "social insurance policies." We may argue for and against proposed paternalistic measures in terms of what fully rational individuals would accept as forms of protection. Now, clearly since the initial agreement is not about specific measures we are dealing with a more-or-less blank check and therefore there have to be carefully defined limits. What I am looking for are certain kinds of conditions which make it plausible to suppose that rational men could reach agreement to limit their liberty even when other men's interests are not affected.

Of course as in any kind of agreement schema there are great difficulties in deciding what rational individuals would or would not accept. Particularly in sensitive areas of personal liberty, there is always a danger of the dispute over agreement and rationality being a disguised version of evaluative and normative disagreement.

Having considered cases where people consent to having their future autonomy limited in the present, i.e., "Odysseus" and "You'll thank me later" cases, Dworkin now considers classes of interference where the person does not give consent but would likely do so if they valued their life in a rational way or if they had the ability to follow through with their own rational desires. In other words, "You'll thank me later." Ask yourself how some medical decisions could also fit into Dworkin's examples of permissible paternalism.

Let me suggest types of situations in which it seems plausible to suppose that fully rational individuals would agree to having paternalistic restrictions imposed upon them. It is reasonable to suppose that there are "goods" such as health which any person would want to have in order to pursue his own good— no matter how that good is conceived. This is an argument that is used in connection with compulsory education for children but it seems to me that it can be extended to other goods which have this character. Then one could agree that the attainment of such goods should be promoted even when not recognized to be such, at the moment, by the individuals concerned.

An immediate difficulty that arises stems from the fact that men are always faced with competing goods and that there may be reasons why even a value such as health—or indeed life—may be overridden by competing values. Thus the problem with the Christian Scientist and blood transfusions. It may be more important for him to reject "impure substances" than to go on living. The difficult problem that must be faced is whether one can give sense to the notion of a person irrationally attaching weights to competing values.

Consider a person who knows the statistical data on the probability of being injured when not wearing seat belts in an automobile and knows the types and gravity of the various injuries. He also insists that the inconvenience attached to fastening the belt every time he gets in and out of the car outweighs for him the possible risks to himself. I am inclined in this case to think that such a weighing is irrational. Given his life-plans which we are assuming are those of the average person, his interests and commitments already undertaken, I think it is safe to predict that we can find inconsistencies in his calculations at some point. I am assuming that this is not a man who for some conscious or unconscious reasons is trying to injure himself nor is he a man who just likes to "live dangerously." I am assuming that he is like us in all the relevant respects but just puts an enormously high negative value on inconvenience—one which does not seem comprehensible or reasonable.

It is always possible, of course to assimilate this person to creatures like myself. I, also, neglect to fasten my seat belt and I concede such behavior is not rational but not because I weigh the inconvenience differently from those who fasten the belts. It is just that having made (roughly) the same calculation as everybody else I ignore it in my actions. [Note: a much better case of weakness of the will than those usually given in ethics texts.] A plausible explanation for this deplorable habit is that although I know in some intellectual sense what the probabilities and risks are I do not fully appreciate them in an emotionally genuine manner.

We have two distinct types of situation in which a man acts in a non-rational fashion. In one case he attaches incorrect weights to some of his values; in the other he neglects to act in accordance with his actual preferences and desires. Clearly there is a stronger and more persuasive argument for paternalism in the latter situation. Here we are really not—by assumption—imposing a good on another person. But why may we not extend our interference to what we might call evaluative delusions? After all in the case of cognitive delusions we are prepared, often, to act against the expressed will of the person involved. If a man believes that when he jumps out the window he will float upwards—Robert Nozick's [1938–2002] example—would not we detain him, forcibly if necessary? The reply will be that this man doesn't wish to be injured and if we could convince him that he is mistaken as to the consequences of his action he would not wish to perform the action. But part of what is involved in claiming that a man who doesn't fasten his seat-belts is attaching an irrational weight to the inconvenience of fastening them is that if he were to be involved in an accident and severely injured he would look back and admit that the inconvenience wasn't as bad as all that. So there is a sense in which if I could convince him of the consequences of his action he also would not wish to continue his present course of action. Now the notion of consequences being used here is covering a lot of ground. In one case it's being used to indicate what will or can happen as a result of a course of action and in the other it's making a prediction about the future evaluation of the consequences—in the first sense—of a course of action. And whatever the difference between facts and values—whether it be hard and fast or soft and slow—we are genuinely more reluctant to consent to interferences where evaluative differences are the issue. Let me now consider another factor which comes into play in some of these situations which may make an important difference in our willingness to consent to paternalistic restrictions.

Some of the decisions we make are of such a character that they produce changes which are in one or another way irreversible. Situations are created in which it is difficult or impossible to return to anything like the initial stage at which the decision was made. In particular some of these changes will make it impossible to continue to make reasoned choices in the future. I am thinking specifically of decisions which involve taking drugs that are physically or psychologically addictive and those which are destructive of one's mental and physical capacities.

I suggest we think of the imposition of paternalistic interferences in situations of this kind as being a kind of insurance policy which we take out against making decisions which are far-reaching, potentially dangerous and irreversible. Each of these factors is important. Clearly there are many decisions we make that are relatively irreversible. In deciding to learn to play chess I could predict in view of my general interest in games that some portion of my free-time was going to be pre-empted and that it would not be easy to give up the game once I acquired a certain competence. But my whole life-style was not going to be jeopardized in an extreme manner. Further it might be argued that even with addictive drugs such as heroin one's normal life plans would not be seriously interfered with if an inexpensive and adequate supply were readily available. So this type of argument might have a much narrower scope than appears to be the case at first.

> There is an old saying: "If the camel's nose gets into the tent, then the rest of it will quickly follow." It is a form of a "slippery slope" objection (see Chapter 7 for more on slippery slopes). Dworkin argues that paternalism is justifiable when someone weighs risk poorly or when they just cannot follow through with their stated preferences. Is this argument like the nose of the camel? Does it logically entail almost any medical paternalism provided we can show that the patient is acting irrational? Dworkin adds a new set of decisions that justify paternalism: when the person is under societal or psychological pressure.

A second class of cases concerns decisions which are made under extreme psychological and sociological pressures. I am not thinking here of the making of the decision as being something one is pressured into—e.g., a good reason for making duelling illegal is that unless this is done many people might have to manifest their courage and integrity in ways in which they would rather not do so—but rather of decisions such as that to commit suicide which are usually made at a point where the individual is not thinking clearly and calmly about the nature of his decision. In addition, of course, this comes under the previous heading of all-too-irrevocable decision. Now there are practical steps which a society could take if it wanted to decrease the possibility of suicide—for example not paying social security benefits to the survivors or as religious institutions do, not allowing such persons to be buried with the same status as natural deaths. I think we may count these as interferences with the liberty of persons to attempt suicide and the question is whether they are justifiable.

Using my argument schema the question is whether rational individuals would consent to such limitations. I see no reason for them to consent to an absolute prohibition but I do think it is reasonable for them to agree to some kind of enforced waiting period. Since we are all aware of the possibility of temporary states, such as great fear or depression, that are inimical to the making of well-informed and rational decisions, it would be prudent for all of us if there were some kind of institutional arrangement whereby we were restrained from making a decision which is (all too) irreversible. What this would be like in practice is difficult to envisage and it may be that if no practical arrangements were feasible then we would have to conclude that there should be no restriction at all on this kind of action. But we might have a "cooling off" period, in much the same way that we now require couples who file for divorce to go through a waiting period. Or, more far-fetched, we might imagine a Suicide Board composed of a psychologist and another member picked by the applicant. The Board would be required to meet and talk with the person proposing to take his life, though its approval would not be required.

A third class of decisions—these classes are not supposed to be disjoint—involves dangers which are either not sufficiently understood or appreciated correctly by the persons involved. Let me illustrate, using the example of cigarette smoking, a number of possible cases.

1. A man may not know the facts—e.g., smoking between 1 and 2 packs a day shortens life expectancy 6.2 years, the costs and pain of the illness caused by smoking, etc.

2. A man may know the facts, wish to stop smoking, but not have the requisite will-power.

3. A man may know the facts but not have them play the correct role in his calculation because, say, he discounts the danger psychologically because it is remote in time and/or inflates the attractiveness of other consequences of his decision which he regards as beneficial.

> Do 1–3 represent a third class of decisions or are they just more examples of deficient reasoning or weakness of will?

In case 1 what is called for is education, the posting of warnings, etc. In case 2 there is no theoretical problem. We are not imposing a good on someone who rejects it. We are simply using coercion to enable people to carry out their own goals. (Note: There obviously is a difficulty in that only a subclass of the individuals affected wish to be prevented from doing what they are doing.) In case 3 there is a sense in which we are imposing a good on someone since given his current appraisal of the facts he doesn't wish to be restricted. But in another sense we are not imposing a good since what is being claimed—and what must be shown or at least argued for—is that an accurate accounting on his part would lead him to reject his current course of action. Now we all know that such cases exist, that we are prone to disregard dangers that are only possibilities, that immediate pleasures are often magnified and distorted.

If in addition the dangers are severe and far-reaching we could agree to allowing the state a certain degree of power to intervene in such situations. The difficulty is in specifying in advance, even vaguely, the class of cases in which intervention will be legitimate.

A related difficulty is that of drawing a line so that it is not the case that all ultra-hazardous activities are ruled out, e.g., mountain-climbing, bull-fighting, sports-car racing, etc. There are some risks—even very great ones—which a person is entitled to take with his life.

> Because these activities represent a form of life (not just a one-time decision) and a life that a person has consented to, they are permissible. Dworkin now considers how we can be paternalistic using the least restrictive means.

A good deal depends on the nature of the deprivation—e.g., does it prevent the person from engaging in the activity completely or merely limit his participation—and how important to the nature of the activity is the absence of restriction when this is weighed against the role that the activity plays in the life of the person. In the case of automobile seat belts, for example, the restriction is trivial in nature, interferes not at all with the use or enjoyment of the activity, and does, I am assuming, considerably reduce a high risk of serious injury. Whereas, for example, making mountain climbing illegal prevents completely a person engaging in an activity which may play an important role in his life and his conception of the person he is.

In general the easiest cases to handle are those which can be argued about in the terms which Mill thought to be so important—a concern not just for the happiness or welfare, in some broad sense, of the individual but rather a concern for the autonomy and freedom of the person. I suggest that we would be most likely to consent to paternalism in those instances in which it preserves and enhances for the individual his ability to rationally consider and carry out his own decisions.

I have suggested in this essay a number of types of situations in which it seems plausible that rational men would agree to granting the legislative powers of a society the right to impose restrictions on what Mill calls "self-regarding" conduct. However, rational men knowing something about the resources of ignorance, ill-will and stupidity available to the law-makers of a society—a good case in point is the history of drug legislation in the United States—will be concerned to limit such intervention to a minimum. I suggest in closing two principles designed to achieve this end.

In all cases of paternalistic legislation there must be a heavy and clear burden of proof placed on the authorities to demonstrate the exact nature of the harmful effects (or beneficial consequences) to be avoided (or achieved) and the probability of their occurrence. The burden of proof here is twofold—what lawyers distinguish as the burden of going forward and the burden of persuasion. That the authorities have the burden of going forward means that it is up to them to raise the question and bring forward evidence of the evils to be avoided. Unlike the case of new drugs where the manufacturer must produce some evidence that the drug has been tested and found not harmful, no citizen has to show with respect to self-regarding conduct that it is not harmful or promotes his best interests. In addition the nature and cogency of the evidence for the harmfulness of the course of action must be set at a high level. To paraphrase a formulation of the burden of proof for criminal proceedings—better 10 men ruin themselves than one man be unjustly deprived of liberty.

Finally I suggest a principle of the least restrictive alternative. If there is an alternative way of accomplishing the desired end without restricting liberty then although it may involve great expense, inconvenience, etc. the society must adopt it.

Notes

1. J.S. Mill, *Utilitarianism* and *On Liberty* (Fontana Library Edition, ed. by Mary Warnock, London, 1962), p. 135. All further quotes from Mill are from this edition unless otherwise noted.
2. J.S. Mill, *Principles of Political Economy* (New York: P.F. Collier and Sons, 1900), p. 442.
3. Mill, *Utilitarianism* and *On Liberty*, p. 197.
4. Ibid., p. 186.
5. Ibid., pp. 235–36.

Reading 3.2: Aanand D. Naik, Carmel B. Dyer, Mark. E Kunik, and Laurence B. McCullough, "Patient Autonomy for the Management of Chronic Conditions: A Two-Component Re-Conceptualization"

Most of the time, when we talk about patient autonomy we are concerned with the patient's ability to make a decision about treatment. This is decisional autonomy. The execution (carrying out) of that treatment is what the medical providers do for the patient in acute care, where a patient is treated for a time and gets better (we hope). What happens, though, when the illness isn't acute but chronic? The patient has to execute the doctor's treatment (e.g., take the pills every day). Naik et al. think that our concept of patient autonomy in medicine is too vague. They present us with situations where a patient has decisional autonomy but not executive autonomy. They can make decisions but have trouble carrying out the doctor's orders. This complication in the concept of autonomy has practical implications because doctors will assess whether the patient has decisional capacity based solely on decisional autonomy.

... Patients can and do electively choose to ignore physicians' recommendations, even in acute settings; and some may be in denial about their conditions and limit the effort needed to manage them. Physicians, reared in the acute-care paradigm, typically perceive non-adherence as a challenging but salient reflection of a patient's decisional autonomy (Anderson and Funnell 2005). Some patients with chronic conditions may articulate understanding of the management plan and appear non-adherent when actually they are unable to implement the steps necessary to meet the treatment objectives. This is an underappreciated ethical challenge to the patient-physician relationship: the need for an expansion of the concept of patient autonomy to include, not only decisional autonomy, but also the patient's capacity to execute complex self-management tasks, i.e., *executive autonomy*. Patients with intact decisional autonomy may nevertheless have unappreciated physical, educational, and cognitive barriers that impair executive autonomy, i.e., their capacity to plan, sequence, and carry out tasks associated with the management of their chronic conditions....

The Two-Component Concept of Patient Autonomy

The concept of patient autonomy was developed in the context of acute care and rightly has centered on decisional autonomy, the patient's capacity to understand information and to make voluntary decisions. This is because, in acute care, the patient's role is to authorize intervention after a deliberative process. Clinicians largely perform the implementation or execution of that decision. The clinical benchmark for evaluating patient autonomy in this paradigm focuses on the patient's capacity to participate in the informed consent process, through which authorization is given or withheld (McCullough, Molinari and Workman 2001). After consenting, patients are only expected to comply with short-term therapy (e.g., 7 days of antibiotics), attend regular clinic appointments, or present on the day of surgery and not leave the hospital until discharged.

There is ample evidence of a consistent trend in the bioethics literature to equate autonomy with autonomous decision-making, i.e., with decisional autonomy....

> The concept of autonomy in moral philosophy and bioethics recognizes the human capacity for self-determination, and puts forward a principle that the autonomy of persons ought to be respected. (Miller 1995, 215)

[...]

Patient preferences are ethically significant because they make explicit the values of self-determination and personal autonomy that are deeply rooted in the ethics of our culture. Autonomy is the moral right to choose and follow one's own plan of life and action. (Jonsen et al. 1982, 53)

[Faden and Beauchamp] proposed a theory of autonomous action comprising three aspects: understanding, intentionality, and voluntariness (Table 1).

Understanding requires that a patient have sufficient knowledge of the situation and the available options or choices, as well as an appreciation of how these affect the patient on a personal level. To exhibit appreciation, a patient should demonstrate some rational process for weighing options and choices and their application to his or her circumstances. The requirement for understanding does not prohibit a patient from making unorthodox or even unreasonable choices as long as the criteria for understanding are fulfilled.

Intentionality requires that actions are initiated and performed according to a patient's goals and plan. At a minimum, patients should articulate their preferences and then settle on a course of action that implements their preferences. In the outpatient setting, intentionality also requires that patients participate in the development of the treatment plan and then execute the plan (Grimes et al. 2000). The third aspect is *voluntariness* or the ability to act without substantially controlling influences. These include external influences, such as those arising from coercion or manipulation, and internal impairments like hearing loss, pain or unreasonable fear that inhibit voluntary actions or compel involuntary actions.

TABLE 1

Faden and Beauchamp's Theory of Autonomous Action

1. Understanding: Actions based on understanding of the situation and choices
   a. Capacity to comprehend the circumstances and facts of a situation
   b. Appreciation of the personal consequences of each choice and/or action
   c. Evidence of a rational process for choosing one versus another option

2. Intentionality: Actions are willed and performed according to one's plan
   a. Capacity to make and express preferences and choose a single option
   b. Development of strategies and tactics for the execution of a choice
   c. Performance of strategies and adaptations to changing circumstances

3. Voluntariness: Ability to act without controlling influences
   a. Actions free of external coercion or manipulation
   b. Actions not compelled or substantially inhibited by internal impairments

... The importance of the executive component of autonomy has become apparent with the shift from acute care, in which the patient authorizes and the clinical team executes a plan of care, to chronic care, in which the patient authorizes and then plays an essential role in executing the plan of care. Most recently, Lai and Karlawish (2007) have proposed a "new approach to assessing everyday decision-making capacity" (2007, 105) that does make reference to executive function but not executive autonomy....

The nature and exercise of the patient's autonomy in the management of chronic conditions cannot be adequately conceptualized or clinically assessed by appealing to a concept of autonomy that includes only decisional autonomy. Chronic care models focus on the self-management of chronic conditions and adaptation to problems as they arise. In doing so, these approaches make an implicit appeal to an expanded concept of autonomy that we propose to make explicit, autonomous decision-making (decisional autonomy) plus executive autonomy, the capacity to perform complex self-management tasks, especially those related to treatment planning and implementation.

Faden and Beauchamp's (1986) theory of autonomous action remains salient for the task of explicating this expanded concept of autonomy (Table 2). In the context of the self-management of chronic conditions, intentionality should be updated to include the patient's capacities to develop a treatment plan, to implement and monitor the plan, and to amend the treatment plan effectively in response to changing circumstances (Faden and Beauchamp 1986; Grimes et al. 2000). Furthermore, voluntariness in the context of chronic illness should be updated to include freedom, not just from external coercion, but also from internal impairments that inhibit goal-directed or compel goal-antagonizing actions. Impairments of intentionality or voluntariness can manifest as impairments of executive autonomy that threaten the patient's ability to adhere to an agreed-upon treatment plan. Furthermore, impairments of executive autonomy can occur independently of or in conjunction with impairments of decisional autonomy.

TABLE 2

Dimensions of Decisional and Executive Autonomy Using Faden and Beauchamp's Theory of Autonomous Action

Decisional Autonomy	Executive Autonomy
UNDERSTANDING	
Comprehension of circumstances and facts regarding a treatment decision	Comprehension of tasks required for treatment performance
Appreciation of personal consequences of a treatment decision	—
Having a rational process for choosing one versus another option	—
INTENTIONALITY	
Capacity to make and express a choice	—
Development of a treatment plan	Identify strategies and surrogates (when appropriate) to implement plan
—	Perform strategies and make adaptations to changing circumstances
VOLUNTARINESS	
Actions free of external coercion	Actions free of external coercion
—	Actions not compelled or inhibited by internal impairments

Evaluating Decisional and Executive Autonomy: Mrs. Brown

Mrs. Brown is a 68-year-old widow with type 2 diabetes mellitus, congestive heart failure, osteoarthritis, and hypertension who lives alone in her home. She had been taking oral medications for diabetes but was switched to insulin-based therapy due to hyperglycemia despite her medications. She appeared willing to perform her diabetes treatments, including home glucose monitoring, after detailed discussions and training with her physician and a diabetes health educator. However, over time Mrs. Brown's physician begins to question her adherence to the treatment plan due to repeated office and emergency room visits for hyper- and hypoglycemia, shortness of breath and the development of a new foot ulcer.

Understanding:

1. She is aware of the health consequences of diabetes and the importance of managing blood glucose to control diabetes.
2. She appreciates that her diabetes is advanced, with retinopathy and neuropathy, and that oral medications are no longer effective.
3. Mrs. Brown concedes the need to take insulin injections given the risk of serious morbidity from uncontrolled diabetes.

Intentionality:

1. She expresses a preference for improved diabetes control and chooses an aggressive treatment plan using insulin injections.
2. Mrs. Brown constructs a treatment plan with her physician and diabetes educator that involves monitoring her daily blood glucose, aggressively adjusting her insulin, and regularly observing her feet.
3. Despite several months of treatment, Mrs. Brown's blood sugar remains poorly controlled. She has difficulty performing daily measurements, makes frequent errors in insulin dosing, and develops a new foot ulcer.

Voluntariness:

1. Her decision to change treatment plans was free of coercion.
2. Mrs. Brown's impaired vision and limitations in executive cognitive functions may be internal inhibitors to performing her treatment plan.

... Any clinician who engages Mrs. Brown would find a patient adequately aware of the risks of her diabetes and eager to participate in the active treatment of her condition. Over several months, however, it has become clear that her capacity to perform her treatment plan is limited by her endogenous impairments, including diminished executive cognitive functions, and complicated by the demands of a rigorous treatment plan. In terms of the expanded, two-component concept of autonomy, she should be understood to exhibit deficits in intentionality and voluntariness, producing limitations in her executive autonomy that may be overlooked using assessments of decisional autonomy alone. Had Mrs. Brown's physician performed a screening evaluation for executive cognitive impairments after she was deemed non-adherent, appropriate changes to the treatment plan might have avoided further morbidity by simplifying the regimen to match the patient's executive capacities. Ongoing morbidity threatens her health and functional status and, therefore, her remaining autonomy.

Mrs. Brown's case highlights a persistent conceptual gap in how patients and clinicians plan and implement treatments for chronic diseases. Physicians focus almost exclusively on discussions of risk, expectations for treatment, and their own knowledge about best treatments. Physicians take on the responsibility for educating their patients and obtaining agreement regarding the scope and bounds of treatment. Since decision-making capacity is the primary basis for establishing patient autonomy, voluntary non-adherence is often the default assumption for patients' failure to comply with the treatment plan, especially when that plan was collaboratively developed. Anderson and Funnell (2005) have described how this dysfunctional model of adherence in chronic care leads to the ethically flawed assumptions that patients' motivations are the source of treatment failure and that the best solution is for patients "to defer to the expertise (and authority derived from it) of clinicians and to follow the recommendations they have been given" (2005, 154). Without a comprehensive conceptual and clinical appreciation for both decisional and executive autonomy in chronic care, this paradigm of non-adherence threatens the decisional autonomy and health outcomes of patients.

As the case of Mrs. Brown demonstrates, patients may be capable of engaging in robust deliberations about treatment goals and processes but physically or cognitively unable (and at times unaware of their inability) to participate in the implementation of the treatment plan. This incapacity is ethically and clinically significant because the patient's executive autonomy may be essential to effectively monitor and execute the treatment plan (Glasgow and Anderson 1999). Clinicians' awareness of these impairments, especially those linked to executive cognitive abilities, is underappreciated and not actively considered when developing treatment plans. In addition to the clinical realities of chronic care, the biological and psychological processes that govern behavior influence the two-component concept of patient autonomy....

Assessment and Management of Deficits in Executive Autonomy

In clinical assessments, decisional autonomy is treated as a threshold phenomenon: a judgment must be reached that either the patient has decisional capacity or does not. Access to treatment, participation in a trial, or even legal rights can be taken away if an individual lacks decisional autonomy. Executive autonomy, on the other hand, should be understood and clinically assessed along a clinical gradient rather than as a threshold phenomenon (in contrast to Faden and Beauchamp's account of intentionality as an either/or phenomenon). This distinction is important to avoid unnecessary infringements of patients' rights and simultaneously add a huge physical and financial burden on healthcare and social service providers....

Conclusion

The one-component concept of patient autonomy as decisional autonomy is deeply rooted in the capacity to make informed choices regarding acute healthcare decisions. As physicians and patients co-manage chronic conditions and implement care plans, an expanded concept of patient autonomy that includes both decisional and executive autonomy is required. The two-component conceptualization of patient autonomy adapts the Faden and Beauchamp (1986) approach, to fashion a model of autonomy that integrates decisional and executive domains into all assessments of a patient's capacity to make and implement decisions for her care....

References [to this extract]

Anderson, R.M. and Funnell, M.M. 2005. Patient empowerment: Reflections on the challenge of fostering the adoption of a new paradigm. *Patient Education and Counseling*, 57(2): 153–57.

Faden, R.R. and Beauchamp, T.L. 1986. *A History and Theory of Informed Consent*, New York, NY: Oxford University Press.

Glasgow, R.E. and Anderson, R.M. 1999. In diabetes care, moving from compliance to adherence is not enough. Something entirely different is needed. *Diabetes Care*, 22(12): 2090–92.

Grimes, A.L., McCullough, L.B., Kunik, M.E., Molinari, V. and Workman, R.H. 2000. Informed consent and neuroanatomic correlates of intentionality and voluntariness among psychiatric patients. *Psychiatric Services*, 51(12): 1561–67.

Jonsen, A.R., Siegler, M. and Winslade, W.J. 1982. *Clinical Ethics*, New York, NY: Macmillan.

Lai, J.M. and Karlawish, J. 2007. Assessing the capacity to make everyday decisions: A guide for clinicians and an agenda for future research. *American Journal of Geriatric Psychiatry*, 15(2): 101–11.

McCullough, L.B., Molinari, V. and Workman, R.H. 2001. Implications of impaired executive control functions for patient autonomy and surrogate decision making. *Journal of Clinical Ethics*, 12(4): 397–405.

Miller, B. 1995. "Autonomy." In *Encyclopedia of Bioethics*, 2nd ed., Edited by: Reich, W.T. 215–20. New York, NY: Macmillan.

Reading 3.3: Camilla Scanlan and Ian H. Kerridge, "Autonomy and Chronic Illness: Not Two Components but Many"

Naik and colleagues questioned the one-dimensional assessment of autonomy and suggested that autonomy is more complex. Scanlan and Kerridge respond by saying, in essence, "Oh it's far more complicated than even the distinction between decisional and executive autonomy."

The authors start by acknowledging Naik et al.'s article (see this chapter) and agree with them. They then use a study with patients who had bone marrow transplants and did not exactly follow doctor's orders.

... The primacy of autonomy in medical care has been extensively critiqued over the past two decades. Naik and colleagues (2009) provide yet another reason to be skeptical of simplistic formulations of autonomy and decision-making in medicine. At the same time, however, we believe that the authors continue to overemphasize rationality, deemphasize the social and relational basis of autonomy and agency, and provide an insufficiently complete model of capacity in chronic illness....

We report the results of on-going qualitative research with patients undergoing allogeneic hematopoietic stem cell transplant ("bone marrow transplant") for a range of hematologic malignancies [bone cancer] that suggest that the reasons for non-adherence may be much more complex than that provided by Naik and colleagues (2009). The participants in our study were aged from their mid-twenties to sixty and none had any history of concomitant psychiatric disorders, or of diminished decisional capacity. All had received extensive education regarding transplantation. In each case, allogeneic stem cell transplant provided the only, or the greatest chance of long-term survival. One might assume, therefore, that these people would be highly motivated to adhere with the established management plan. In fact, a number of the participants in this study chose to "go against" the established treatment regime; some chose not to take antibiotics, others refused to remain in isolation at the time when they were at high risk of infection due to lowered immunity, some continued to smoke during the transplant period when they were at high risk of serious respiratory infections, others took up their pre-transplant social and occupational "roles" when this may have posed an infection risk, with one man carrying out physically demanding work including deconstructing an old shed and several cars soon after discharge from hospital and against medical advice. Given that none had educational or cognitive barriers to executing their management plan, were their actions really a deficit in executive autonomy, or perhaps related to something else?

One of the problems with autonomy is that it fails to account for the moral significance of vulnerability in the setting of serious illness and dependency on healthcare and assumes that decisions are, and even should be rational. For in the context of chronic illness a person may be judged to do:

- the "right thing" for the "right reason,"
- the "right thing" for the "wrong reason,"
- the "wrong thing" for the "right reason,"
- the "wrong thing" for the "wrong reason,"

and still be acting autonomously.

> Can you think of examples of how someone who is chronically ill might do each of these? Do you agree that someone can do the wrong thing for the wrong reason and still be acting with decisional capacity (autonomy)? Can you think of some examples outside of the medical context where this might be true?

Patients choosing not to adhere with the agreed management plan were acting against their "medical best interests" but were arguably acting in a way that restored control over their lives, and their illness (Seeman and Seeman 1983). We would argue that if a patient elects to "take control" the only way he/she knows, or the only way that he/she can, by choosing to "do things their way," as some patients in our study reported, then they may be acting autonomously, with capacity, and with rationality, insofar as their actions are consistent with their belief system and with the choices open to them.

> So do the authors want us to believe that patients will sometimes auton-omously choose not to comply with doctors' recommendations as a way of gaining control (agency) and "sticking it to" the situation they are in? The authors do not give us details about their communication with their doctors with regard to this non-compliance. What do you think are the ethical duties in this situation?

In other words, assessments of an individual's capacity to plan, sequence and carry out tasks only makes sense within the context of their life's narrative and their illness experience and may be better understood through a broad construction of agency than through executive autonomy.

This is not, however, inconsistent with theories of autonomy, as there is frequently overlap between agency and autonomy, and autonomy may include reference to: 1) sovereignty over him/herself; 2) "capacity" to reflect on and identify his/her desires or preferences; 3) "agency" i.e. is capable of rationally guiding one's reasoned desires into actions; and 4) free will.

Benson (1983) defined the autonomous person as one who is able to:

> ... trust one's own powers and to have a disposition to use them, to be able to resist the fear of failure, ridicule or disapproval that threatens to drive one into reliance on the guidance of others (9).

While this seems clear, this idea is challenged by the context of serious illness, as patients have little choice but to rely upon medical expertise for their survival.

Dworkin (1993) and Frankfurt (1971) amongst others, believe that autonomy is a matter of the patient having capacity to reflectively control and identify with one's basic (first order) desires through higher-level (second order) desires. This may be logical but it also assumes that anxiety, fear, or the desire to avoid death, all diminish functional autonomy—a rather narrow reading of the existential impact of serious illness.

First order desires are simply those things we want. Second-order desires is a fancy term (coined by Frankfurt, name-dropped above) for those things we want to want. I may not want to exercise. I do not desire it like my health-conscious neighbor who actually enjoys jogging. I only run when chased. However, I do have a second-order desire about exercise. I want to be the sort of person who wants to exercise. Some people think that being able to form second-order desires is a sign of rational/autonomous thinking even if we do not always follow through.

Agency can be constructed purely in terms of rational choice (Feinberg 1986, 28). People may act in certain ways because it is the only thing that they can do, and patients may, for example, choose to undergo transplant not because their choice is a logically considered assessment of the burdens and benefits of treatment, but because, in the face of death, they believe they have no option. Likewise, non-adherence may, to others, seem completely irrational, but when one cannot do anything else to regain a sense of control over one's life, then it becomes completely explicable. In this way, actions that seem entirely out of step with an agreed management plan may be entirely consistent with free will, according to Frankfurt's construction of free will as the harmony between desires and volition of one's values (Frankfurt 1971), or the subject of control by unconscious fear or desires.

Thus, while a patient's non-adherence with management plans may be frustrating for their healthcare team (and sometimes for the patient's family) we need to make a serious attempt to understand their situation and their perspective given that the choices that a person makes are only comprehensible within their individual, social, cultural and institutional context. Any useful conception of autonomy must therefore acknowledge the impact of illness on choice and behavior and the influences, constraints and obligation that arise from the network of social relationships that envelope us.

Should we, as Naik and colleagues (2009) suggest, develop a means for testing the executive autonomy, resolve or intentionality of every patient prior to their commencing treatment for a chronic or serious illness? And what would we do if we identified a patient who appeared to have "weakness of will" or who appeared more likely to have difficulty with adherence?

> If you buy Scanlan and Kerridge's argument that patients are non-compliant for rational reasons, then should we expand the definition of autonomy even further than Naik et al. (2009) did? Should we change the way in which we assess a patient's decisional capacity yet again? "Not really," Scanlan and Kerridge say. Instead of tweaking our tests for capacity yet again, we should just listen to the patient and communicate better rather than make assumptions about decisional capacity based on non-compliance.

We would suggest that rather than developing more complex neurobiological or neuropsychiatric assessments, what is required is closer attention to a patient's narrative and to the way in which acute or chronic illness may disrupt this narrative. This may both enable members of the healthcare team to understand why patients may act in the ways that they do and also assist them to construct a management plan more consistent with the patient's particular goals, needs and capabilities. At times this may mean that health professionals will have to accept that non-adherence is a meaningful expression of a patient's autonomy, and at times they may need to encourage patients to accept care and guidance from others (Benson 1983). We would also suggest that while Naik and colleagues (2009) are right to broaden the scope of thinking about autonomy, what is ultimately required is acknowledgement of the impact of illness on independence and social relationships and the importance of trust, the provision of care and compassion (Kerridge et al. 2005; Little 2002).

Do you agree with the conclusion? Assessing decisional capacity (autonomy) is important for how paternalistic a health-care provider can be with a patient. However, if autonomy is not really measurable in terms of decisions and compliance, then where does that leave medical providers?

References [to this extract]

Benson, J. 1983. Who is the autonomous man? *Philosophy* 58(223): 5–17.

Dworkin, R. 1993. *Life's Dominion*. London, UK: HarperCollins.

Frankfurt, H.G. 1971. Freedom of the will and the concept of a person. *Journal of Philosophy* 68: 5–20.

Feinberg, J. 1986. *Harm to Self*. New York, NY: Oxford University Press, 28.

Kerridge, I.H., Lowe, M., and McPhee, J. 2005. *Ethics and Law for the Health Professions*. Sydney, Australia: Federation Press.

Little, J.M. 2002. The fivefold root of an ethics of surgery. *Bioethics* 16(3): 183–201.

Naik, A.D., Dyer, C.B., Kunik, M.E., and McCullough, L.B. 2009. Patient autonomy for the management of chronic conditions: A two-component re-conceptualization. *American Journal of Bioethics* 9(2): 23–30.

Seeman, M., and Seeman, T.E. 1983. Health behavior and personal autonomy: A longitudinal study of the sense of control in illness. *Journal of Health and Social Behavior* 24(2): 144–60.

ETHICS COMMITTEE

The Anxious Patient

A thirty-year-old man comes to an internal medicine specialist complaining of daily fevers, joint pain, and night sweats. After several tests indicating an enlarged spleen and elevated white blood-cell counts, infection is ruled out. The physician suspects that the patient has some form of cancer, possibly Hodgkin's lymphoma. The patient suffers from anxiety and is extremely nervous about diagnosis. Nurse Jackie, while taking yet another vial of blood, overhears the doctor tell the young man that he is being referred to a "liver specialist" who will probably do a biopsy of his liver. The young man is noticeably concerned but accepts that this is necessary. The nurse leaves the room and hears the receptionist scheduling an appointment for the young man with a local oncologist two weeks from now. Later, while the young man is still in the treatment room, the nurse asks the doctor about this. The doctor sighs. "Yeah. He has such anxiety. He requested a valium just to do those blood draws earlier. I didn't want him worrying about a cancer diagnosis that may or may not be confirmed for two weeks. Can you imagine, knowing I'm sending him to an oncologist, what his mind will dream up for the next two weeks?" "But he will find out as soon as he gets there that you lied to him," the nurse says. "Yeah, and I'll have to repair that trust. But I've been seeing him now for a month and I think he will understand. It's better for him."

> Discuss as a group whether the doctor is doing something morally permissible. Is this a morally licit example of therapeutic privilege? Why or why not? Discuss what Nurse Jackie should do.

CHAPTER 4

Dilemmas in Medical Research

Fruit from the Poisonous Tree?

Eduard Pernkopf was professor of anatomy at the University of Vienna, a thorough researcher, and a Nazi. Pernkopf is famous for producing a very detailed anatomy textbook complete with pictures. This anatomy text has been enormously influential in modern medicine. A review of the text in the *New England Journal of Medicine* called the atlas outstanding, "in a class of its own," a book that "will continue to be valued as a reference work even if its prohibitive cost and great detail makes it unsuitable for purchase by medical students."

The bodies used for Pernkopf's anatomy paintings were likely the victims of Nazi terror, although there is little evidence they are from concentration-camp victims. In the original paintings, the illustrator used Nazi symbols in his signature, and Pernkopf did as well. In later editions, these were airbrushed out. The American publisher for the text has promised that if the identities of the models can be ascertained, the victims will be acknowledged and honored in any new editions.

Dr. Howard Israel, an oral surgeon, has a slightly different take. Dr. Israel wants any future editions to contain a full disclosure of the history of the *Pernkopf Anatomy* in the book so that readers can make up their own mind about whether to use the text. Israel will not use the book because the models for the paintings were the victims of Nazi evil.

Ask yourself this: Should medical schools use the Pernkopf text to teach students? Should the text be altered? Should the publisher include a foreword explaining the circumstances?

WHAT'S AT STAKE?

The history of research ethics is largely a history of moral failures and lessons learned from those failures. Nazi doctors did unspeakable experiments on concentration-camp victims. From this travesty of justice came the Nuremberg Code, which mandated, among other things, informed and voluntary consent to participate in a research trial. Later, the Helsinki Declaration built upon the Nuremberg Code, establishing institutional review boards (IRBs), independent committees which ensure that researchers conduct human experiments ethically.

By far one of the most infamous failures of research ethics was the Tuskegee syphilis study. US government researchers studied four hundred African-American men with syphilis. Researchers misled the subjects about every aspect of the study. From this egregious violation came the *Belmont Report*, which not only established the necessity of IRBs but also provided three ethical principles that should inform any research protocol: respect for persons (autonomy), beneficence, and justice. Those principles clash with the principle of utility embodied in the drive to advance medical science in order to save lives and make people healthier.

There is an inherent conflict in research for medical purposes between the duties of a medical provider and the duties of a scientist. Medical providers have an obligation to care for their patients; scientists have an obligation to further science. Thus there is a dilemma between the duties of beneficence/non-maleficence and utility. The study of research ethics is concerned with this dilemma. The history of research ethics is a study of the failures of beneficence/non-maleficence in pursuit of utility. So how do we correct such things? What do we do with the fruit of medical progress when it comes from the poisonous tree of harm to patients? Do we still use it?

This conundrum does not apply just to the Nazis. One of the major objections to COVID-19 vaccination is that each one (Moderna, Pfizer, and Johnson and Johnson) uses stem-cell lines grown from aborted fetuses in testing vaccines. Johnson and Johnson uses fetal stem cells in the manufacture of its vaccine. To staunch anti-abortion advocates, taking the vaccine is participating in a wrong, just like using the Pernkopf Anatomy text. Does the analogy hold?

How consistent is that request for religious exemption?

Administration at a hospital in Arkansas wanted to make sure that those who applied for a religious exemption on the basis that COVID vaccines use fetal stem cells know just what they are getting into. When 5% of the hospital applied for religious exemption citing use of fetal cells in the research that led to a vaccine, the administration said that they would grant the exemption as long as the employees pledged to refrain from any products that use fetal stem cells in their production. The list included ibuprofen, Tylenol, Zoloft, Benadryl, and Pepto-Bismol. According to CEO Mike Troup, "The intent of the religious attestation form is twofold: to ensure staff requesting exemption are sincere in their beliefs and to educate staff who might have requested an exemption without understanding the full scope of how fetal cells are used in testing and development in common medicines."

Source: Parris Kane, "Conway Regional CEO says COVID-19 religious exemption isn't an attempt to shame employees," *KATV*, Sept. 14, 2021, https://katv.com/news/local/conway-regional-ceo-says-covid-19-religious-exemption-isnt-an-attempt-to-shame-employees.

Along with worries about fruit from the poisonous tree, medical research can be exploitative. Exploitation is defined as something like taking advantage of someone for your own benefit. It is usually considered unfair. You can see this intuition in Immanuel Kant's categorical imperative. Kant says, "Never treat others including yourself as merely a means to your end but always as an end in themselves." In other words, don't treat people as things or instruments for your own ends, but treat them as persons with their own ends. But what does it mean to treat others merely as a means? (See box.)

What is a means? What is an end?

Let's play a game. Why did you decide to take this course? You needed it for your major. Fine. Why did you pick your major? You wanted a job? Fantastic. Really practical of you. Why do you want a job? Silly question? Maybe, but humor me. You want to make money? Why? We could keep going with this. All of these reasons, especially the one about money, are what Kant meant by "merely a means." You value them merely because they are a means to an end. Money is a means to an end, namely paying for the things you like. The end is the goal, or what the means gets you.

Those ends can also be a means. The means of money, for example, gets you stuff that could make you happy. However, some things are merely a means to another end. Money is just paper we all agree to value and exchange. It's not valuable in itself. Don't believe me? In a post-apocalyptic world where there is no government (*Walking Dead* anyone?), how valuable is that money? Right. Bullets and vegetable seeds are much more important. When Kant says we should never treat others (or yourself) as merely a means to an end, he's saying, "Don't treat people as if they are just valuable as a means to something else."

Don't make the mistake of thinking you won't use people as a means. We do that all the time. You are using the instructor of this course as a means to getting your degree. The instructor is using you as a means to make a living. I'm using you as a means to my end of being an author. However, we should never treat each other as *merely* a means—like pieces of paper we exchange. Rather, we should treat others as an end in themselves, valuable not just because of what they can do for us, but valuable in their own right.

Nuremberg and Helsinki and Belmont: The Trend toward Beneficence

In first-world countries there are laws that prevent pharmaceutical companies from mistreating research subjects. In North America, the FDA and Health Canada monitor how human research participants are treated. While the World Health Organization monitors research trials, each country has its own standards for such trials. Therein lies the problem: Whose standards should apply? Those of the host country or those of the country where the research is done? If we rely on the home country's protocols, then research in third-world countries becomes much more attractive to pharmaceutical companies because complying with first-world regulations often costs money.

Consider non-therapeutic trials. Therapeutic trials are trials where the research subject receives some sort of treatment to determine whether the drug is effective. Non-therapeutic trials, on the other hand, are studies where the subjects receive no treatment at all. The goal is to study the disease to reveal its pathology or learn more about how the body responds to the disease. Non-therapeutic trials are the most problematic because researchers must refrain from interfering even when they have reason to believe they could do something to help the patient, because any interference would skew the data they are collecting.

The Tuskegee syphilis study was the longest non-therapeutic trial in US history. Four hundred African-American men from the poorest part of Macon County, Alabama, were studied to see how syphilis progressed through the body. The study was started in 1932 and continued into the 1970s. Even after the FDA approved a treatment for syphilis, the participants were not given any treatment. The researchers even went so far as to note on medical records that doctors should not treat the subjects who joined the military because they were part of a study. The justification given was that this sort of non-therapeutic trial would never be able to be done again. Much like the justifications for the Pernkopf anatomy text, the hope was that something good would come from the study. However, there is no evidence that the Tuskegee syphilis study ever produced research that helped advance the treatment and prevention of syphilis which wasn't obtained by other more ethical studies.

To complicate matters, the Tuskegee men were told they were being treated for syphilis. Vanessa Northington Gamble points out that when the men were given spinal taps (a risky and painful procedure) to test for the spread of neurosyphilis, they were told they were receiving shots for their syphilis.[*] In fact, there was little about the Tuskegee syphilis study that was ethical at all.

As a result of this awful history, research ethics has become a major issue. The record of Nazi experiments and abuses led to the Nuremberg Code (see box).

Ten Points of the Nuremberg Code

1. The voluntary consent of the human subject is absolutely essential.

    This means that the person involved should have legal capacity to give consent; should be so situated as to be able to exercise free power of choice, without the intervention of any element of force, fraud, deceit, duress, over-reaching, or other ulterior form of constraint or coercion; and should have sufficient knowledge and comprehension of the elements of the subject matter involved as to enable him to make an understanding and enlightened decision. This latter element requires that before the acceptance of an affirmative decision by the experimental subject there should be made known to him the nature, duration, and purpose of the experiment; the method and means by which it is to be conducted; all

---

[*] "It's Not Just About Tuskegee: The History of African Americans and Medicine," *YouTube*, https://www.youtube.com/watch?v=6_lowoAfGho.

inconveniences and hazards reasonably to be expected; and the effects upon his health or person which may possibly come from his participation in the experiment.

The duty and responsibility for ascertaining the quality of the consent rests upon each individual who initiates, directs or engages in the experiment. It is a personal duty and responsibility which may not be delegated to another with impunity.

2. The experiment should be such as to yield fruitful results for the good of society, unprocurable by other methods or means of study, and not random and unnecessary in nature.

3. The experiment should be so designed and based on the results of animal experimentation and a knowledge of the natural history of the disease or other problem under study that the anticipated results will justify the performance of the experiment.

4. The experiment should be so conducted as to avoid all unnecessary physical and mental suffering and injury.

5. No experiment should be conducted where there is an a priori reason to believe that death or disabling injury will occur; except, perhaps, in those experiments where the experimental physicians also serve as subjects.

6. The degree of risk to be taken should never exceed that determined by the humanitarian importance of the problem to be solved by the experiment.

7. Proper preparations should be made and adequate facilities provided to protect the experimental subject against even remote possibilities of injury, disability, or death.

8. The experiment should be conducted only by scientifically qualified persons. The highest degree of skill and care should be required through all stages of the experiment of those who conduct or engage in the experiment.

9. During the course of the experiment the human subject should be at liberty to bring the experiment to an end if he has reached the physical or mental state where continuation of the experiment seems to him to be impossible.

10. During the course of the experiment the scientist in charge must be prepared to terminate the experiment at any stage, if he has probable cause to believe, in the exercise of the good faith, superior skill and careful judgment required of him that a continuation of the experiment is likely to result in injury, disability, or death to the experimental subject.

Source: United States Holocaust Memorial Museum, "Nuremberg Code," https://www.ushmm.org/information/exhibitions/online-exhibitions/special-focus/doctors-trial/nuremberg-code.

In the Nuremberg Code there are elements of non-maleficence (minimizing risks and harm) and autonomy (informed consent) taking precedence over utility. However, there is little there about beneficence. There is no discussion about whether the experiments should actually help the patients. The Nuremberg Code says nothing about therapeutic trials, only that the expected utility to the body of medical knowledge should justify the risks to the patients. If the benefits are great enough and the patient's consent is valid, then the experiments are permissible.

Is progress in medicine sufficient to override patient beneficence? Philosopher of medicine Hans Jonas (1903–93) says no. In fact, Jonas goes so far as to say that medical progress is optional and should always take a back seat to patient care (i.e., beneficence). In the clash between beneficence and utility in medical research, Jonas says beneficence has priority.* This seems to be the trend in medical research documents. The "Declaration of Helsinki" and the "Belmont Report" (see the What's the Debate section) show a trend toward the priority of beneficence and non-maleficence over utility, as if Jonas is right that medical progress is optional. This sentiment seems colored by the horrible ethical abuses of the past, including Nazi experiments and Tuskegee.

Tuskegee illustrates what can happen to vulnerable populations (the poor, minorities, the mentally handicapped, and children) when there is no strict oversight of medical research, especially non-therapeutic trials. This brings us to the problem of third-world countries, where the poor and the disenfranchised

---

* Hans Jonas, "Philosophical Reflections on Experimenting with Human Subjects," *Daedalus, Journal of the American Academy of Arts and Sciences* 98 (Spring 1969), 219–47.

make up the bulk of research participants. Why would we even think of using research participants from the third world? One good reason is that they ask for it. Many countries in Africa have requested that pharmaceutical companies test new HIV drugs in their countries. Why would a country do this? The same reason an individual would: with the hope that some new drug will make a breakthrough and make things better.

In HIV research in third-world countries, we have a conflict between beneficence and utility. What is good for the subjects, as HIV sufferers, is to get well. However, what researchers need is a population on which they can try experimental drugs. What's good for the research and therefore the greatest number of people overall (utility) is bad for the people suffering from HIV in Africa. What is good for the patients (beneficence) is bad for the research overall (utility).

This clash happens a lot in research studies. If we honor the patient's beneficence and give them treatment, then we will skew or invalidate the scientific data. On the other hand, if we keep the integrity of the data in order to advance medical science, we may harm the patient or at the very least not do them very much good.

A way to resolve this dilemma is to invoke another principle from the last chapter—autonomy via informed consent. Ethicist Alan Wertheimer (1942–2015) says that informed consent is morally transformative; it transforms actions that might be unethical into permissible ones. Consent may not be sufficient to make something unethical into something ethically required, but it can make an action permissible. If research subjects understand that the drug being tested may not do anything to their disease or that they may receive a placebo because they are part of the control group, then preventing them from being part of the research trial just because it is risky would violate their right to direct their own lives, would it not?

Clinical Trials

Clinical trials, especially those involving experimental drugs, tend to follow a certain set of protocols that the US Food and Drug Administration calls the "Gold Standard" for clinical research. The gold standard is a double-blind, placebo-controlled, randomized clinical trial. These terms need unpacking.

Double blind means that neither the research participants nor the researchers know who is getting the experimental drug and who is getting the standard treatment or the placebo. Neither the researchers nor the participants know who is in the control group and who is in the experimental group. Once the study is considered complete, the study may become "unblinded."

The purpose here is to maintain *clinical equipoise*. Equipoise is a term meaning balance. In this case, the balance is in the uncertainty of the effectiveness of an experimental drug and the standard treatment (including no treatment at all). If a researcher is also a physician (as is sometimes the case), it is important that there be uncertainty about whether an experimental drug is more effective than a placebo or a standard treatment, because if a physician had reason to believe that an experimental drug was more effective and did not give it to someone who was suffering from a disease, they would be violating the principle of beneficence. If the patient was in pain and the researcher/physician knew they might receive a placebo (i.e., no treatment at all), it could also violate the principle of non-maleficence. The double-blind part of the study is designed to keep the researcher in a state of equipoise about the effectiveness of the drug to prevent any knowing violation of beneficence or non-maleficence.

Of course, one might argue that such concerns about equipoise are misguided. Franklin Miller and Howard Brody argue that it is a mistake to rely on clinical equipoise as a concept in clinical research. In fact, it is comparable to the error of research participants thinking that the experiment they are part of is no different from clinical treatment from a doctor. Brody and Miller argue that the ethics of treatment and the ethics of clinical trials are two different standards, and one should not be confused with the other.[*]

The term *placebo controlled* refers to the use of placebos in the clinical trial. A placebo is a substance that has no therapeutic value and is used in a research trial to correct for the *placebo effect*. Researchers need to know if a drug is better than no treatment at all in order to honor the principle of beneficence. If a research participant is given a placebo and thinks they may be getting the experimental treatment, the placebo effect may make them improve or show symptoms.

What to know and ask if you are part of a research trial

The National Cancer Institute has a website for patients who are considering being part of a clinical trial. Here are some questions patients should ask before volunteering for a clinical trial.[†]

---

[*] F.G. Miller and H. Brody, "Clinical Equipoise and the Incoherence of Research Ethics," *Journal of Medical Philosophy* 32, no. 2 (2007): 151–65.

[†] From "Questions to Ask Your Doctor About Treatment Clinical Trials," https://www.cancer.gov/about-cancer/treatment/clinical-trials/questions.

Questions about the Trial

- What is the purpose of the trial?
- Why do the researchers believe that the treatment being studied may be better than the one being used now? Why may it not be better?
- How long will I be in the trial?
- What kinds of tests and treatments are involved?
- How will the doctor know if the treatment is working?
- How will I be told about the trial's results?
- How long do I have to make up my mind about joining this trial?
- Who can I speak with about questions I have during and after the trial?
- Who will be in charge of my care?
- Is there someone I can talk to who has been in the trial?

Questions about Risks and Benefits

- What are the possible side effects or risks of the new treatment?
- What are the possible benefits?
- How do the possible risks and benefits of this trial compare to those of the standard treatment?

Questions about Your Rights

- How will my health information be kept private?
- What happens if I decide to leave the trial?

Questions about Costs

- Which costs do I have to pay if I take part in the trial?
- What costs will my health insurance cover?
- Who pays if I'm injured in the trial?
- Who can help answer questions from my insurance company?
- Who can I talk with about costs and payments?

Questions about Daily Life

- How could the trial affect my daily life?
- How often will I have to come to the hospital or clinic?
- Will I have to stay in the hospital during the clinical trial? If so, how often and for how long?
- How far will I need to travel to take part in the trial?
- Will I have check-ups after the trial?

Questions about Comparing Choices

▣ What are my other treatment choices, including standard treatments?

▣ How does the treatment I would receive in this trial compare with the other treatment choices?

▣ What will happen to my [condition] without treatment?

One reason that third-world research trials are problematic is that often the language barrier can cause doubt about the "informed" part of informed consent. Does the subject really understand the risks, benefits, and alternatives? What if there is not a word for "placebo" in the subject's language? There is room for a great deal of abuse.

In addition, if you are so desperate for medical treatment or the conditions in the research trial are so much better than the ones you live in, you might not deliberate too much over the risks or benefits when the alternatives look so bad. Call this the "Offer too good to refuse problem." Two conditions might make the offer to enter a research trial "too good to refuse" and therefore make consent invalid. The status quo conditions for the subject might be so bad that the conditions of a research subject are far better than their day-to-day lives. After all, research subjects often get free medical care and nicer conditions than the everyday conditions of prison or poverty. Alternatively, research trial conditions might be so good that no rational person would refuse a way to make their lives better, and this too could invalidate consent and make the study unethical.

In 1996, Lilly Pharmaceuticals paid healthy volunteers $85 a day to test drugs in a Phase I clinical trial.* Word of mouth spread throughout the homeless community near the Indianapolis clinic run by the company. The volunteers were given housing, an ID card that made it easier for them to cash checks, and a place to shower and shave. All this was light years better than living on the streets. All subjects signed a consent to be part of the study, even though many could not name the drug when asked the drug they were being tested with.

Is this ethical? It depends on whether you think consent is informed and voluntary. If you think informed and voluntary consent is "morally transformative," then even if Lilly's offer is too good to refuse, there is reason to think it is morally permissible, even though it is unfortunate that homeless men need this money. Economist Michael Munger calls this "euvoluntary" exchange: It is not

---

* Rick Callahan, "Drug Firm Defends Use of Homeless as Subjects in Pharmaceutical Tests," *Seattle Times*, Nov. 21, 1996, https://archive.seattletimes.com/archive/?date=19961121&slug=2361031.

ideal, but it should not be prohibited because there is consent.* Both parties will be better off than they would be otherwise.

> ## Clinical Trial Phases
>
> Phase I studies assess the safety of a drug or device. This initial phase of testing, which can take several months to complete, usually includes a small number of healthy volunteers (20 to 100) who are generally paid for participating in the study. The study is designed to determine the effects of the drug or device on humans, including how it is absorbed, metabolized, and excreted. This phase also investigates the side-effects that occur as dosage levels are increased. About 70 per cent of experimental drugs pass this phase of testing.
>
> Phase II studies test the efficacy of a drug or device. This second phase of testing can last from several months to two years and involves up to several hundred patients. Most Phase II studies are randomized trials, where one group of patients receives the experimental drug while a second, "control" group receives a standard treatment or placebo. Often these studies are "blinded," which means that neither the patients nor the researchers know who has received the experimental drug. This allows investigators to provide the pharmaceutical company and the FDA with comparative information about the relative safety and effectiveness of the new drug. About one-third of experimental drugs successfully complete both Phase I and Phase II studies.
>
> Phase III studies involve randomized and blind testing in several hundred to several thousand patients. This large-scale testing, which can last several years, provides the pharmaceutical company and the FDA with a more thorough understanding of the effectiveness of the drug or device, the benefits, and the range of possible adverse reactions. Some 70 to 90 per cent of drugs that enter Phase III studies successfully complete this phase of testing. Once Phase III is complete, a pharmaceutical company can request FDA approval for marketing the drug.
>
> Phase IV studies, often called post marketing surveillance trials, are conducted after a drug or device has been approved for consumer sale. Pharmaceutical companies have several objectives at this stage: (1) to compare a drug with other drugs already in the market; (2) to monitor a

---

* Michael C. Munger, "Euvoluntary or Not, Exchange Is Just," *Social Philosophy and Policy* 28, no. 2 (2011): 192–211.

drug's long-term effectiveness and impact on a patient's quality of life; and (3) to determine the cost-effectiveness of a drug therapy relative to other traditional and new therapies. Phase IV studies can result in a drug or device being taken off the market, or restrictions of use could be placed on the product, depending on the findings in the study.

Source: "Overview of Clinical Trials," https://www.centerwatch.com/clinical-trials/overview.aspx/.

Philosopher Michael Sandel (b. 1953) argues that some things simply shouldn't involve money or goods because it creates perverse vices of character.* Indeed, the homeless in the Lilly study admitted they often lied about when they had their last drink. Many used all manner of home remedies, from drinking vinegar to drinking two gallons of water, to fool the liver tests needed to qualify for the trial.

Still, both parties were arguably better off. Several of the homeless subjects credit the study with giving them the means to stop drinking and buy a car or needed clothing. When you consider the subjects stood to make an average of $4,500 for their stay at the clinic, it seems rational for them to consent. But just because someone will consent to a study to make their lives better does not mean it is ethical to offer them a chance to be part of the study itself. Just as physicians are not obligated to do a procedure just because a patient consents to it, neither are research companies obligated to sweeten the deal for research subjects.

Paying research participants presents a problem for research ethics because it presents a problem for informed consent. If an offer to be part of a research study is "too good to refuse," that any rational person would participate given their circumstances, then is consent sufficient? Maybe consent is necessary to prevent doing things to people without their approval, but in the case of "too good to refuse," someone might argue that consent is not so much inadequate in this sort of case as it is irrelevant. It may be that researchers have an obligation beyond their duty to autonomy. This will be explored in the readings.

---

* Michael Sandel, *What Money Can't Buy: The Moral Limits of Markets* (New York, NY: Farrar, Straus and Giroux, 2013).

WHAT'S THE DEBATE?

Reading 4.1: World Medical Association, "Declaration of Helsinki"

Ethical Principles for Medical Research Involving Human Subjects

Adopted by the 18th WMA General Assembly, Helsinki, Finland, June 1964; amended by the 29th WMA General Assembly, Tokyo, Japan, October 1975; 35th WMA General Assembly, Venice, Italy, October 1983; 41st WMA General Assembly, Hong Kong, September 1989; 48th WMA General Assembly, Somerset West, Republic of South Africa, October 1996; and the 52nd WMA General Assembly, Edinburgh, Scotland, October 2000

A. INTRODUCTION

1. The World Medical Association has developed the Declaration of Helsinki as a statement of ethical principles to provide guidance to physicians and other participants in medical research involving human subjects. Medical research involving human subjects includes research on identifiable human material or identifiable data.

2. It is the duty of the physician to promote and safeguard the health of the people. The physician's knowledge and conscience are dedicated to the fulfillment of this duty.

3. The Declaration of Geneva of the World Medical Association binds the physician with the words, "The health of my patient will be my first consideration," and the International Code of Medical Ethics declares that, "A physician shall act only in the patient's interest when providing medical care which might have the effect of weakening on the physical and mental condition of the patient."

4. Medical progress is based on research which ultimately must rest in part on experimentation involving human subjects.

5. In medical research on human subjects, considerations related to the well-being of the human subject should take precedence over the interests of science and society.

6. The primary purpose of medical research involving human subjects is to improve prophylactic, diagnostic and therapeutic procedures and the understanding of the aetiology and pathogenesis of disease. Even the best proven prophylactic, diagnostic, and therapeutic methods must continuously be challenged through research for their effectiveness, efficiency, accessibility and quality.

7. In current medical practice and in medical research, most prophylactic, diagnostic and therapeutic procedures involve risks and burdens.

8. Medical research is subject to ethical standards that promote respect for all human beings and protect their health and rights. Some research populations are vulnerable and need special protection. The particular needs of the economically and medically disadvantaged must be recognized. Special attention is also required for those who cannot give or refuse consent for themselves, for those who may be subject to giving consent under duress, for those who will not benefit personally from the research and for those for whom the research is combined with care.

9. Research Investigators should be aware of the ethical, legal and regulatory requirements for research on human subjects in their own countries as well as applicable international requirements. No national ethical, legal or regulatory requirement should be allowed to reduce or eliminate any of the protections for human subjects set forth in this Declaration.

B. BASIC PRINCIPLES FOR ALL MEDICAL RESEARCH

10. It is the duty of the physician in medical research to protect the life, health, privacy, and dignity of the human subject.

11. Medical research involving human subjects must conform to generally accepted scientific principles, be based on a thorough knowledge of the scientific literature, other relevant sources of information, and on adequate laboratory and, where appropriate, animal experimentation.

12. Appropriate caution must be exercised in the conduct of research which may affect the environment, and the welfare of animals used for research must be respected.

13. The design and performance of each experimental procedure involving human subjects should be clearly formulated in an experimental protocol. This protocol should be submitted for consideration, comment, guidance, and where appropriate, approval to a specially appointed ethical review committee, which must be independent of the investigator, the sponsor or any other kind of undue influence. This independent committee should be in conformity with the laws and regulations of the country in which the research experiment is performed. The committee has the right to monitor ongoing trials. The researcher has the obligation to provide monitoring information to the committee, especially any serious adverse events. The researcher should also submit to the committee, for review, information regarding funding, sponsors, institutional affiliations, other potential conflicts of interest and incentives for subjects.

14. The research protocol should always contain a statement of the ethical considerations involved and should indicate that there is compliance with the principles enunciated in this Declaration.

15. Medical research involving human subjects should be conducted only by scientifically qualified persons and under the supervision of a clinically competent medical person. The responsibility for the human subject must always rest with a medically qualified person and never rest on the subject of the research, even though the subject has given consent.

16. Every medical research project involving human subjects should be preceded by careful assessment of predictable risks and burdens in comparison with foreseeable benefits to the subject or to others. This does not preclude the participation of healthy volunteers in medical research. The design of all studies should be publicly available.

17. Physicians should abstain from engaging in research projects involving human subjects unless they are confident that the risks involved have been adequately assessed and can be satisfactorily managed. Physicians should cease any investigation if the risks are found to outweigh the potential benefits or if there is conclusive proof of positive and beneficial results.

18. Medical research involving human subjects should only be conducted if the importance of the objective outweighs the inherent risks and burdens

to the subject. This is especially important when the human subjects are healthy volunteers.

19. Medical research is only justified if there is a reasonable likelihood that the populations in which the research is carried out stand to benefit from the results of the research.

20. The subjects must be volunteers and informed participants in the research project.

21. The right of research subjects to safeguard their integrity must always be respected. Every precaution should be taken to respect the privacy of the subject, the confidentiality of the patient's information and to minimize the impact of the study on the subject's physical and mental integrity and on the personality of the subject.

22. In any research on human beings, each potential subject must be adequately informed of the aims, methods, sources of funding, any possible conflicts of interest, institutional affiliations of the researcher, the anticipated benefits and potential risks of the study and the discomfort it may entail. The subject should be informed of the right to abstain from participation in the study or to withdraw consent to participate at any time without reprisal. After ensuring that the subject has understood the information, the physician should then obtain the subject's freely-given informed consent, preferably in writing. If the consent cannot be obtained in writing, the non-written consent must be formally documented and witnessed.

23. When obtaining informed consent for the research project the physician should be particularly cautious if the subject is in a dependent relationship with the physician or may consent under duress. In that case the informed consent should be obtained by a well-informed physician who is not engaged in the investigation and who is completely independent of this relationship.

24. For a research subject who is legally incompetent, physically or mentally incapable of giving consent or is a legally incompetent minor, the investigator must obtain informed consent from the legally authorized representative in accordance with applicable law. These groups should not be included in research unless the research is necessary to promote the health

of the population represented and this research cannot instead be performed on legally competent persons.

25. When a subject deemed legally incompetent, such as a minor child, is able to give assent to decisions about participation in research, the investigator must obtain that assent in addition to the consent of the legally authorized representative.

26. Research on individuals from whom it is not possible to obtain consent, including proxy or advance consent, should be done only if the physical/mental condition that prevents obtaining informed consent is a necessary characteristic of the research population. The specific reasons for involving research subjects with a condition that renders them unable to give informed consent should be stated in the experimental protocol for consideration and approval of the review committee. The protocol should state that consent to remain in the research should be obtained as soon as possible from the individual or a legally authorized surrogate.

27. Both authors and publishers have ethical obligations. In publication of the results of research, the investigators are obliged to preserve the accuracy of the results. Negative as well as positive results should be published or otherwise publicly available. Sources of funding, institutional affiliations and any possible conflicts of interest should be declared in the publication. Reports of experimentation not in accordance with the principles laid down in this Declaration should not be accepted for publication.

C. ADDITIONAL PRINCIPLES FOR MEDICAL RESEARCH COMBINED WITH MEDICAL CARE

28. The physician may combine medical research with medical care, only to the extent that the research is justified by its potential prophylactic, diagnostic or therapeutic value. When medical research is combined with medical care, additional standards apply to protect the patients who are research subjects.

29. The benefits, risks, burdens and effectiveness of a new method should be tested against those of the best current prophylactic, diagnostic, and therapeutic methods. This does not exclude the use of placebo, or no treatment, in studies where no proven prophylactic, diagnostic or therapeutic method exists.

30. At the conclusion of the study, every patient entered into the study should be assured of access to the best proven prophylactic, diagnostic and therapeutic methods identified by the study.

31. The physician should fully inform the patient which aspects of the care are related to the research. The refusal of a patient to participate in a study must never interfere with the patient–physician relationship.

32. In the treatment of a patient, where proven prophylactic, diagnostic and therapeutic methods do not exist or have been ineffective, the physician, with informed consent from the patient, must be free to use unproven or new prophylactic, diagnostic and therapeutic measures, if in the physician's judgement it offers hope of saving life, re-establishing health or alleviating suffering. Where possible, these measures should be made the object of research, designed to evaluate their safety and efficacy. In all cases, new information should be recorded and, where appropriate, published. The other relevant guidelines of this Declaration should be followed.

Reading 4.2: National Commission for the Protection of Human Subjects of Biomedical and Behavioral Research, "The Belmont Report"

Office of the Secretary

Ethical Principles and Guidelines for the Protection of Human Subjects of Research

The National Commission for the Protection of Human Subjects of Biomedical and Behavioral Research

April 18, 1979

Ethical Principles & Guidelines for Research Involving Human Subjects

Scientific research has produced substantial social benefits. It has also posed some troubling ethical questions. Public attention was drawn to these questions by reported abuses of human subjects in biomedical experiments, especially during the Second World War. During the Nuremberg War Crime Trials, the

Nuremberg code was drafted as a set of standards for judging physicians and scientists who had conducted biomedical experiments on concentration camp prisoners. This code became the prototype of many later codes[1] intended to assure that research involving human subjects would be carried out in an ethical manner.

The codes consist of rules, some general, others specific, that guide the investigators or the reviewers of research in their work. Such rules often are inadequate to cover complex situations; at times they come into conflict, and they are frequently difficult to interpret or apply. Broader ethical principles will provide a basis on which specific rules may be formulated, criticized and interpreted.

Three principles, or general prescriptive judgments, that are relevant to research involving human subjects are identified in this statement. Other principles may also be relevant. These three are comprehensive, however, and are stated at a level of generalization that should assist scientists, subjects, reviewers and interested citizens to understand the ethical issues inherent in research involving human subjects. These principles cannot always be applied so as to resolve beyond dispute particular ethical problems. The objective is to provide an analytical framework that will guide the resolution of ethical problems arising from research involving human subjects.

This statement consists of a distinction between research and practice, a discussion of the three basic ethical principles, and remarks about the application of these principles.

Part A: Boundaries Between Practice & Research

It is important to distinguish between biomedical and behavioral research, on the one hand, and the practice of accepted therapy on the other, in order to know what activities ought to undergo review for the protection of human subjects of research. The distinction between research and practice is blurred partly because both often occur together (as in research designed to evaluate a therapy) and partly because notable departures from standard practice are often called "experimental" when the terms "experimental" and "research" are not carefully defined.

For the most part, the term "practice" refers to interventions that are designed solely to enhance the well-being of an individual patient or client and that have a reasonable expectation of success. The purpose of medical or behavioral practice is to provide diagnosis, preventive treatment or therapy to particular individuals.[2] By contrast, the term "research" designates an activity designed to test an hypothesis, permit conclusions to be drawn, and thereby to develop or contribute to generalizable knowledge (expressed, for example, in theories, principles, and statements of relationships). Research is usually described in a formal protocol that sets forth an objective and a set of procedures designed to reach that objective.

When a clinician departs in a significant way from standard or accepted practice, the innovation does not, in and of itself, constitute research. The fact that a procedure is "experimental," in the sense of new, untested or different, does not automatically place it in the category of research. Radically new procedures of this description should, however, be made the object of formal research at an early stage in order to determine whether they are safe and effective. Thus, it is the responsibility of medical practice committees, for example, to insist that a major innovation be incorporated into a formal research project.[3]

Research and practice may be carried on together when research is designed to evaluate the safety and efficacy of a therapy. This need not cause any confusion regarding whether or not the activity requires review; the general rule is that if there is any element of research in an activity, that activity should undergo review for the protection of human subjects.

Part B: Basic Ethical Principles

The expression "basic ethical principles" refers to those general judgments that serve as a basic justification for the many particular ethical prescriptions and evaluations of human actions. Three basic principles, among those generally accepted in our cultural tradition, are particularly relevant to the ethics of research involving human subjects: the principles of respect of persons, beneficence and justice.

1. Respect for Persons. — Respect for persons incorporates at least two ethical convictions: first, that individuals should be treated as autonomous agents, and second, that persons with diminished autonomy are entitled to protection. The principle of respect for persons thus divides into two separate moral requirements: the requirement to acknowledge autonomy and the requirement to protect those with diminished autonomy.

   An autonomous person is an individual capable of deliberation about personal goals and of acting under the direction of such deliberation. To respect autonomy is to give weight to autonomous persons' considered opinions and choices while refraining from obstructing their actions unless they are clearly detrimental to others. To show lack of respect for an autonomous agent is to repudiate that person's considered judgments, to deny an individual the freedom to act on those considered judgments, or to withhold information necessary to make a considered judgment, when there are no compelling reasons to do so.

However, not every human being is capable of self-determination. The capacity for self-determination matures during an individual's life, and some individuals lose this capacity wholly or in part because of illness, mental disability, or circumstances that severely restrict liberty. Respect for the immature and the incapacitated may require protecting them as they mature or while they are incapacitated.

Some persons are in need of extensive protection, even to the point of excluding them from activities which may harm them; other persons require little protection beyond making sure they undertake activities freely and with awareness of possible adverse consequence. The extent of protection afforded should depend upon the risk of harm and the likelihood of benefit. The judgment that any individual lacks autonomy should be periodically reevaluated and will vary in different situations.

In most cases of research involving human subjects, respect for persons demands that subjects enter into the research voluntarily and with adequate information. In some situations, however, application of the principle is not obvious. The involvement of prisoners as subjects of research provides an instructive example. On the one hand, it would seem that the principle of respect for persons requires that prisoners not be deprived of the opportunity to volunteer for research. On the other hand, under prison conditions they may be subtly coerced or unduly influenced to engage in research activities for which they would not otherwise volunteer. Respect for persons would then dictate that prisoners be protected. Whether to allow prisoners to "volunteer" or to "protect" them presents a dilemma. Respecting persons, in most hard cases, is often a matter of balancing competing claims urged by the principle of respect itself.

2. Beneficence. — Persons are treated in an ethical manner not only by respecting their decisions and protecting them from harm, but also by making efforts to secure their well-being. Such treatment falls under the principle of beneficence. The term "beneficence" is often understood to cover acts of kindness or charity that go beyond strict obligation. In this document, beneficence is understood in a stronger sense, as an obligation. Two general rules have been formulated as complementary expressions of beneficent actions in this sense: (1) do not harm and (2) maximize possible benefits and minimize possible harms.

The Hippocratic maxim "do no harm" has long been a fundamental principle of medical ethics. Claude Bernard extended it to the realm of research, saying that one should not injure one person regardless of the benefits that might come to others. However, even avoiding harm requires learning what is harmful; and, in the process of obtaining this information, persons may be exposed to risk of harm. Further, the Hippocratic Oath requires physicians to benefit their patients "according to their best judgment." Learning what will in fact benefit may require exposing persons to risk. The problem posed by these imperatives is to decide when it is justifiable to seek certain benefits despite the risks involved, and when the benefits should be foregone because of the risks.

The obligations of beneficence affect both individual investigators and society at large, because they extend both to particular research projects and to the entire enterprise of research. In the case of particular projects, investigators and members of their institutions are obliged to give forethought to the maximization of benefits and the reduction of risk that might occur from the research investigation. In the case of scientific research in general, members of the larger society are obliged to recognize the longer term benefits and risks that may result from the improvement of knowledge and from the development of novel medical, psychotherapeutic, and social procedures.

The principle of beneficence often occupies a well-defined justifying role in many areas of research involving human subjects. An example is found in research involving children. Effective ways of treating childhood diseases and fostering healthy development are benefits that serve to justify research involving children—even when individual research subjects are not direct beneficiaries. Research also makes it possible to avoid the harm that may result from the application of previously accepted routine practices that on closer investigation turn out to be dangerous. But the role of the principle of beneficence is not always so unambiguous. A difficult ethical problem remains, for example, about research that presents more than minimal risk without immediate prospect of direct benefit to the children involved. Some have argued that such research is inadmissible, while others have pointed out that this limit would rule out much research promising great benefit to children in the future. Here again, as with all hard cases, the different claims covered by the principle of beneficence may come into conflict and force difficult choices.

3. Justice. — Who ought to receive the benefits of research and bear its burdens? This is a question of justice, in the sense of "fairness in distribution" or "what is deserved." An injustice occurs when some benefit to which a person is entitled is denied without good reason or when some burden is imposed unduly. Another way of conceiving the principle of justice is that equals ought to be treated equally. However, this statement requires explication. Who is equal and who is unequal? What considerations justify departure from equal distribution? Almost all commentators allow that distinctions based on experience, age, deprivation, competence, merit and position do sometimes constitute criteria justifying differential treatment for certain purposes. It is necessary, then, to explain in what respects people should be treated equally. There are several widely accepted formulations of just ways to distribute burdens and benefits. Each formulation mentions some relevant property on the basis of which burdens and benefits should be distributed. These formulations are (1) to each person an equal share, (2) to each person according to individual need, (3) to each person according to individual effort, (4) to each person according to societal contribution, and (5) to each person according to merit.

Questions of justice have long been associated with social practices such as punishment, taxation and political representation. Until recently these questions have not generally been associated with scientific research. However, they are foreshadowed even in the earliest reflections on the ethics of research involving human subjects. For example, during the 19th and early 20th centuries the burdens of serving as research subjects fell largely upon poor ward patients, while the benefits of improved medical care flowed primarily to private patients. Subsequently, the exploitation of unwilling prisoners as research subjects in Nazi concentration camps was condemned as a particularly flagrant injustice. In this country, in the 1940's, the Tuskegee syphilis study used disadvantaged, rural black men to study the untreated course of a disease that is by no means confined to that population. These subjects were deprived of demonstrably effective treatment in order not to interrupt the project, long after such treatment became generally available.

Against this historical background, it can be seen how conceptions of justice are relevant to research involving human subjects. For example, the selection of research subjects needs to be scrutinized in order to determine whether some classes (e.g., welfare patients, particular racial and ethnic minorities, or persons confined to institutions) are being systematically selected simply because of their easy availability, their compromised position, or their manipulability, rather than for reasons directly related to the problem being studied. Finally, whenever research supported by public funds leads to the development of therapeutic devices and procedures, justice demands both that these not provide advantages only to those who can afford them and that such research should not unduly involve persons from groups unlikely to be among the beneficiaries of subsequent applications of the research.

Part C: Applications

Applications of the general principles to the conduct of research leads to consideration of the following requirements: informed consent, risk/benefit assessment, and the selection of subjects of research.

1. Informed Consent. — Respect for persons requires that subjects, to the degree that they are capable, be given the opportunity to choose what shall or shall not happen to them. This opportunity is provided when adequate standards for informed consent are satisfied.

   While the importance of informed consent is unquestioned, controversy prevails over the nature and possibility of an informed consent. Nonetheless, there is widespread agreement that the consent process can be analyzed as containing three elements: information, comprehension and voluntariness.

   Information. Most codes of research establish specific items for disclosure intended to assure that subjects are given sufficient information. These items generally include: the research procedure, their purposes, risks and anticipated benefits, alternative procedures (where therapy is involved), and a statement offering the subject the opportunity to ask questions and to withdraw at any time from the research. Additional items have been proposed, including how subjects are selected, the person responsible for the research, etc.

   However, a simple listing of items does not answer the question of what the standard should be for judging how much and what sort of information should be provided. One standard frequently invoked in medical practice, namely the information commonly provided by practitioners in the field or in the locale, is inadequate since research takes place precisely when a common understanding does not exist. Another standard, currently popular in malpractice law, requires the practitioner to reveal the information that reasonable persons would wish to know in order to make a decision regarding their care. This, too, seems insufficient since the research subject, being in essence a volunteer, may wish to know considerably more about risks gratuitously undertaken than do patients who deliver themselves into the hand of a clinician for needed care. It may be that a standard of "the reasonable volunteer" should be proposed: the extent and nature of information should be such that persons, knowing that the procedure is neither necessary for their care nor perhaps fully understood, can decide whether they wish to participate in the furthering of knowledge. Even when some direct benefit to them is anticipated, the subjects should understand clearly the range of risk and the voluntary nature of participation.

A special problem of consent arises where informing subjects of some pertinent aspect of the research is likely to impair the validity of the research. In many cases, it is sufficient to indicate to subjects that they are being invited to participate in research of which some features will not be revealed until the research is concluded. In all cases of research involving incomplete disclosure, such research is justified only if it is clear that (1) incomplete disclosure is truly necessary to accomplish the goals of the research, (2) there are no undisclosed risks to subjects that are more than minimal, and (3) there is an adequate plan for debriefing subjects, when appropriate, and for dissemination of research results to them. Information about risks should never be withheld for the purpose of eliciting the cooperation of subjects, and truthful answers should always be given to direct questions about the research. Care should be taken to distinguish cases in which disclosure would destroy or invalidate the research from cases in which disclosure would simply inconvenience the investigator.

Comprehension. The manner and context in which information is conveyed is as important as the information itself. For example, presenting information in a disorganized and rapid fashion, allowing too little time for consideration or curtailing opportunities for questioning, all may adversely affect a subject's ability to make an informed choice.

Because the subject's ability to understand is a function of intelligence, rationality, maturity and language, it is necessary to adapt the presentation of the information to the subject's capacities. Investigators are responsible for ascertaining that the subject has comprehended the information. While there is always an obligation to ascertain that the information about risk to subjects is complete and adequately comprehended, when the risks are more serious, that obligation increases. On occasion, it may be suitable to give some oral or written tests of comprehension.

Special provision may need to be made when comprehension is severely limited—for example, by conditions of immaturity or mental disability. Each class of subjects that one might consider as incompetent (e.g., infants and young children, mentally disabled patients, the terminally ill and the comatose) should be considered on its own terms. Even for these persons, however, respect requires giving them the opportunity to choose to the extent they are able, whether or not to participate in research. The objections of these subjects to involvement should be honored, unless the research entails providing them a therapy unavailable elsewhere. Respect for persons also requires seeking the permission of other parties in order to protect the subjects from harm. Such persons are thus respected both by acknowledging their own wishes and by the use of third parties to protect them from harm.

The third parties chosen should be those who are most likely to understand the incompetent subject's situation and to act in that person's best interest. The person authorized to act on behalf of the subject should be given an opportunity to observe the research as it proceeds in order to be able to withdraw the subject from the research, if such action appears in the subject's best interest.

Voluntariness. An agreement to participate in research constitutes a valid consent only if voluntarily given. This element of informed consent requires conditions free of coercion and undue influence. Coercion occurs when an overt threat of harm is intentionally presented by one person to another in order to obtain compliance. Undue influence, by contrast, occurs through an offer of an excessive, unwarranted, inappropriate or improper reward or other overture in order to obtain compliance. Also, inducements that would ordinarily be acceptable may become undue influences if the subject is especially vulnerable.

Unjustifiable pressures usually occur when persons in positions of authority or commanding influence—especially where possible sanctions are involved—urge a course of action for a subject. A continuum of such influencing factors exists, however, and it is impossible to state precisely where justifiable persuasion ends and undue influence begins. But undue influence would include actions such as manipulating a person's choice through the controlling influence of a close relative and threatening to withdraw health services to which an individual would otherwise be entitled.

2. Assessment of Risks and Benefits. — The assessment of risks and benefits requires a careful arrayal of relevant data, including, in some cases,

alternative ways of obtaining the benefits sought in the research. Thus, the assessment presents both an opportunity and a responsibility to gather systematic and comprehensive information about proposed research. For the investigator, it is a means to examine whether the proposed research is properly designed. For a review committee, it is a method for determining whether the risks that will be presented to subjects are justified. For prospective subjects, the assessment will assist the determination whether or not to participate.

The Nature and Scope of Risks and Benefits. The requirement that research be justified on the basis of a favorable risk/benefit assessment bears a close relation to the principle of beneficence, just as the moral requirement that informed consent be obtained is derived primarily from the principle of respect for persons. The term "risk" refers to a possibility that harm may occur. However, when expressions such as "small risk" or "high risk" are used, they usually refer (often ambiguously) both to the chance (probability) of experiencing a harm and the severity (magnitude) of the envisioned harm.

The term "benefit" is used in the research context to refer to something of positive value related to health or welfare. Unlike, "risk," "benefit" is not a term that expresses probabilities. Risk is properly contrasted to probability of benefits, and benefits are properly contrasted with harms rather than risks of harm. Accordingly, so-called risk/benefit assessments are concerned with the probabilities and magnitudes of possible harm and anticipated benefits. Many kinds of possible harms and benefits need to be taken into account. There are, for example, risks of psychological harm, physical harm, legal harm, social harm and economic harm and the corresponding benefits. While the most likely types of harms to research subjects are those of psychological or physical pain or injury, other possible kinds should not be overlooked.

Risks and benefits of research may affect the individual subjects, the families of the individual subjects, and society at large (or special groups of subjects in society). Previous codes and Federal regulations have required that risks to subjects be outweighed by the sum of both the anticipated benefit to the subject, if any, and the anticipated benefit to society in the form of knowledge to be gained from the research. In balancing these different elements, the risks and benefits affecting the immediate research subject will normally carry special weight. On the other hand, interests other than those of the subject may on some occasions be sufficient by themselves to justify the risks involved in the research, so long as the subjects' rights have been protected. Beneficence thus requires that we protect against risk of harm to subjects and also that we be concerned about the loss of the substantial benefits that might be gained from research.

The Systematic Assessment of Risks and Benefits. It is commonly said that benefits and risks must be "balanced" and shown to be "in a favorable ratio." The metaphorical character of these terms draws attention to the difficulty of making precise judgments. Only on rare occasions will quantitative techniques be available for the scrutiny of research protocols. However, the idea of systematic, nonarbitrary analysis of risks and benefits should be emulated insofar as possible. This ideal requires those making decisions about the justifiability of research to be thorough in the accumulation and assessment of information about all aspects of the research, and to consider alternatives systematically. This procedure renders the assessment of research more rigorous and precise, while making communication between review board members and investigators less subject to misinterpretation, misinformation and conflicting judgments. Thus, there should first be a determination of the validity of the presuppositions of the research; then the nature, probability and magnitude of risk should be distinguished with as much clarity as possible. The method of ascertaining risks should be explicit, especially where there is no alternative to the use of such vague categories as small or slight risk. It should also be determined whether an investigator's estimates of the probability of harm or benefits are reasonable, as judged by known facts or other available studies.

Finally, assessment of the justifiability of research should reflect at least the following considerations: (i) Brutal or inhumane treatment of human subjects is never morally justified. (ii) Risks should be reduced to those necessary to achieve the research objective. It should be determined whether it is in fact necessary to use human subjects at all. Risk can perhaps never be entirely eliminated, but it can often be reduced by careful attention to alternative procedures. (iii) When research involves significant risk of serious impairment, review committees should be extraordinarily insistent on the justification of the risk (looking usually to the likelihood of benefit to the subject—or, in some rare cases, to the manifest voluntariness of the participation). (iv) When vulnerable populations are involved in research, the appropriateness of involving them should itself be demonstrated. A number of variables go into such judgments, including the nature and degree of risk, the condition of the particular population involved, and the nature and level of the anticipated benefits. (v) Relevant

risks and benefits must be thoroughly arrayed in documents and procedures used in the informed consent process.

3. Selection of Subjects. — Just as the principle of respect for persons finds
expression in the requirements for consent, and the principle of beneficence in risk/benefit assessment, the principle of justice gives rise to moral
requirements that there be fair procedures and outcomes in the selection
of research subjects.

Justice is relevant to the selection of subjects of research at two levels: the social and the individual. Individual justice in the selection of subjects would require that researchers exhibit fairness: thus, they should not
offer potentially beneficial research only to some patients who are in their
favor or select only "undesirable" persons for risky research. Social justice
requires that distinction be drawn between classes of subjects that ought,
and ought not, to participate in any particular kind of research, based on
the ability of members of that class to bear burdens and on the appropriateness of placing further burdens on already burdened persons. Thus, it
can be considered a matter of social justice that there is an order of preference in the selection of classes of subjects (e.g., adults before children) and
that some classes of potential subjects (e.g., the institutionalized mentally
infirm or prisoners) may be involved as research subjects, if at all, only on
certain conditions.

Injustice may appear in the selection of subjects, even if individual subjects are selected fairly by investigators and treated fairly in the course of
research. Thus injustice arises from social, racial, sexual and cultural biases
institutionalized in society. Thus, even if individual researchers are treating their research subjects fairly, and even if IRBs are taking care to assure
that subjects are selected fairly within a particular institution, unjust social
patterns may nevertheless appear in the overall distribution of the burdens
and benefits of research. Although individual institutions or investigators
may not be able to resolve a problem that is pervasive in their social setting, they can consider distributive justice in selecting research subjects.

Some populations, especially institutionalized ones, are already burdened in many ways by their infirmities and environments. When research
is proposed that involves risks and does not include a therapeutic component, other less burdened classes of persons should be called upon first to
accept these risks of research, except where the research is directly related
to the specific conditions of the class involved. Also, even though public
funds for research may often flow in the same directions as public funds for

health care, it seems unfair that populations dependent on public health care constitute a pool of preferred research subjects if more advantaged populations are likely to be the recipients of the benefits.

One special instance of injustice results from the involvement of vulnerable subjects. Certain groups, such as racial minorities, the economically disadvantaged, the very sick, and the institutionalized may continually be sought as research subjects, owing to their ready availability in settings where research is conducted. Given their dependent status and their frequently compromised capacity for free consent, they should be protected against the danger of being involved in research solely for administrative convenience, or because they are easy to manipulate as a result of their illness or socioeconomic condition.

Notes

1. Since 1945, various codes for the proper and responsible conduct of human experimentation in medical research have been adopted by different organizations. The best known of these codes are the Nuremberg Code of 1947, the Helsinki Declaration of 1964 (revised in 1975), and the 1971 Guidelines (codified into Federal Regulations in 1974) issued by the U.S. Department of Health, Education, and Welfare. Codes for the conduct of social and behavioral research have also been adopted, the best known being that of the American Psychological Association, published in 1973.

2. Although practice usually involves interventions designed solely to enhance the well-being of a particular individual, interventions are sometimes applied to one individual for the enhancement of the well-being of another (e.g., blood donation, skin grafts, organ transplants) or an intervention may have the dual purpose of enhancing the well-being of a particular individual, and, at the same time, providing some benefit to others (e.g., vaccination, which protects both the person who is vaccinated and society generally). The fact that some forms of practice have elements other than immediate benefit to the individual receiving an intervention, however, should not confuse the general distinction between research and practice. Even when a procedure applied in practice may benefit some other person, it remains an intervention designed to enhance the well-being of a particular individual or groups of individuals; thus, it is practice and need not be reviewed as research.

3. Because the problems related to social experimentation may differ substantially from those of biomedical and behavioral research, the Commission specifically declines to make any policy determination regarding such research at this time. Rather, the Commission believes that the problem ought to be addressed by one of its successor bodies.

Reading 4.3: Marcia Angell, "The Ethics of Clinical Research in the Third World"

In this article, taken from the New England Journal of Medicine, *Marcia Angell (b. 1939) argues against different standards for research trials in third-world countries. It is a violation of the principle of justice, she argues, for researchers to design research protocols for third-world clinical research that they could not use in the industrial world.*

An essential ethical condition for a randomized clinical trial comparing two treatments for a disease is that there be no good reason for thinking one is better than the other.[1,2] Usually, investigators hope and even expect that the new treatment will be better, but there should not be solid evidence one way or the other. If there is, not only would the trial be scientifically redundant, but the investigators would be guilty of knowingly giving inferior treatment to some participants in the trial. The necessity for investigators to be in this state of equipoise[2] applies to placebo-controlled trials, as well. Only when there is no known effective treatment is it ethical to compare a potential new treatment with a placebo. When effective treatment exists, a placebo may not be used. Instead, subjects in the control group of the study must receive the best known treatment. Investigators are responsible for all subjects enrolled in a trial, not just some of them, and the goals of the research are always secondary to the well-being of the participants. Those requirements are made clear in the Declaration of Helsinki of the World Health Organization (WHO), which is widely regarded as providing the fundamental guiding principles of research involving human subjects.[3] It states, "In research on man [*sic*], the interest of science and society should never take precedence over considerations related to the wellbeing of the subject," and "In any medical study, every patient—including those of a control group, if any—should be assured of the best proven diagnostic and therapeutic method."

Can you spot the references to our ethical principles in this quote from the "Declaration of Helsinki"? Can you put the dilemma in your own words? In the next section, can you spot Angell's mention of Kantian theory?

One reason ethical codes are unequivocal about investigators' primary obligation to care for the human subjects of their research is the strong temptation to subordinate the subjects' welfare to the objectives of the study. That is partic-ularly likely when the research question is extremely important and the answer would probably improve the care of future patients substantially. In those cir-cumstances, it is sometimes argued explicitly that obtaining a rapid, unambig-uous answer to the research question is the primary ethical obligation. With the most altruistic of motives, then, researchers may find themselves slipping across a line that prohibits treating human subjects as means to an end. When that line is crossed, there is very little left to protect patients from a callous disregard of their welfare for the sake of research goals. Even informed consent, important though it is, is not protection enough, because of the asymmetry in knowledge and authority between researchers and their subjects. And approval by an institutional review board, though also important, is highly variable in its responsiveness to patients' interests when they conflict with the interests of researchers.

A textbook example of unethical research is the Tuskegee Study of Untreated Syphilis.[4] In that study, which was sponsored by the U.S. Public Health Service and lasted from 1932 to 1972, 412 poor African-American men with untreated syphilis were followed and compared with 204 men free of the disease to determine the natural history of syphilis. Although there was no very good treatment available at the time the study began (heavy metals were the standard treatment), the research continued even after penicillin became widely available and was known to be highly effective against syphilis. The study was not terminated until it came to the attention of a reporter and the outrage pro-voked by front-page stories in the *Washington Star* and *New York Times* embar-rassed the Nixon administration into calling a halt to it.[5] The ethical violations were multiple: Subjects did not provide informed consent (indeed, they were deliberately deceived); they were denied the best known treatment; and the study was continued even after highly effective treatment became available. And what were the arguments in favor of the Tuskegee study? That these poor African-American men probably would not have been treated anyway, so the investigators were merely observing what would have happened if there were no study; and that the study was important (a "never-to-be-repeated opportunity," said one physician after penicillin became available).[6]

Defenders of the Tuskegee study appeal to which principles/ethical the-ories to justify not treating Tuskegee syphilis patients? Do these appeals seem particularly compelling? Why not?

Ethical concern was even stood on its head when it was suggested that not only was the information valuable, but it was especially so for people like the subjects—an impoverished rural population with a very high rate of untreated syphilis. The only lament seemed to be that many of the subjects inadvertently received treatment by other doctors.

> The author draws a parallel between what happened at Tuskegee (where patients were not treated at all, even though a treatment existed) with several placebo-controlled trials in third-world countries where some of the patients receive a placebo rather than a treatment.

Some of these issues are raised by Lurie and Wolfe elsewhere in this issue of the *Journal* [i.e., *The New England Journal of Medicine*, in which this op-ed appears]. They discuss the ethics of ongoing trials in the Third World of regimens to prevent the vertical transmission of human immunodeficiency virus (HIV) infection.[7] All except one of the trials employ placebo-treated control groups, despite the fact that zidovudine has already been clearly shown to cut the rate of vertical transmission greatly and is now recommended in the United States for all HIV-infected pregnant women. The justifications are reminiscent of those for the Tuskegee study: Women in the Third World would not receive antiretroviral treatment anyway, so the investigators are simply observing what would happen to the subjects' infants if there were no study. And a placebo-controlled study is the fastest, most efficient way to obtain unambiguous information that will be of greatest value in the Third World. Thus, in response to protests from Wolfe and others to the secretary of Health and Human Services, the directors of the National Institutes of Health (NIH) and the Centers for Disease Control and Prevention (CDC)—the organizations sponsoring the studies—argued, "It is an unfortunate fact that the current standard of perinatal care for the HIV-infected pregnant women in the sites of the studies does not include any HIV prophylactic intervention at all," and the inclusion of placebo controls "will result in the most rapid, accurate, and reliable answer to the question of the value of the intervention being studied compared to the local standard of care."[8]

...

Here Angell states her thesis. We should not decide that a research study is ethical based on local standards of care (i.e., in sub-Saharan Africa) but on the best current treatment. Why does she think this is so important?

Although I believe an argument can be made that a placebo-controlled trial was ethically justifiable because it was still uncertain whether prophylaxis would work, it should not be argued that it was ethical because no prophylaxis is the "local standard of care" in sub-Saharan Africa. For reasons discussed by Lurie and Wolfe, that reasoning is badly flawed.[7] As mentioned earlier, the Declaration of Helsinki requires control groups to receive the "best" current treatment, not the local one. The shift in wording between "best" and "local" may be slight, but the implications are profound. Acceptance of this ethical relativism could result in widespread exploitation of vulnerable Third World populations for research programs that could not be carried out in the sponsoring country.[9] Furthermore, it directly contradicts the Department of Health and Human Services' own regulations governing U.S.-sponsored research in foreign countries,[10] as well as joint guidelines for research in the Third World issued by WHO and the Council for International Organizations of Medical Sciences,[11] which require that human subjects receive protection at least equivalent to that in the sponsoring country....

The *Journal* has taken the position that it will not publish reports of unethical research, regardless of their scientific merit.[12,9] After deliberating at length about the study by Whalen et al., the editors concluded that publication was ethically justified, although there remain differences among us. The fact that the subjects gave informed consent and the study was approved by the institutional review board at the University Hospitals of Cleveland and Case Western Reserve University and by the Ugandan National AIDS Research Subcommittee certainly supported our decision but did not allay all our misgivings. It is still important to determine whether clinical studies are consistent with preexisting, widely accepted ethical guidelines, such as the Declaration of Helsinki, and with federal regulations, since they cannot be influenced by pressures specific to a particular study.

Quite apart from the merits of the study by Whalen et al., there is a larger issue. There appears to be a general retreat from the clear principles enunciated in the Nuremberg Code and the Declaration of Helsinki as applied to research in the Third World. Why is that? Is it because the "local standard of care" is different? I don't think so. In my view, that is merely a self-serving justification after the fact. Is it because diseases and their treatments are very different in the Third World, so that information gained in the industrialized world has no relevance and we have to start from scratch? That, too, seems an unlikely explanation, although here again it is often offered as a justification. Sometimes there may be relevant differences between populations, but that cannot be assumed. Unless there are specific indications to the contrary, the safest and most reasonable position is that people everywhere are likely to respond similarly to the same treatment.

I think we have to look elsewhere for the real reasons. One of them may be a slavish adherence to the tenets of clinical trials. According to these, all trials should be randomized, double-blind, and placebo-controlled, if at all possible. That rigidity may explain the NIH's pressure on Marc Lallemant to include a placebo group in his study, as described by Lurie and Wolfe.[7] Sometimes journals are blamed for the problem, because they are thought to demand strict conformity to the standard methods. That is not true, at least not at this journal. We do not want a scientifically neat study if it is ethically flawed, but like Lurie and Wolfe we believe that in many cases it is possible, with a little ingenuity, to have both scientific and ethical rigor.

> Here Angell gets at what she thinks is the real reason for the shift to "local standards" rather than "best standards." Which ethical principle does she think research in third-world countries really violates according to this last paragraph?

The retreat from ethical principles may also be explained by some of the exigencies of doing clinical research in an increasingly regulated and competitive environment. Research in the Third World looks relatively attractive as it becomes better funded and regulations at home become more restrictive. Despite the existence of codes requiring that human subjects receive at least the same protection abroad as at home, they are still honored partly in the breach. The fact remains that many studies are done in the Third World that simply could not be done in the countries sponsoring the work. Clinical trials have become a big business, with many of the same imperatives. To survive, it is necessary to get the work done as quickly as possible, with a minimum of obstacles. When these considerations prevail, it seems as if we have not come very far from Tuskegee after all. Those of us in the research community need to redouble our commitment to the highest ethical standards, no matter where the research is conducted, and sponsoring agencies need to enforce those standards, not undercut them....

Notes

1. Angell M. Patients' preferences in randomized clinical trials. *N Engl J Med* 1984;310:1385–7.
2. Freedman B. Equipoise and the ethics of clinical research. *N Engl J Med* 1987;317:141–5.
3. Declaration of Helsinki IV, 41st World Medical Assembly, Hong Kong, September 1989. In: Annas GJ, Grodin MA, eds. *The Nazi doctors and the Nuremberg Code: human rights in human experimentation.* New York: Oxford University Press, 1992:339–42.
4. Twenty years after: the legacy of the Tuskegee syphilis study. *Hastings Cent Rep* 1992;22(6):29–40.
5. Caplan AL. When evil intrudes. *Hastings Cent Rep* 1992;22(6):29–32.
6. The development of consent requirements in research ethics. In: Faden RR, Beauchamp TL. *A history and theory of informed consent.* New York: Oxford University Press, 1986:151–99.
7. Lurie P, Wolfe SM. Unethical trials of interventions to reduce perinatal transmission of the human immunodeficiency virus in developing countries. *N Engl J Med* 1997;337:853–6.
8. *The conduct of clinical trials of maternal–infant transmission of HIV supported by the United States Department of Health and Human Services in developing countries.* Washington, D.C.: Department of Health and Human Services, July 1997.
9. Angell M. Ethical imperialism? Ethics in international collaborative clinical research. *N Engl J Med* 1988;319:1081–3.
10. Protection of human subjects, 45 CFR § 46 (1996).
11. *International ethical guidelines for biomedical research involving human subjects.* Geneva: Council for International Organizations of Medical Sciences, 1993.
12. Angell M. The Nazi hypothermia experiments and unethical research today. *N Engl J Med* 1990;322:1462–4.

Reading 4.4: Baruch A. Brody, "Ethical Issues in Clinical Trials in Developing Countries"

Baruch Brody (1943–2018) responds to Marcia Angell's claim that placebo-controlled trials are unjust for the third-world subjects. Informed consent is the reason such trials are ethical. Brody begins by noting that the "Declaration of Helsinki" rejected one version of the patient's right to the "best proven method" that Angell discussed in her article.

... Despite this scientific value, the critics have argued that it was wrong to use a placebo control arm because the patients in that arm were being denied a proven therapy (the 076 regimen) and were being offered nothing in its place.[1] The critics claim that this did not meet the standard found in earlier versions of the Declaration of Helsinki (World Medical Association, Declaration of Helsinki, Principle II.3) "In any medical study, every patient, including those of a control group, if any, should be assured of the best proven diagnostic and therapeutic method."

Defenders of these trials quite properly note that none of the participants in these trials would otherwise have received any antiretroviral therapy, so nothing was being denied to them that they would otherwise have received. How then, ask the defenders, can the members of the control group have been treated unjustly? This led to a proposed, very controversial and eventually rejected, revision of the Declaration of Helsinki which read: "In any biomedical research protocol every patient-subject, including those of a control group, if any, should be assured that he or she will not be denied access to the best proven diagnostic, prophylactic, or therapeutic method that would otherwise be available to him or her."[2] The point is then that the justice or injustice of what is done to the control group depends on what the members of that group would have received if the trial had not been conducted.

> If Brody is correct that justice or injustice depends on what the people in the study would have had access to otherwise, then it is not wrong to do placebo-controlled clinical trials in third-world countries that would be unethical in first-world countries (e.g., the U.S., Britain) because there was access to proven therapies not available in, say, sub-Saharan Africa. What counts as fair access depends on the baseline where one lives, and pharmaceutical companies are not obligated to provide above that baseline. Do you agree with this? Why or why not?

While the reality of what the members of the control group would have received is obviously relevant, I am not satisfied that this proposed revision would have properly taken that into account. Would it be just, for example, to use such a placebo control group in a trial in a developed country where the antiretroviral therapy is widely available except to members of some persecuted minority from whom the control group is drawn? They would not have received the treatment if the trial had not been conducted, although they should have given the resources available in the developed country. Their use in a placebo control group is not therefore justified. The proposed revision made too much reference to what would have occurred and not enough to what should have occurred.

> Brody says we could have situations where there was unjust distribution of what should be available goods in a fair society. If some tribe was discriminated against when it comes to a certain treatment, then it would be wrong to use that discriminated baseline as a justification for not testing experimental drugs against a proven therapy. But couldn't the same be said for the larger unfair access of first-world countries to the latest treatments that the third-world countries don't have? Could we say that all of sub-Saharan Africa for example is a "persecuted minority"?

A recent workshop proposed instead that "study participants should be assured the highest standard of care practically attainable in the country in which the trial is being carried out."[3] This seems better, although it may suggest too much. Suppose that the treatment is practically attainable but only by inappropriately cutting corners on other forms of health care which may have a higher priority. I would suggest therefore that the normative nature of the standard be made explicit. It would then read that all participants in the study, including those in the control group, should not be denied any treatment that should otherwise be available to him or her in light of the practical realities of health care resources available in the country in question. The question for IRBs reviewing proposals for such research is then precisely the question of justice.

On that standard, the trials in question were probably not unjust.... Such trials will be harder to justify in the future given the current availability of proven much less expensive therapies which should be available even in some of the poorest countries....

> Even if you buy Brody's argument about justice, there are still the worries about people being unfairly forced into these studies because of their health problems and the exploitation of poor people to benefit much wealthier countries that Marcia Angell mentioned. In this next section Brody considers both.

Coercive Offers

It has been suggested by other critics that the participants in these trials were coerced into participating because of their desperation. "The very desperation of women with no alternatives to protect their children from HIV infection can be extremely coercive," argue one set of critics.[4] One of the requirements of an ethical trial is that the participants voluntarily agree to participate, and how can their agreement to participate be voluntary if it was coerced?

This line of thinking is analogous to the qualms that many have about paying research subjects substantial sums of money for their participation in research. Such inducements are often rejected on the grounds that they are coercive, because they are too good to refuse....

Normally, coercion involves a threat to put someone below their baseline unless they co-operate with the demands of the person issuing the threat.[5] As the researchers were not going to do anything to those who chose not to participate, they were clearly not threatening them. Further evidence of this comes from the reflection that threats are unwelcome to the parties being threatened, and there is no reason to suppose that the potential subjects saw the request to participate as something unwelcome. Even the critics recognize this. The potential subjects were being offered an opportunity that might improve their situation. This was an offer "too good to refuse," not a threat.

Should we expand the concept of coercion to include these very favourable offers? There are several reasons for thinking that we should not. First, it is widely believed that offering people valuable new opportunities is desirable. Moreover, the individuals in question want to receive these offers, and denying them the opportunity to receive them seems paternalistic or moralistic.[6] It is important that participants understand that what they are being offered is a chance to receive a treatment that may reduce transmission (since this is a randomized placebo controlled trial of a new regimen), and ensuring that is essential for the consent to be informed. As long as care is taken to ensure that this information is conveyed in a culturally sensitive fashion, and is understood, then there seems to be little reason to be concerned about coercion simply because a good opportunity is being offered to those with few opportunities....

Exploitation of Subjects

The final criticism of the trials is that they are exploitative of developing countries and their citizens because the interventions in question, even if proven successful, will not be available in these countries. To quote one of the critics: "To use a population as research subjects because of its poverty and its inability to obtain care, and then to not use that knowledge for the direct benefit of that population, is the very definition of exploitation. This exploitation is made worse by the fact that richer nations will unquestionably benefit from this research ... [they] will begin to use these lower doses, thereby receiving economic benefit."[7]

There are really two claims being advanced in that quotation. The second, that the developed countries ran these trials to discover cheaper ways of treating their own citizens, is very implausible since pregnant women in developed countries are receiving even more expensive cocktails of drugs both to treat the woman and to reduce transmission. The crucial issue is whether the trials are exploitative of the developing countries.

There seems to be a growing consensus that they are exploitative unless certain conditions about future availability in the country in question are met. The Council for International Organizations of Medical Sciences (CIOMS) is the source of this movement, as it declared in its 1992 guidelines that "as a general rule, the initiating agency should insure that, at the completion of successful testing, any products developed will be made reasonably available to residents of the host community or country."[8] A slightly weaker version of this requirement was adopted by a recent workshop which concluded that "studies are only appropriate if there is a reasonable likelihood that the populations in which they are carried out stand to benefit from successful results."[9]

This growing consensus is part of what lies behind the effort to secure these benefits by negotiating more favourable prices for the use of the tested drugs in developing countries. It seems highly desirable that this goal be achieved, but I want to suggest that it should be viewed as an aspiration, rather than a requirement, and that a different more modest requirement must be met to avoid charges of exploitation.

A good analysis of exploitation is that it is a wrong done to individuals who do not receive a fair share of the benefits produced by an activity in which they take part, even if they receive some benefit.[10] This is why a mutually beneficial activity, one from which both parties will be better off, can still be exploitative if one of the parties uses their greater bargaining power to harvest most of the benefits and the other party agrees because they need whatever modest benefit is being left for them.

As we apply this concept to the trials in question, we need to ask who needs to be protected from being exploited by the trials in question. It would seem that it is the participants. Are they getting a fair share of the benefits from the trial if it proves successful? This is a particularly troubling question when we consider those in the control group, whose major benefit from participation may have been an unrealized possibility of getting treated. If we judge that the participants have not received enough, then it is they who must receive more. An obvious suggestion is that they be guaranteed access to any regimen proved efficacious in any future pregnancies (or perhaps even that they be granted access to antiretroviral therapy for their own benefit). This would be analogous to familiar concepts of subjects receiving continued access to treatment after their participation in a trial is completed.

I certainly support every reasonable effort to increase access to treatments which will reduce vertical transmission, but imposing the types of community-wide requirements that have been suggested, but not necessarily justified if the above analysis is correct, may prevent important trials from being run because of the potential expense. Such proposals should be treated as moral aspirations, and exploitation should be avoided by focusing on what is owed to the subjects who have participated in the trials. It is they, after all, who are primarily at risk for being exploited....

Notes

1. Lurie P, Wolfe SM. Unethical trials of interventions to reduce perinatal transmission of the human immunodeficiency virus in developing countries. *New England Journal of Medicine* 1997; 337:853–56.
2. Proposed revision of the Declaration of Helsinki. *Bulletin of Medical Ethics* 1999; 18–21.
3. Perinatal HIV Intervention Research in Developing Countries Workshop Participants. Science ethics and the future of research into maternal infant transmission of HIV-1. *Lancet* 1999; 353:832–35.
4. Tafesse E, Murphy. Letter. *New England Journal of Medicine* 1998; 338:838.
5. Nozick R. Coercion. In *Philosophy, Science, and Method*, Morgenbesser S (ed.). St Martin's: New York, 1969.
6. Wilkinson M, Moore A. Inducement in research. *Bioethics* 1997; 11:373–89.
7. Glantz L, Grodin M. Letter. *New England Journal of Medicine* 1998; 338:839.
8. CIOMS. International Ethical Guidelines for Biomedical Research Involving Subjects. *CIOMS*, 1992; 68.
9. Perinatal HIV Intervention Research in Developing Countries Workshop Participants. Science ethics and the future of research into maternal infant transmission of HIV-1. *Lancet* 1999; 353:832–35.
10. Wertheimer A. *Exploitation*. Princeton University Press: Princeton, 1996.

Reading 4.5: Christine Grady, "Money for Research Participation: Does It Jeopardize Informed Consent?"

Christine Grady (b. 1952) answers those like Marcia Angell who are concerned that some kinds of offers to research subjects might invalidate informed consent. Grady signals her thesis by saying, "I argue that...." Ask yourself if she is for or against paying research subjects.

Some are concerned about the possibility that offering money for research participation can constitute coercion or undue influence capable of distorting the judgment of potential research subjects and compromising the voluntariness of their informed consent. The author recognizes that more often than not there are multiple influences leading to decisions, including decisions about research participation. The concept of undue influence is explored, as well as the question of whether or not there is something uniquely distorting about money as opposed to a chance for treatment or medical care. An amount of money that is not excessive and is calculated on the basis of time or contribution may, rather than constitute an undue inducement, be an indication of respect for the time and contribution that research subjects make.

Advertisements similar to these are increasingly common in newspapers around the United States, where, every day, people receive money for their participation in clinical research designed to test new drugs or devices or to learn more about human health and illness. Money is offered to research subjects as reimbursement for their expenses, compensation or reward for their time and effort, and/or as an incentive for studies that might otherwise have difficulty recruiting. Even though the practice of paying subjects is quite common, attitudes among investigators, members of Institutional Review Boards (IRBs) and others diverge, with some defending payment to research subjects as fair and appropriate and others condemning it as problematic and possibly even offensive or unethical.

Some of those uncomfortable with paying subjects are concerned that payment could jeopardize informed consent. Specifically, the concern is that money is potentially coercive or could cause "undue inducement." Coercion and undue inducement are threats to the possibility of voluntary informed consent, a tenet of ethical research as described in guidelines and codes of research ethics. The U.S. Common Rule for the Protection of Human Subjects (1991) states:

> An investigator shall seek consent only under circumstances that provide the prospective subject or representative sufficient opportunity to consider whether or not to participate *and that minimize the possibility of coercion or undue influence* (emphasis added)

The U.S. Food and Drug Administration (FDA) requires IRBs to "review both the amount of payment and the method and timing of disbursement *to assure that neither are coercive or present undue influence*" (1998, emphasis added). In this article I will briefly explore the concepts of coercion and undue influence as they have been applied to paying research subjects. I argue that the offer of payment to research subjects is not coercive, and that although in rare circumstances money could possibly constitute an undue inducement, prohibiting the use of money for research subjects is not the solution.

Grady offers a short summary of informed consent (see Chapter 3 for discussion) before making her case for why money is not unduly influential.

An individual's agreement to participate in research after deciding—based on information about the study—that it is compatible with his or her interests is an informed consent, widely accepted as central to the ethical conduct of clinical research. Informed consent is a process that includes several elements. In this process a potential research subject who is capable of making decisions is provided with information about a proposed study in an amount and manner

sufficient to promote a thorough understanding of the purpose, risks, benefits, alternatives, and requirements of the study. Given the information, a subject then voluntarily decides whether or not he or she wants to participate.
Voluntariness is understood, as suggested above, as free from coercion and
undue influence. Under what circumstances or conditions might the offer of
money be coercive or unduly influential and thereby limit voluntariness?

> Compare Grady's definition of coercion with Brody's in this chapter. How
> do they compare?

Although in common usage "coercion" is often meant to include much more,
coercion is, by definition, the intentional use of a credible and severe threat
of harm or force to control another or compel him or her to do something
(Beauchamp and Childress 1994, 165). Coercion, although certainly possible in
research, is not very probable under the current system of checks and balances.
Threatening someone who refuses to participate in a research study with punishment or retaliation (for example, by a military officer, a professor, employer, warden, or even a doctor) would be coercive. Coercion may also occur if
someone who refused to participate was threatened with physical or other harm
(e.g., injury or loss of promotion or a job). However, since the offer of money
is not a threat of punishment or harm, but rather an offer, it is hard to see how
money as payment for research participation is or could be coercive (Faden and
Beauchamp 1986, ch. 10; Wilkinson and Moore 1997). But what about money as
undue influence?

Undue influence might be thought of as too much or excessive influence.
Therefore it is worth briefly considering the nature of influence more generally.
Most decisions that a person makes, including the decision whether to participate in a research study, are susceptible to multiple influences. People usually
choose and act in accordance with their wants and needs, influenced by their
physical, psychological, social, economic, and cultural experiences and circumstances. Ruth Faden and Tom Beauchamp in their landmark work, *A History and
Theory of Informed Consent*, recognize that "influences come in many forms, and
from many sources.... They can vary dramatically in degree of influence actually
exerted" (1986, 256). Some influences are strong enough to serve as inducements, motivations, or stimuli for action.

However, inducements—many of which are nonmonetary—do not necessarily invalidate or preclude voluntary choice. We welcome and respond to

inducements all of the time in many areas of life, including selecting employment, making purchases, and other choices. For example, even if we are attracted to a job by a higher salary, we still generally choose a job based on a number of other factors, including what we feel qualified for, what would be satisfying, as well as where, with whom, and what hours we would work. Since human motivation is complex and almost always involves multiple considerations, there is rarely a single reason for doing something. In the same way, being attracted to the money offered for research participation does not necessarily negate the possibility of other influential motivations and considerations. Subjects participate in research for multiple reasons. For some subjects money may be one reason among others. If inducements can be compatible with voluntary choice, then money, as an inducement, does not inherently obviate or compromise voluntariness.

Payment for research participation has been objected to, however, not simply because it is an inducement, but because it can be an undue inducement or influence. In Faden and Beauchamp's analysis, influences exist along a continuum from controlling to noncontrolling. Control beyond a certain point is not compatible with voluntary autonomous decision making and action. The control of influences found "irresistible" by an individual might compel unwelcome choices and in this sense compromise voluntariness (Faden and Beauchamp 1986, 256). These influences might be regarded as "undue" or excessively influential. On this analysis individuals who find participation in a particular research study unwelcome yet are unable to refuse because of the influence or inducement of money could be "unduly induced." Presumably, most subjects attracted to research by money, or subjects who choose to participate in research partly because of the money, do have the freedom to refuse.

Prospective subjects are reminded of their right to exercise this freedom in the process of obtaining informed consent. They are advised that participation is their choice and they have the right to refuse or withdraw at any time without penalty. In addition, many people who are attracted to research because of the money (including students, people looking for a little extra income, or even the "professional guinea pig") generally do have additional options for obtaining money, usually from other full or part-time unskilled jobs. Perhaps they select research participation because it has more flexible hours, is time limited, or seems more interesting or easier. In addition, research volunteers can and do exercise their freedom to refuse when they decide participating in the particular study is not in their interests.

Perhaps the potential for undue inducement—in the sense that money literally makes research an offer that one cannot refuse—is a worry when a person is economically destitute and truly has no other options for acquiring comparable amounts of money. Even then, do we protect such people by allowing them to participate in (the same kind of) research without receiving money or by not allowing them to participate at all? In fact, denying the possibility of financial payment to a research subject may serve only to eliminate an option—the option of obtaining money through research participation. Careful attention, in the process of obtaining informed consent, to a subject's reasons for participating, his or her understanding and expectations of research, and his or her sense of freedom to choose to participate or not seems more appropriate and may be more effective than eliminating the opportunity to receive money. The offer of money for research participation may actually expand options for some people, while not restricting their options to do anything else they could otherwise have done (Wilkinson and Moore 1999).

> You could summarize Grady's argument so far by saying money usually isn't an undue influence (it wouldn't make informed consent invalid), and even if it is in some situations, this is not a reason to prevent people from getting money for research studies for their own good. Ask yourself this: Do you agree with this assessment or do you think it is possible for someone to be so desperate for money that their participation in research shows they are not really consenting?

If a principal concern with respect to undue influence is a limited freedom to refuse research participation because of the lack of other available money-making options, we ought to be at least as or more concerned about other influences on research subjects with other types of need and limited options. These influences include: the promise of treatment, albeit investigational, for the desperately ill who have exhausted other treatment options; access to care or medications or other treatment for those who cannot afford these on their own or have no or inadequate healthcare coverage; the advice from a trusted physician or healthcare provider that the study is the best or only hope; or course credit for student participants. People in these situations may find research participation extremely difficult to resist or refuse. However, as Wilkinson and Moore (1997) argue, there may be a distinction between autonomy—understood as the ability to decide what to do for oneself—and freedom—the presence of more than one acceptable option. According to their analysis, even people who are unfree, in that they have no other good options, may still be capable of autonomous consent. A nonresearch example of this is our acceptance of individuals' right to refuse life-sustaining therapy, based on respect for their autonomy, knowing that, in many cases, their options are limited to either accepting the therapy or death. There are few data on the extent to which research participants feel free to refuse or withdraw from research within the context of their often limited options, and the extent to which some actually do agree to participate in research that compromises their values or interests. Of note is data collected in the Subject Interview Survey by the Advisory Committee on Human Radiation Experiments. They report that 31% of responding patients felt they had no choice but to participate because of their few medical alternatives (1996, 469). Nevertheless, greater than 98% felt that "the decision to participate had been theirs to make and that they had not felt pressured into that decision" (472). Further empirical research would help us to better understand these issues.

> Ask yourself, what is the distinction Grady makes between autonomy and freedom? Do you agree that one could have autonomy without freedom in this sense? Can you think of some other examples? In the next section, what is the distinction Grady makes between excessive influence and inappropriate influence? Why is this important to her argument?

According to the Belmont Report, an influence may be *undue* not only when it is *excessive*, but also when it is *inappropriate* or improper (National Commission for the Protection of Human Subjects of Biomedical Behavioral Research 1979). Some may believe that money, unlike the need for treatment or care, is an *inappropriate* influence in decisions about research participation. It is sometimes argued that since research participants volunteer with altruistic motives of contributing to science and society, money has no place in this arrangement. The ethical concern, then, is not simply that some might find the offer of money irresistible, but also that money is simply an inappropriate motivating factor for research participation.

Money certainly has a reputation for getting people to do things they otherwise would not do, and, in some cases, for getting people to do something they know is wrong. Hence, we see daily newspaper accounts of scandals, bribes, and extortion. Money is also believed capable of inappropriately distorting people's judgments and motivations. The U.S. Office of Protection from Research Risks (OPRR, replaced in 2000 by the Office of Human Research Protections [OHRP]) says that money as a possible undue inducement for research is problematic because it can impair an individual's judgment regarding what is at stake in the research or blind him or her to the potential risks of research participation (1993, 3–44). OPRR further notes that offers of money could cause potential participants to misrepresent something about themselves in order to gain or maintain enrollment in a study and receive the money. Misrepresentation may not only jeopardize the participant's informed consent, but possibly also his or her well-being as well as the integrity of the study. An individual's susceptibility to distorted judgment because of money is relative to his or her particular circumstances, but importantly also to his or her values, as some people even in very desperate straits cannot be "bought."

Presumably, however, the larger the sum of money involved, the greater the potential for distorting judgment or prompting potential participants to lie or ignore risks. Commentators and common wisdom have argued that limiting the amount of payment offered for research participation minimizes the possibility that money will distort judgment and push people towards deception (Levine 1986; Macklin 1981). Payment as recognition of the research participant's contribution and calculated according to some regularly applied and locally acceptable standard (per day, visit, or procedure) is likely to be more modest and less likely to distort judgment than amounts designed solely to attract subjects and outperform the competition in terms of recruitment (Dickert and Grady 1999). Arbitrary or large amounts of money designed simply to entice, to outbid other studies, or to make up for risk should not be allowed. Modest payment thought of as remuneration for the participant's contribution minimizes the possibility of undue inducement, because the offer of money is neither excessive nor inappropriate.

On the other hand, it is not clear that money is uniquely capable of distorting judgment about the risks and benefits of research. Again, a person with few or no other treatment options might also be prompted to conceal something about past medical history or current behaviors that would otherwise disqualify him or her from the option he or she perceives as the best "treatment" or only hope. In the process of obtaining informed consent, particular care should be taken with people who might be feeling desperate. In order to assess comprehension and ensure an adequate voluntary informed consent, reasons for participating should be carefully assessed, as well as participants' understanding of the research risks and benefits and the alternatives available to them. Information about the potential for therapeutic benefit or lack thereof in any particular study should be presented clearly and accurately. In addition, the threshold of understanding should be higher for those who are invited to participate in risky, uncomfortable, or even inconvenient research without the prospect of direct benefit to them, whether they be healthy students looking for a little extra cash or chronically ill and vulnerable patients dependent on us for their treatment and care.

> What do you think of Grady's claim that money need be no more distorting of consent than any other incentive if the patient is desperate? Do you think there is something about money that makes it more unsavory than, say, a last-ditch experimental treatment for a patient who is out of options? Why or why not?

Some may object that careful evaluation of a research participant's motivations for participating and his or her understanding of risks, benefits, and alternatives puts too much additional burden on the process of obtaining informed consent—a process which is already less than ideal. In my view, by focusing less on the details and words in written documents and focusing more time and attention assuring that research subjects understand and feel confident that the choice about participation is theirs, we could improve the reality of informed consent.

Summary

A decision about whether or not to participate in research is subject to many influences, of various forms and degrees and from different sources. Money may be one of these influences, although it is often just one among several other factors that an individual will consider in making a decision. In asking prospective research participants to give informed consent for research participation, it is incumbent upon us not only to provide clear and honest information about the study and assess how well they understand the information provided, but also to assess their reasons for participating and whether they feel free to refuse. Particular attention should be given to the informed consent of individuals who perceive they have no other choice because they need the money or the "treatment" or something else available to them only through the research. In these cases extra effort to assure that they understand the nature, risks, benefits, alternatives, and requirements of the study is warranted. In addition, the amount of money offered through research participation should be standardized and calculated so that it is more or less comparable to that available through other similar unskilled moneymaking opportunities in the relevant community. In these ways the potential that money will unduly influence an individual to participate in a research study against his or her interests, or with a distorted view of what is at stake, is minimized.

Research participants volunteer and sacrifice their time and effort to generate knowledge that is helpful to others and society, often with little or uncertain benefit for themselves. Rather than an undue inducement, money to reimburse research participants for their expenses and compensate them in some way for their time and effort may be a demonstration of respect and appreciation for these generous individuals.

References

Advisory Committee on Human Radiation Experiments. 1996. *Final report.* New York: Oxford University Press.

Beauchamp, T., and J. Childress. 1994. *Principles of biomedical ethics,* 4th ed. New York: Oxford University Press.

Common Rule for the Protection of Human Subjects. 1991. *U.S. Code of Federal Regulations.* Title 45, pt. 46, sec. 116.

Dickert, N., and C. Grady. 1999. What's the price of a research subject? Approaches to payment for research participation. *The New England Journal of Medicine* 341:198–203.

Faden, R., and T. Beauchamp. 1986. *A history and theory of informed consent.* New York: Oxford University Press.

Levine, R. 1986. *Ethics and regulation of clinical research,* 2nd ed. New Haven: Yale University Press.

Macklin, R. 1981. "Due" and "undue" inducements: On paying money to research subjects. *IRB: A Review of Human Subjects Research* 3(5):1–6.

U.S. Department of Health and Human Services. Office of Protection from Research Risks. 1993. *Protecting human research subjects: IRB guidebook.* Washington: GPO.

U.S. Food and Drug Administration. 1998. *Payment to research subjects.* Guidance for Investigational Review Boards and clinical investigators. Washington: GPO.

U.S. National Commission for the Protection of Human Subjects of Biomedical and Behavioral Research. 1979. *The Belmont report.* Washington: GPO.

Wilkinson, M., and A. Moore. 1997. Inducement in research. *Bioethics* 11:373–89.

——.1999. Inducements revisited. *Bioethics* 13:114–30.

Reading 4.6: Mark Kuczewski, "Is Informed Consent Enough? Monetary Incentives for Research Participation and the Integrity of Biomedicine"

Continuing the conversation, Kuczewski does not dispute Christine Grady's claim that money doesn't necessarily invalidate consent to be a research subject; however, he still thinks that offering money is inappropriate and this shows that informed consent is not as morally transformative as we think it is.

... Christine Grady's (2001) analysis of the coercive power of money on research subjects is fairly persuasive. She establishes that monetary payment to the subject does not intrinsically undermine the process of informed consent. Regarding this central thesis, I believe she is correct. However, there are other good reasons to prohibit payment to subjects. Grady has inadvertently underscored the inadequacy of the informed consent doctrine to do as much moral work as we'd like.

... Grady believes our concern for coercion due to a lack of options implies that we should be very concerned about other undue influences, such as the desperation of persons in need of a cure for a terminal condition that is currently untreatable. Money is no more likely than illness to undermine freedom and distort judgment. In both cases Grady argues that what is needed is demonstrable evidence that the subject truly understands the risks and benefits (or lack thereof) as a result of the information-giving process. Grady allows that some reasonable restrictions on the amount of money offered for participation in research may be in order. But, these offers should be calibrated based on alternative opportunities in the community for money making, not indexed to the earnings and opportunities forfeited by the subject. Does Grady's analogy between those who enroll for money and those who enroll due to lack of treatment options demonstrate what she had hoped?

> Grady's argument depended on the similarity between desperate patients seeking a cure through experimental treatment and people volunteering for research for money. Kuczewski questions this in the next section.

Experimental Exploitation versus Dying Well

Grady's analogy between the influence money has on a choice to participate in research and the influence of a terminal illness with no effective standard of care is instructive. In each case, she finds the level of influence may be acceptable. Of particular note is that she points out that research ethics usually focuses on the forms that get signed rather than whether the subject really appreciates the implications of enrollment in the protocol and the potential alternatives. The profundity of this point is only beginning to be appreciated by the bioethics community and has not been adequately studied.

What information subjects learn during the informed consent process has been studied (Braddock et al. 1997). Other studies have examined whether subjects know they are involved in research and often measure the retention of risks and benefits and whether memory can be enhanced (Anonymous 1976; Aaronson et al. 1996). Many have focused on the fact that although research subjects may be informed that a trial is not designed to benefit them, e.g., a phase I trial, they nevertheless enroll because they believe it might help them. This is sometimes called the "therapeutic misconception" (Applebaum, Roth, and Lidz 1982; Daugherty et al. 1995).

What the example of subjects who are desperate for an effective treatment shares with the example of subjects who enroll only for payment is that the autonomy of the subjects seems to be compromised in similar ways. Neither is coerced but both raise the concern that the transaction is still not morally acceptable. Somehow the subject's situation is being taken advantage of in a way that seems inappropriate. They are making a deal that more fortunate people would find repugnant. They are being exploited.

The recruitment of desperately ill subjects has been under scrutiny, but in recent years the concern has been about inclusion rather than exploitation. The AIDS crisis shifted the regulatory emphasis from protecting human subjects against risky, nonbeneficial research to ensuring access to the potential benefits of clinical research (Jonsen and Stryker 1993). According to some, the main thing desperately ill volunteers needed protection against was a placebo (Minogue et al. 1995). [That is, a placebo-controlled trial.]

... [A]t this point we find that we may not be so much concerned with free and informed consent as with making sure that medicine is true to its ideals. Medicine is often conceived in teleological terms (Pellegrino and Thomasma 1981), i.e. is about curing illness and aiding the healing process. However, when these goals are not possible, it is about relieving pain and suffering and helping the patient to achieve the best quality of life possible. To allow a part of the biomedical enterprise to exploit the illness is to undermine the integrity of contemporary medicine. Because the integrity of a profession such as medicine is a sketchier concept than patient autonomy, it has been less often invoked in these debates. However, interest in professional integrity probably provides the best reasons to be concerned about patient exploitation.

> Kuczewski summarizes his thesis in the above paragraph. Can you find it?

The Integrity of the Biomedical Enterprise

The advertisement tag line with which Grady begins her article seems repugnant and likely to elicit disdain. However, I doubt that the average person would begin to explain what is wrong with it by arguing that those who might respond to such an advertisement are coerced. When one watches an analogous advertisement on television for personal injury attorneys, the common response is to note how the professionals are demeaning themselves. Certainly, their self-degradation is linked to the fact that they are preying upon certain vulnerable populations. But, this does not entail that these populations literally have no choice but to seek the assistance of the attorneys. If pressed, the average person might say something about how those advertisements give all attorneys "a bad name." In effect, the common response is about the integrity of the professions involved and the fact that they are not aiming at their loftier goals.

Research and medical treatment are, in theory, separable. Researchers seek knowledge, medical professionals seek the well-being of their patients. In recent years, this line has become increasingly blurred (Eichenwald and Kolata 1999; Department of Health and Human Services 2000). As a result, if biomedical researchers invite public scorn, this disdain is likely to spill over to all medical professions. Thus, preventing such offers from being made is a legitimate interest of the medical professions, even if they are not strictly coercive.

Here the analogy between the cases of those who are exploited through monetary offers and those whose autonomy is compromised by desperation breaks down. Enrolling desperately ill patients does not compromise the integrity of the biomedical enterprise in the same way as exploiting relatively healthy volunteers by means of monetary rewards. I believe there is simply something more unseemly about the latter than the former. In the case of desperately ill volunteers, the research is at least related to the patients' condition.

Is the author's statement above more like a reason based on evidence or an emotional appeal? If more like a reason, what is the evidence he offers to support his claim?

Even if they strongly overestimate the likelihood that the protocol will help them, the protocol is at least part of a process that is designed eventually to help people like them. There is an intrinsic relationship between the ends of the researcher and the patients' wellbeing, even if this relationship is not likely to be presently realized. Thus, in such a situation our concern about their compromised autonomy must be balanced with a concern for the justice of excluding potential beneficiaries of the research. In the case of those who enroll in a protocol solely or mainly for money, no such balancing of legitimate concerns obtains.

In sum, one's immediate revulsion at monetary inducements for research participation is probably best conceived as a concern for the integrity of the medical profession, not as a concern about coercion or compromised autonomy. It is a concern that, once the general public sees biomedical researchers as mercenary in the pursuit of their agenda, the trust of the medical professions will similarly erode. Of course, a concept such as the integrity of the medical profession is not a concept that is as readily accepted as that of patient autonomy. However, as the biomedical establishment is directly and indirectly heavily subsidized by public funds, the public has a right to hold that establishment to relatively high standards and ideals.

References [to this extract]

Aaronson, N. K., E. Visser-Pol, G. H. Leenhouts et al. 1996. Telephone-based nursing intervention improves the effectiveness of the informed consent process in cancer clinical trials. *Journal of Clinical Oncology* 14(3):984–86.

Anonymous. 1976. Patient consent given—but forgotten. *Medical World News* 17(4):26.

Appelbaum, P. S., L. H. Roth, and C. Lidz. 1982. The therapeutic misconception: Informed consent in psychiatric research. *International Journal of Law and Psychiatry* 5:319–29.

Braddock, C. H. III, S. D. Finn, W. Levinson et al. 1997. How doctors and patients discuss routine clinical decisions: Informed decision making in the outpatient setting. *Journal of General Internal Medicine* 12(6):339–45.

Daugherty, C., M.J. Retain, E. Grochowski et al. 1995. Perceptions of cancer patients and their physicians involved in Phase I clinical trials. *Journal of Clinical Oncology* 13(5):1062–72.

Eichenwald, K., and G. Kolata. 1999. Drug trials hide conflicts for doctors. *New York Times*, 16 May.

Grady, C. 2001. Money for research participation: Does it jeopardize informed consent? *American Journal of Bioethics* 1(2):40–44.

Jonsen, A. R., and J. Stryker, eds. 1993. *The social impact of AIDS in the United States*. Washington: National Academy Press.

Minogue, B., G. Palmer-Fernandez et al. 1995. Individual autonomy and the double-blind controlled experiment: The case of desperate volunteers. *Journal of Medicine and Philosophy* 20:43–55.

Pellegrino, E. O., and D. C. Thomasma. 1981. *A philosophical basis of medical practice: Toward a philosophy and ethic of the healing professions*. New York: Oxford University Press.

U.S. Department of Health and Human Services. Office of the Inspector General. 2000. *Recruiting human subjects: Pressures in industry-sponsored clinical research*. Washington: GPO.

ETHICS COMMITTEE

African HIV Trials

The following is a fictional case based on actual clinical trials.

Africa has one of the largest populations of HIV-positive people in the world. The World Health Organization estimates that as of 2020 over 25 million Africans live with HIV.[*] The president of South Africa has pleaded with US pharmaceutical companies to begin fast-tracking HIV drug trials. Normally clinical trials of HIV drugs can take years. The South African Minister of National Health, Nuala Olwendo, invited Veritan pharmaceuticals to begin trials in three South African villages where FDA rules do not apply.

Veritan agreed to one trial study in the tribal village of Shangana and began double-blind studies with 500 men, women, and infants with HIV. Some received placebos, while others received a new experimental treatment code-named EXHIV. This was explained thoroughly using interpreters. However some difficulty was reported regarding translation of the term "placebo" since there is no equivalent in the tribal dialect of Shangana. No infants were tested without the consent of both the parents. As a precaution, Veritan enlisted the help of the International Red Cross to monitor the treatment of patients.

As you can imagine, this decision was not without criticism. The following are quotes from critics and defenders of Vertian's clinical trial.

> "It is a moral outrage to conduct placebo-controlled clinical trials of EXHIV in countries like South Africa. We know that there are other drugs like AZT that are proven effective. To enroll people who may get a placebo is denying them treatment for their disease."
> —Roberto Garza, US Undersecretary for Health and Human Services

---

[*] World Health Organization, "Estimated Number of People (All Ages) Living with HIV," https://www.who.int/data/gho/data/indicators/indicator-details/GHO/estimated-number-of-people–living-with-hiv.

"Veritan is deceiving South Africans into thinking they are getting treated when they aren't. At least Veritan should test the effectiveness of EXHIV against proven therapies like AZT. As it stands, I'm sorry to say, the Veritan study is little different from Tuskegee or Willowbrook."

—Brett Hopper M.D., *New England Journal of Medicine*

"You can't compare what's standard in the US with practices in African countries. The history here is so much different from in the States. Thanks to Apartheid, almost no one who isn't white trusts a foreign doctor. In the outlying villages almost no one gets treatment for HIV unless they can find a clinic that isn't over-flowing with typhoid or dysentery. The South African study gives a 50/50 chance of getting HIV treatment. Even those who get the placebo get unprecedented medical care, including regular medical exams, antibiotics for infections in a country where such drugs are rare, and food supplements from the clinics. That is hardly Tuskegee. Furthermore, AZT has a complicated dosing schedule requiring specific pills at specific times. Most of the potential subjects don't even own wrist-watches. EXHIV consists simply of two quick dissolve tablets per day, a far easier dosing schedule."

—Charlene Stein, M.D. FACCP, Chief Investigator assigned to EXHIV for Veritan

"Critics shouldn't discount the importance of the EXHIV trials. If EXHIV performs as the early data indicates, we will be able to provide poor Africans with an inexpensive drug with less complicated regimens than AZT. EXHIV has the potential to save millions of lives. We applaud Veritan's resourcefulness and leadership."

—Jeremy Chapley, M.D., *British Journal of Medicine*

> Analyze the justifications given for the trial and the objections in the quotes below. As a group project, decide, if you were on an IRB, would you have allowed the trial to go forward as described, would you have insisted on changes to the research protocols, or would you have stopped the trial altogether?

CHAPTER 5

Dilemmas at the End of Life

Mr. Perry Wants It ALL Unplugged[*]

Mr. Perry (not his real name) was 83 years old and had several medical problems. He had spent the past several months in and out of hospitals and rehab. Prior to that, he lived independently in a small Midwestern town. Widowed many years ago, he subsequently enjoyed the company of a lovely lady friend who lived down the street from the Perry home. He had five adult children and numerous grandchildren.

Life should have been relatively good for this octogenarian. But life was not good. Not anymore. "My body is all worn out. I'm worn out. Don't want to do this anymore, Doc. They say I can't go home and be safe. And I'm NOT going to a nursing home. No way! Just stop that little gadget that shocks me and the part that keeps my heart going. I want them stopped. Yes, the pacemaker, too. A magnet will stop it, right? Just do it. Please." ...

Mr. Perry had a cardiac resynchronization therapy defibrillator (CRT-D) implanted a few years ago. It included an electrical pacing component for heart rhythms, on which the patient was 100% dependent. The defibrillator had shocked him, more than once, just before he came to the hospital E.R. with this request. That was the last straw for Mr. Perry. No more shocks for him.

---

[*] Excerpted from Tarris Rosell, "A Good Death or Assisted Suicide," *Practical Bioethics: A Blog for Practical Bioethics*, June 6, 2017.

No nursing home or rehab or hospitalizations or medications. And no more mechanical pacing either. "I'm tired of fighting."

Deactivating an internal defibrillator is one thing. The patient's cardiologist didn't need an ethics consultation for that decision. "If he doesn't want to be shocked again, that's his decision. And if it went off again after he'd requested it stopped, that could be a kind of torture," she reasoned. Deactivation happened quickly after admission from the Emergency Department. A "Do Not Attempt Resuscitation" order was placed in the chart.

But the pacemaker, also? He wanted it stopped. Ought we do so? Would that be ethically respectful of this patient's autonomy? Or would it be physician-technician assisted suicide?

"If we stop the pacemaker, Mr. Perry, you will die within a few minutes."

"Yes, I know. I'm tired of fighting. Please."

WHAT'S AT STAKE?

If autonomy means anything for patients, it means the right to refuse treatment. Patients do not have full control over what they can request in terms of treatment. Just because a 30-year-old will consent to her twelfth face-lift surgery does not mean a surgeon has a duty to do what she asks. However, the right to refuse treatment has been, from the beginning of medical ethics, one of the most important rights of all.

Treating people for something against their will, even for their own good, can be construed as assault. This is what makes Mr. Perry's case a dilemma. Mr. Perry is refusing a treatment that he consented to before—the pacemaker; however, since he cannot remove it himself, his choice requires others to be complicit in his decision. That means Mr. Perry's choice is not just one of personal autonomy; it requires others to do something they may find morally objectionable.

When medical staff are asked to do things by administration or patients that make them feel they are engaging in something immoral, they experience what is called moral distress. The doctors in the scenario are fine with deactivating the defibrillator because it is analogous to not using an external defibrillator (those paddles and "clear!" routine you see on TV and movies). However, the medical staff experience moral distress when Mr. Perry asks them to deactivate the pacemaker. Why? Interestingly enough, a survey shows that providers make an intuitive distinction between medical devices that are external (machines the patient is "hooked up" to) and internal medical devices (e.g., pacemakers).

Providers are much more likely to think removal of an external device is more permissible than an internal device.

Is this just an intuition, or are there principled reasons we might make this distinction?

It may just be an intuition. Most of us have a picture of what a "good death" looks like. If I asked you to picture a "good death" and then list the common factors in any sort of "good death," I would bet your pictures might have the following features:

1. As little pain as possible (not prolonged suffering until death)
2. All affairs in order (not leaving things undone)
3. The result of an illness (not the result of some violence)
4. Under your own terms (peaceful, not scared and fighting)

Now some people might object that the best death is quick and unexpected—"I just want to get hit by a truck one day and never see it coming"—but why is the quick and surprised death so desirable? Because it is without prolonged pain, and you are not scared because you never see it coming?

Now consider the providers attending to Mr. Perry and their concerns about deactivating a pacemaker. Which of the elements of a good death does not quite fit within the frame of the case study? If you said number 3 (and possibly 1) then you might be getting somewhere. The doctors and nurses are concerned because deactivating a pacemaker seems like they, not his heart condition, would be the cause of Mr. Perry's death. On the other hand, deactivating the defibrillator seems more like preventing a machine from extending Mr. Perry's life, something they do all the time.

So we have a clash between patient autonomy (Mr. Perry has the right to refuse treatment, even treatment he consented to in the past) and duty not to harm (turning off the pacemaker will make staff complicit in Mr. Perry's death).

Killing and Letting Die

Is there a moral difference between killing and letting die? This is a vigorous debate in bioethics about the distinction between killing someone and letting them die. Just on the surface, I can bet you thought "killing" must be wrong and "letting die" elicited a sense of "might be morally permissible."

Is this just an intuition? Can we think of examples of "killing" that are morally permissible, such as what happens with soldiers in combat? Could we think of examples of "letting die" that would be morally impermissible? Such as when a person stands by while another drowns because they hate them? These two examples show that "killing" and "letting die" are not terms that are synonymous with "immoral" and "moral," respectively.

Moral philosopher James Rachels (1941–2003) claimed there is no definitive *moral* distinction between killing and letting die. There are instances of moral "killing" and immoral "letting die," such that the terms are meaningless without other moral considerations like the intent of the one intervening (see this chapter's What's the Debate?).

Consider the act of removing a breathing tube, or "extubation," that ends in a patient's death. This is a procedure that happens in hospitals across the world every day, and it is considered ethical. A patient who is breathing on a ventilator (breathing machine) is extubated; the tube is taken out, and because they cannot breathe on their own due to some underlying illness, they die. Such actions are considered moral and compassionate to prevent prolonged suffering. Suppose, however, a greedy nephew who stands to gain an inheritance sneaks into the room of a patient dependent on a ventilator and removes the breathing tube because his intent is to kill his aunt and get the money right away. He performs exactly the same action as doctors, and his action does prevent her prolonged suffering. Still, it does seem intuitive that what the nephew does is wrong.

From the ethical theories covered in Chapter 2, consequentialists cannot say that what makes the greedy nephew's action wrong is intent. Only consequences are wrong making for consequentialists. A consequentialist might have to say that what is wrong is that a bad person gets an inheritance and that this might lead to other bad actions. In addition, the action might be wrong because it violates a rule that leads to better consequences, namely that only medical staff should extubate someone.

Deontologists, however, can say that regardless of the consequences, the extubation is immoral because the intent was to take a life without the patient's consent, and that is murder. Intent is what separates killing and letting die, not action and inaction. Isn't there a reason to think that the action (hastening death through a lethal dose) is usually worse than inaction (withholding CPR)? At least, isn't there a reason for our intuitions on this matter? One explanation given by Daniel Callahan (1930–2019) is that the real distinction between killing and letting die is the cause of death. When we remove a breathing tube, the cause of death is ultimately the underlying disease.

In contrast, when we give someone a lethal dose of morphine or withhold food or hydration, the cause of death is not the underlying illness but the intervention itself. If this is true, then turning off Mr. Perry's defibrillator is tantamount to withholding CPR on someone with a Do Not Resuscitate order, allowing him to die.

What about the pacemaker? It depends on what you think the pacemaker is doing. If you think it is sustaining Mr. Perry's life by correcting his underlying heart rhythm when it goes out of whack, then shutting it off means he would die as a result of withdrawing that support. In this case it is treatment, and Mr. Perry can refuse treatment, whether we agree or not, because of his right to self-determination (autonomy).

However, you might think the pacemaker is really just supporting his heart function and shutting it off is like shutting off his heart. The pacemaker function of the device is part of ongoing care, not an extraordinary intervention. On this interpretation, it is immoral to shut off the pacemaker since doing so would become the cause of Mr. Perry's death.

For the medical staff, complying with his wishes to end his life would make them, rather than his underlying illness, complicit in his death. It is one thing for Mr. Perry to want to cease treatment and let his disease take his life; it is another for him to want to shut off his pacemaker so he can die more quickly than he would when his heart needed a jolt from his CRT-D. That would be a kind of active killing on this account.

Often, the term "euthanasia" is synonymous with mercy killing or hastening someone's death. It is considered immoral, and in most states it is illegal. However, medical providers also use it to describe end-of-life interventions that are legal and considered ethical. Thus "voluntary, passive euthanasia" describes a patient's request to remove a breathing tube and be allowed to die, not "kept on machines," as family members often say. So let's get clear on the terms.

Voluntary, Non-Voluntary, and Involuntary

The distinction between voluntary, non-voluntary, and involuntary turns on the wishes of the patient. In voluntary euthanasia, the patient has clearly consented to the withdrawing of treatment or the active intervention of some drug to hasten death. Non-voluntary euthanasia refers to instances where the patient's wishes are not known or they cannot consent because they lack decisional capacity. If someone with no next of kin is allowed to die rather than be actively resuscitated because the doctor believed it was in the patient's best interest, the intervention would be non-voluntary.

Involuntary euthanasia refers to allowing a patient to die or actively intervening to kill them against their express wishes. Involuntary euthanasia would be considered homicide by any medical community and is the chief reason that professional medical associations have discouraged or banned medical personnel from participating in lethal injections as capital punishment.

Active and Passive

The distinction between active and passive euthanasia is a far more controversial distinction than the voluntary/non-voluntary distinction. Is there a moral difference between active intervention and passive withholding or withdrawing of treatment when both are the cause of a patient's death? Rachels thinks not, while Callahan says there is a distinction in cause of death. Active interventions in medicine would include administering a drug through an IV or writing a prescription for a lethal dose of a barbiturate for those seeking voluntary active euthanasia.

Passive interventions would include withdrawing of life support (e.g., a ventilator) or withholding lifesaving treatment like CPR or cardiac stimulation, as in the standard "do not resuscitate" order. There is a sense in which both active and passive interventions are still the cause of a person's death, but in the active intervention, the person might remain alive until the disease progresses, were it not for the intervention. In the passive intervention, what is preventing the person from dying of their underlying disease state is withheld or withdrawn and the disease is allowed to continue.

As Rachels argues, both active and passive interventions can be immoral if the intent is wrongful. However, it is not clear whether there is anything morally permissible about passive interventions that should make them more likely to be moral without appeal to other principles like autonomy, beneficence, and non-maleficence. In practical terms, the traditional preference for passive euthanasia as being "morally okay" can be transformed if we consider "preventing prolonged suffering" a greater value than the "killing/letting die" distinction.

This tension was never clearer than in the case of Brittany Maynard. Brittany was 29 years old when she was diagnosed with an aggressive form of brain cancer. She had a partial craniotomy as treatment, but in April of that same year, her cancer returned. Doctors gave her six months to live. She moved to Oregon to take advantage of Oregon's death with dignity act. Ethicist Arthur Caplan notes that Brittany did not look like the typical patient seeking physician-assisted suicide. She was young, vibrant, and dying. What made her decision significant is that with only six months to live, Brittany could have died in a hospice care situation. However, she feared the loss of cognitive function in the six months she had left.

"Because the rest of my body is young and healthy, I am likely to physically hang on for a long time even though cancer is eating my mind. I probably would have suffered in hospice care for weeks or even months. And my family would have had to watch that." Faced with prolonged suffering or physician-assisted suicide in Oregon, Brittany chose Oregon, where a physician wrote her a prescription for a lethal dose of medication.

Brittany Maynard's case forces us to confront the clash between beneficence, non-maleficence, and autonomy. Specifically, we confront the choice between the harm of killing and the harm of continued suffering. If Rachels is right, preventing prolonged suffering could outweigh the moral concerns about giving someone in Brittany's situation access to lethal doses of drugs. Preventing prolonged suffering seems morally praiseworthy. It is true that Brittany could have been made comfortable using palliative medications, and this would have been a way to honor non-maleficence/beneficence without being complicit in her death. Brittany considers this in an article she wrote for CNN.com:

> I considered passing away in hospice care at my San Francisco Bay-area home. But even with palliative medication, I could develop potentially morphine-resistant pain and suffer personality changes and verbal, cognitive and motor loss of virtually any kind.[*]

In other words, palliative pain management would not have lessened the cognitive effects of her brain cancer.

This brings up an important distinction that is ethically relevant between "pain" and "suffering" when discussing end of life. The sensations of pain are physical and can be alleviated with medication. However, suffering is thought to be subjective. Brittany considered the loss of cognitive function to be excessive suffering, a suffering that could not be alleviated with opioids. It is true that she could have been put into a coma for her last few months to alleviate pain. Would that have been a reasonable alternative to physician-assisted suicide, where she could have died at home surrounded by her family? Notice, when presented with the choice between pain management—albeit with cognitive debilitation—as an alternative to assisted suicide, Brittany ultimately appealed to autonomy to make her case:

> I would not tell anyone else that he or she should choose death with dignity. My question is: Who has the right to tell me that I don't

---

* Brittany Maynard, "My right to die with dignity at 29," *CNN*, Nov. 2, 2014.

deserve this choice? That I deserve to suffer for weeks or months in tremendous amounts of physical and emotional pain? Why should anyone have the right to make that choice for me?

While Brittany appealed to beneficence and non-maleficence at first, when others objected that there was an alternative, namely pain management coupled with cognitive debilitation, she fell back on autonomy to justify her decision to end her life.

Brittany's case is important for two reasons. First, it highlights the distinction between suffering and pain. Second, if we accept her moral justification then there is good reason for people diagnosed with Alzheimer's to qualify for physician-assisted suicide. After all, the cognitive debilitation with Alzheimer's is arguably the same or worse than the last stages of Brittany's brain cancer.

Alzheimer's is not curable, progressively debilitating, and ultimately terminal. If Brittany's death was justified, wouldn't the same be true for an Alzheimer's patient who requests physician-assisted suicide when they get the diagnosis? Brittany's argument was that she had the right to end her life *before* the brain cancer took away her cognitive function. If so, an Alzheimer's patient would be justified in requesting lethal medication at diagnosis.

Indeed, why stop with terminal cases? If the justification is alleviating mental suffering (non-maleficence) and the right to die on one's own terms (autonomy), then would a chronic mental condition such as schizophrenia or multiple personality disorder qualify under Brittany's reasoning provided that the condition is resistant to treatment? It would cut short prolonged suffering and would be voluntary. Indeed, such patients could argue that they should be able to end their life before they become so incapacitated that they cannot make their own decisions.

This slippery slope argument is by no means inevitable. I present it only to show that it matters which principle justifies the right to refuse, withdraw, or request active intervention. If autonomy is the guiding principle, then patients and providers are going to have to allow for more leeway in end-of-life decisions, including voluntary active euthanasia. However, if alleviating suffering (non-maleficence) is the guiding principle, then patients and providers can draw the line against active interventions. To do so they will have to distinguish between physical pain, which providers can monitor and treat, and suffering, which is arguably subjective. To do so, however, both sides of the patient-provider relationship will have to hedge against patient autonomy, which argues that suffering is subjective and up to the patient.

Withdrawing and Withholding

Consider two scenarios, both involving ALS patients. ALS (Lou Gehrig's disease) slowly paralyzes a person. This starts usually in the extremities, but eventually it progresses until the ALS patient cannot breathe on their own. From there, the prognosis is dire. Eventually an ALS patient can become so paralyzed that they can only move their eyes, as renowned astrophysicist Stephen Hawking did in his last years of life. Without very special equipment, the person is locked in and cannot communicate.

Understandably, some ALS patients opt not to have artificial breathing devices and die before their ALS progresses to the locked-in phase. They elect to withhold ventilator support and die. What are your intuitions about the morality of withholding breathing devices and allowing the ALS to end the patient's life? Medical providers can make end-stage ALS patients comfortable, and most patients do not report pain during this final stage. Most people consider this sort of withholding treatment to be morally acceptable.

Now, consider a scenario where an ALS patient is *already* on a ventilator that breathes for them. They decide that the prospect of being unable to communicate is too much and ask medical providers to withdraw their breathing tube, knowing they will die. What are your intuitions about this scenario?

If your intuition was that withdrawing life-sustaining treatment is somehow worse than withholding life-sustaining treatment, you wouldn't be alone. Surveys of physicians indicate more moral distress from withdrawing active life support than withholding life support.

Voluntary Active Euthanasia in the United States

Physician-assisted suicide is legal in nine US states and the District of Columbia. It is an option given to individuals by law in the District of Columbia, Hawaii, Maine, New Jersey, Oregon, Vermont, and Washington. It is an option given to individuals in Montana and California via court decision. Individuals must have a terminal illness as well as a prognosis of six months or less to live. Physicians cannot be prosecuted for prescribing medications to hasten death.

Source: CNN Library, "Physician-Assisted Suicide Fast Facts," Aug. 1, 2019.

WHAT'S THE DEBATE?

Reading 5.1: James Rachels, "Active and Passive Euthanasia"

James Rachels seriously questions the distinction between "active euthanasia," which many people think is always immoral, and passive euthanasia (letting someone die), considered permissible in some circumstances.

The distinction between active and passive euthanasia is thought to be crucial for medical ethics. The idea is that it is permissible, at least in some cases, to withhold treatment and allow a patient to die, but it is never permissible to take any direct action designed to kill the patient. This doctrine seems to be accepted by most doctors, and it is endorsed in a statement adopted by the House of Delegates of the American Medical Association on December 4, 1973:

> The intentional termination of the life of one human being by another—mercy killing—is contrary to that for which the medical profession stands and is contrary to the policy of the American Medical Association.
>
> The cessation of the employment of extraordinary means to prolong the life of the body when there is irrefutable evidence that biological death is imminent is the decision of the patient and/or his immediate family. The advice and judgment of the physician should be freely available to the patient and/or his immediate family.

However, a strong case can be made against this doctrine. In what follows I will set out some of the relevant arguments, and urge doctors to reconsider their views on this matter.

To begin with a familiar type of situation, a patient who is dying of incurable cancer of the throat is in terrible pain, which can no longer be satisfactorily alleviated. He is certain to die within a few days, even if present treatment is continued, but he does not want to go on living for those days since the pain is unbearable. So he asks the doctor for an end to it, and his family joins in the request.

Suppose the doctor agrees to withhold treatment, as the conventional doctrine says he may. The justification for his doing so is that the patient is in terrible agony, and since he is going to die anyway, it would be wrong to prolong his suffering needlessly.

Rachels uses a counter-example here to challenge the intuitions about allowing someone to die rather than killing them in order to hasten their death and minimize suffering. Which principles does Rachels appeal to in his argument without stating them?

But now notice this. If one simply withholds treatment, it may take the patient longer to die, and so he may suffer more than he would if more direct action were taken and a lethal injection given. This fact provides strong reason for thinking that once the initial decision not to prolong his agony has been made active euthanasia is actually preferable to passive euthanasia, rather than the reverse. To say otherwise is to endorse the option that leads to more suffering rather than less, and is contrary to the humanitarian impulse that prompts the decision not to prolong his life in the first place.

This article was written at a time when palliative pain management was in its early days. Do you think Rachels would back off his claim if this dying person could be kept relatively pain free through pain-management medications? If not, could there be an unstated assumption that suffering is more than just the experience of pain? Like Brittany Maynard argued, one could be comfortable but still suffer. Does this weaken or strengthen Rachels's argument?

Part of my point is that the process of being "allowed to die" can be relatively slow and painful, whereas being given a lethal injection is relatively quick and painless. Let me give a different sort of example. In the United States about one in 600 babies is born with Down's syndrome. Most of these babies are otherwise healthy—that is, with only the usual pediatric care, they will proceed to an otherwise normal infancy. Some, however, are born with congenital defects such as intestinal obstructions that require operations if they are to live. Sometimes, the parents and the doctor will decide not to operate, and let the infant die. Anthony Shaw describes what happens then:

> ... When surgery is denied, the doctor must try to keep the infant
> from suffering while natural forces sap the baby's life away. As a
> surgeon whose natural inclination is to use the scalpel to fight off

death, standing by and watching a salvageable baby die is the most emotionally exhausting experience I know. It is easy at a conference, in a theoretical discussion, to decide that such infants should be allowed to die. It is altogether different to stand by in the nursery and watch as dehydration and infection wither a tiny being over hours and days. This is a terrible ordeal for me and the hospital staff—much more so than for the parents who never set foot in the nursery.

I can understand why some people are opposed to all euthanasia, and insist that such infants must be allowed to live. I think I can also understand why other people favor destroying these babies quickly and painlessly. But why should anyone favor letting "dehydration and infection wither a tiny being over hours and days?" The doctrine that says that a baby may be allowed to dehydrate and wither, but may not be given an injection that would end its life without suffering, seems so patently cruel as to require no further refutation. The strong language is not intended to offend, but only to put the point in the clearest possible way.

My second argument is that the conventional doctrine leads to decisions concerning life and death made on irrelevant grounds. Consider again the case of the infants with Down's syndrome who need operations for congenital defects unrelated to the syndrome to live. Sometimes, there is no operation, and the baby dies, but when there is no such defect, the baby lives on. Now, an operation such as that to remove an intestinal obstruction is not prohibitively difficult. The reason why such operations are not performed in these cases is, clearly, that the child has Down's syndrome, and the parents and doctor judge that because of that fact it is better for the child to die.

But notice that this situation is absurd, no matter what view one takes of the lives and potentials of such babies. If the life of such an infant is worth preserving, what does it matter if it needs a simple operation? Or, if one thinks it better that such a baby should not live on, what difference does it make that it happens to have an unobstructed intestinal tract? In either case, the matter of life and death is being decided on irrelevant grounds. It is the Down's syndrome, and not the intestines, that is the issue. The matter should be decided, if at all, on that basis, and not be allowed to depend on the essentially irrelevant question of whether the intestinal tract is blocked.

What makes this situation possible, of course, is the idea that when there is an intestinal blockage, one can "let the baby die," but when there is no such defect there is nothing that can be done, for one must not "kill" it. The fact that this idea leads to such results as deciding life or death on irrelevant grounds is another good reason why the doctrine should be rejected.

One reason why so many people think that there is an important moral difference between active and passive euthanasia is that they think killing someone is morally worse than letting someone die. But is it? Is killing, in itself, worse than letting die? To investigate this issue, two cases may be considered that are exactly alike except that one involves killing whereas the other involves letting someone die. Then, it can be asked whether this difference makes any difference to the moral assessments. It is important that the cases be exactly alike, except for this one difference, since otherwise one cannot be confident that it is this difference and not some other that accounts for any variation in the assessment of the two cases. So, let us consider this pair of cases:

In the first, Smith stands to gain a large inheritance if anything should happen to his six-year-old cousin. One evening while the child is taking his bath, Smith sneaks into the bathroom and drowns the child, and then arranges things so that it will look like an accident.

In the second, Jones also stands to gain if anything should happen to his six-year-old cousin. Like Smith, Jones sneaks in planning to drown the child in its bath. However, just as he enters the bathroom Jones sees the child slip and hit his head, and fall face down in the water. Jones is delighted; he stands by, ready to push the child's head back under if it is necessary, but it is not necessary. With only a little thrashing about, the child drowns all by himself, "accidentally," as Jones watches and does nothing.

Now Smith killed the child, whereas Jones "merely" let the child die. That is the only difference between them. Did either man behave better, from a moral point of view? If the difference between killing and letting die were in itself a morally important matter, one should say that Jones's behavior was less reprehensible than Smith's. But does one really want to say that? I think not. In the first place, both men acted from the same motive, personal gain, and both had exactly the same end in view when they acted. It may be inferred from Smith's conduct that he is a bad man, although that judgment may be withdrawn or modified if certain further facts are learned about him for example, that he is mentally deranged. But would not the very same thing be inferred about Jones from his conduct? And would not the same further considerations also be relevant to any, modification of this judgment? Moreover, suppose Jones pleaded, in his own defense, "After all, I didn't do anything except just stand there and watch the child drown. I didn't kill him; I only let him die." Again, if letting die were in itself less bad than killing, this defense should have at least some weight.

But it does not. Such a "defense" can only be regarded as a grotesque perversion of moral reasoning. Morally speaking, it is no defense at all.

Now, it may be pointed out, quite properly, that the cases of euthanasia with which doctors are concerned are not like this at all. They do not involve personal gain or the destruction of normal healthy children. Doctors are concerned only with cases in which the patient's life is of no further use to him, or in which the patient's life has become or will soon become a terrible burden. However, the point is the same in these cases: the bare difference between killing and letting die does not, in itself, make a moral difference. If a doctor lets a patient die, for humane reasons, he is in the same moral position as if he had given the patient a lethal injection for humane reasons. If his decision was wrong—if, for example, the patient's illness was in fact curable—the decision would be equally regrettable no matter which method was used to carry it out. And if the doctor's decision was the right one, the method used is not in itself important.

The AMA policy statement isolates the crucial issue very well; the crucial issue is "the intentional termination of the life of one human being by another." But after identifying this issue, and forbidding "mercy killing," the statement goes on to deny that the cessation of treatment is the intentional termination of a life. This is where the mistake comes in, for what is the cessation of treatment, in these circumstances, if it is not "the intentional termination of the life of one human being by another?" Of course, it is exactly that, and if it were not, there would be no point to it.

Many people will find this judgment hard to accept. One reason, I think, is that it is very easy to conflate the question of whether killing is, in itself, worse than letting die, with the very different question of whether most actual cases of killing are more reprehensible than most actual cases of letting die. Most actual cases of killing are clearly terrible (think, for example, of all the murders reported in the newspapers), and one hears of such crises every day. On the other hand, one hardly ever hears of a case of letting die, except for the actions of doctors who are motivated by humanitarian reasons. So one learns to think of killing in a much worse light than of letting die. But this does not mean that there is something about killing that makes it in itself worse than letting die, for it is not the bare difference between killing and letting die that makes the difference in these cases. Rather, the other factors—the murderer's motive of personal gain, for example, contrasted with the doctor's humanitarian motivation—account for different reactions to the different cases.

I have argued that killing is not in itself any worse than letting die; if my contention is right, it follows that active euthanasia is not any worse than passive euthanasia. What arguments can be given on the other side? The most common, I believe, is the following:

> In this next section, Rachels considers an objection to his own view. He tries out a response to his argument and then offers reasons that this response should not sway you if you agree with his argument. Note that the first paragraph does not represent Rachels's own view but what his opponent might say.

"The important difference between active and passive euthanasia is that, in passive euthanasia, the doctor does not do anything to bring about the patient's death. The doctor does nothing, and the patient dies of whatever ills already afflict him. In active euthanasia, however, the doctor does something to bring about the patient's death: he kills him. The doctor who gives the patient with cancer a lethal injection has himself caused his patient's death; whereas if he merely ceases treatment, the cancer is the cause of the death."

A number of points need to be made here. The first is that it is not exactly correct to say that in passive euthanasia the doctor does nothing, for he does do one thing that is very important: he lets the patient die. "Letting someone die" is certainly different, in some respects, from other types of action—mainly in that it is a kind of action that one may perform by way of not performing certain other actions. For example, one may let a patient die by way of not giving medication, just as one may insult someone by way of not shaking his hand. But for any purpose of moral assessment, it is a type of action nonetheless. The decision to let a patient die is subject to moral appraisal in the same way that a decision to kill him would be subject to moral appraisal: it may be assessed as wise or unwise, compassionate or sadistic, right or wrong. If a doctor deliberately let a patient die who was suffering from a routinely curable illness, the doctor would certainly be to blame for what he had done, just as he would be to blame if he had needlessly killed the patient. Charges against him would then be appropriate. If so, it would be no defense at all for him to insist that he didn't "do anything." He would have done something very serious indeed, for he let his patient die.

Fixing the cause of death may be very important from a legal point of view, for it may determine whether criminal charges are brought against the doctor. But I do not think that this notion can be used to show a moral difference between active and passive euthanasia. The reason why it is considered bad to be the cause of someone's death is that death is regarded as a great evil—and so it is. However, if it has been decided that euthanasia—even passive euthanasia—is desirable in a given case, it has also been decided that in this instance death is no greater an evil than the patient's continued existence. And if this is true, the usual reason for not wanting to be the cause of someone's death simply does not apply.

> Rachels ends by explaining why his point about the morality of killing and letting die is very practical.

Finally, doctors may think that all of this is only of academic interest—the sort of thing that philosophers may worry about but that has no practical bearing on their own work. After all, doctors must be concerned about the legal consequences of what they do, and active euthanasia is clearly forbidden by the law. But even so, doctors should also be concerned with the fact that the law is forcing upon them a moral doctrine that may well be indefensible, and has a considerable effect on their practices. Of course, most doctors are not now in the position of being coerced in this matter, for they do not regard themselves as merely going along with what the law requires. Rather, in statements such as the AMA policy statement that I have quoted, they are endorsing this doctrine as a central point of medical ethics. In that statement, active euthanasia is condemned not merely as illegal but as "contrary to that for which the medical profession stands," whereas passive euthanasia is approved. However, the preceding considerations suggest that there is really no moral difference between the two, considered in themselves (there may be important moral differences in some cases in their consequences, but, as I pointed out, these differences may make active euthanasia, and not passive euthanasia, the morally preferable option). So, whereas doctors may have to discriminate between active and passive euthanasia to satisfy the law, they should not do any more than that. In particular, they should not give the distinction any added authority and weight by writing it into official statements of medical ethics.

Reading 5.2: Daniel Callahan, "When Self-Determination Runs Amok"

Daniel Callahan disagrees with Rachels and the implications of his argument. Callahan thinks there is a way to distinguish morally between killing and letting die and he uses this distinction to argue against euthanasia and assisted suicide. Callahan's argument is not just relevant to the assisted suicide debate but also for all end of life decision-making because it delineates who is responsible for a patient's death when providers remove life-support.

The euthanasia debate is not just another moral debate, one in a long list of arguments in our pluralistic society. It is profoundly emblematic of three important turning points in Western thought. The first is that of the legitimate conditions under which one person can kill another. The acceptance of voluntary active euthanasia would morally sanction what can only be called "consenting adult killing." By that term, I mean the killing of one person by another in the name of their mutual right to be killer and killed if they freely agree to play those roles. This turn flies in the face of a long-standing effort to limit the circumstances under which one person can take the life of another, from efforts to control the free flow of guns and arms, to abolish capital punishment, and to more tightly control warfare. Euthanasia would add a whole new category of killing to a society that already has too many excuses to indulge itself in that way.

The second turning point lies in the meaning and limits of self-determination. The acceptance of euthanasia would sanction a view of autonomy holding that individuals may, in the name of their own private, idiosyncratic view of the good life, call upon others, including such institutions as medicine, to help them pursue that life, even at the risk of harm to the common good. This works against the idea that the meaning and scope of our own right to lead our own lives must be conditioned by, and be compatible with, the good of the community, which is more than an aggregate of self-directing individuals.

The third turning point is to be found in the claim being made upon medicine: it should be prepared to make its skills available to individuals to help them achieve their private vision of the good life. This puts medicine in the business of promoting the individualistic pursuit of general human happiness and well-being. It would overturn the traditional belief that medicine should limit its domain to promoting and preserving human health, redirecting it instead to the relief of that suffering which stems from life itself, not merely from a sick body.

> Before you read further, ask yourself which of Callahan's three moral turning points you find the most compelling. Which do you find the least compelling, and what would Callahan have to do to convince you of this weakest claim?

I believe that, at each of these three turning points, proponents of euthanasia push us in the wrong direction. Arguments in favor of euthanasia fall into four general categories, which I will take up in turn: (1) the moral claim of individual self-determination and well being; (2) the moral irrelevance of the difference between killing and allowing to die; (3) the supposed paucity of evidence to show likely harmful consequences of legalized euthanasia; and (4) the compatibility of euthanasia and medical practice.

Self-Determination

Central to most arguments for euthanasia is the principle of self-determination. People are presumed to have an interest in deciding for themselves, according to their own beliefs about what makes life good, how they will conduct their lives. That is an important value, but the question in the euthanasia context is, What does it mean and how far should it extend? If it were a question of suicide, where a person takes her own life without assistance from another, that principle might be pertinent, at least for debate. But euthanasia is not that limited a matter. The self-determination in that case can only be effected by the moral and physical assistance of another. Euthanasia is thus no longer a matter only of self-determination, but of a mutual, social decision between two people, the one to be killed and the other to do the killing.

How are we to make the moral move from my right of self-determination to some doctor's right to kill me—from my right to his right? Where does the doctor's moral warrant to kill come from? Ought doctors to be able to kill anyone they want as long as permission is given by competent persons? Is our right to life just like a piece of property, to be given away or alienated if the price (happiness, relief of suffering) is right? And then to be destroyed with our permission once alienated?

In answer to all those questions, I will say this: I have yet to hear a plausible argument why it should be permissible for us to put this kind of power in the hands of another, whether a doctor or anyone else. The idea that we can waive our right to life, and then give to another the power to take that life, requires a justification yet to be provided by anyone.

Slavery was long ago outlawed on the ground that one person should not have the right to own another, even with the other's permission. Why? Because it is a fundamental moral wrong for one person to give over his life and fate to another, whatever the good consequences, and no less a wrong for another person to have that kind of total, final power. Like slavery, dueling was long ago banned on similar grounds: even free, competent individuals should not have the power to kill each other, whatever their motives, whatever the circumstances. Consenting adult killing, like consenting adult slavery or degradation, is a strange route to human dignity.

> Callahan says he has yet to hear any justification for why I can give up my right to life by giving someone permission to help me end my life. Could the concept of consent (covered in Chapter 3) serve this function? Why or why not?

There is another problem as well. If doctors, once sanctioned to carry out euthanasia, are to be themselves responsible moral agents—not simply hired hands with lethal injections at the ready—then they must have their own independent moral grounds to kill those who request such services. What do I mean? As those who favor euthanasia are quick to point out, some people want it because their life has become so burdensome it no longer seems worth living.

The doctor will have a difficulty at this point. The degree and intensity to which people suffer from their diseases and their dying, and whether they find life more of a burden than a benefit, has very little directly to do with the nature or extent of their actual physical condition. Three people can have the same condition, but only one will find the suffering unbearable. People suffer, but suffering is as much a function of the values of individuals as it is of the physical causes of that suffering. Inevitably, in that circumstance, the doctor will in effect be treating the patient's values. To be responsible, the doctor would have to share those values. The doctor would have to decide, on her own, whether the patient's life was "no longer worth living."

> In the next paragraph, Callahan references a conference and a report "elsewhere in this issue." Callahan's article originally appeared in the issue of a journal with other articles. The "issue" he refers to is this journal.

But how could a doctor possibly know that or make such a judgment? Just because the patient said so? I raise this question because, while in Holland at the euthanasia conference reported by Maurice de Wachter elsewhere in this issue, the doctors present agreed that there is no objective way of measuring or judging the claims of patients that their suffering is unbearable. And if it is difficult to measure suffering, how much more difficult to determine the value of a patient's statement that her life is not worth living?

However one might want to answer such questions, the very need to ask them, to inquire into the physician's responsibility and grounds for medical and moral judgment, points out the social nature of the decision. Euthanasia is not a private matter of self-determination. It is an act that requires two people to make it possible, and a complicit society to make it acceptable.

Killing and Allowing to Die

Against common opinion, the argument is sometimes made that there is no moral difference between stopping life-sustaining treatment and more active forms of killing, such as lethal injection. Instead, I would contend that the notion that there is no morally significant difference between omission and commission is just wrong. Consider in its broad implications what the eradication of the distinction implies: that death from disease has been banished, leaving only the actions of physicians in terminating treatment as the cause of death. Biology, which used to bring about death, has apparently been displaced by human agency. Doctors have finally, I suppose, thus genuinely become gods, now doing what nature and the deities once did.

What is the mistake here? It lies in confusing causality and culpability, and in failing to note the way in which human societies have overlaid natural causes with moral rules and interpretations. Causality (by which I mean the direct physical causes of death) and culpability (by which I mean our attribution of moral responsibility to human actions) are confused under three circumstances.

They are confused, first, when the action of a physician in stopping treatment of a patient with an underlying lethal disease is construed as causing death. On the contrary, the physician's omission can only bring about death on the condition that the patient's disease will kill him in the absence of treatment. We may hold the physician morally responsible for the death, if we have morally judged such actions wrongful omissions. But it confuses reality and moral judgment to see an omitted action as having the same causal status as one that directly kills. A lethal injection will kill both a healthy person and a sick person. A physician's omitted treatment will have no effect on a healthy person. Turn off the machine on me, a healthy person, and nothing will happen. It will only, in contrast, bring the life of a sick person to an end because of an underlying fatal disease.

Causality and culpability are confused, second, when we fail to note that judgments of moral responsibility and culpability are human constructs. By that I mean that we human beings, after moral reflection, have decided to call some actions right or wrong, and to devise moral rules to deal with them. When physicians could do nothing to stop death, they were not held responsible for it. When, with medical progress, they began to have some power over death—but only its timing and circumstances, not its ultimate inevitability—moral rules were devised to set forth their obligations. Natural causes of death were not thereby banished. They were, instead, overlaid with a medical ethics designed to determine moral culpability in deploying medical power.

To confuse the judgments of this ethics with the physical causes of death which is the connotation of the word kill is to confuse nature and human action. People will, one way or another, die of some disease; death will have dominion over all of us. To say that a doctor "kills" a patient by allowing this to happen should only be understood as a moral judgment about the licitness of his omission, nothing more. We can, as a fashion of speech only, talk about a doctor killing a patient by omitting treatment he should have provided. It is a fashion of speech precisely because it is the underlying disease that brings death when treatment is omitted; that is its cause, not the physician's omission. It is a misuse of the word killing to use it when a doctor stops a treatment he believes will no longer benefit the patient—when, that is, he steps aside to allow an eventually inevitable death to occur now rather than later. The only deaths that human beings invented are those that come from direct killing—when, with a lethal injection, we both cause death and are morally responsible for it. In the case of omissions, we do not cause death even if we may be judged morally responsible for it.

This difference between causality and culpability also helps us see why a doctor who has omitted a treatment he should have provided has "killed" that patient while another doctor—performing precisely the same act of omission on another patient in different circumstances—does not kill her, but only allows her to die. The difference is that we have come, by moral convention and conviction, to classify unauthorized or illegitimate omissions as acts of "killing." We call them "killing" in the expanded sense of the term: a culpable action that permits the real cause of death, the underlying disease, to proceed to its lethal conclusion. By contrast, the doctor who, at the patient's request, omits or terminates unwanted treatment does not kill at all. Her underlying disease, not his action, is the physical cause of death; and we have agreed to consider actions of that kind to be morally licit. He thus can truly be said to have "allowed" her to die.

According to Callahan, the major distinction between killing and letting die is that when a medical provider "lets someone die," the cause of death can be attributed to some underlying illness. When a doctor removes a ventilator because a patient or decision maker agrees to it, the doctor is not properly said to "kill" the patient, though the removal does result in death. However, the patient's underlying illness has killed them.

If we fail to maintain the distinction between killing and allowing to die, moreover, there are some disturbing possibilities. The first would be to confirm many physicians in their already too-powerful belief that, when patients die or when physicians stop treatment because of the futility of continuing it, they are somehow both morally and physically responsible for the deaths that follow. That notion needs to be abolished, not strengthened. It needlessly and wrongly burdens the physician, to whom should not be attributed the powers of the gods. The second possibility would be that, in every case where a doctor judges medical treatment no longer effective in prolonging life, a quick and direct killing of the patient would be seen as the next, most reasonable step, on grounds of both humaneness and economics. I do not see how that logic could easily be rejected.

Callahan now switches from an argument against assisted suicide based on the killing/letting die distinction to a consequentialist argument. If assisted suicide is allowed, it logically leads to non-voluntary euthanasia, as Holland's permissive euthanasia policy shows.

Calculating the Consequences

When concerns about the adverse social consequences of permitting euthanasia are raised, its advocates tend to dismiss them as unfounded and overly speculative. On the contrary, recent data about the Dutch experience suggests that such concerns are right on target. From my own discussions in Holland, and from the articles on that subject in this issue and elsewhere, I believe we can now fully see most of the likely consequences of legal euthanasia.

Three consequences seem almost certain, in this or any other country: the inevitability of some abuse of the law; the difficulty of precisely writing, and then enforcing, the law; and the inherent slipperiness of the moral reasons for legalizing euthanasia in the first place.

Why is abuse inevitable? One reason is that almost all laws on delicate, controversial matters are to some extent abused. This happens because not everyone will agree with the law as written and will bend it, or ignore it, if they can get away with it. From explicit admissions to me by Dutch proponents of euthanasia, and from the corroborating information provided by the Remmelink Report and the outside studies of Carlos Gomez and John Keown, I am convinced that in the Netherlands there are a substantial number of cases of nonvoluntary euthanasia, that is, euthanasia undertaken without the explicit permission of the person being killed. The other reason abuse is inevitable is that the law is likely to have a low enforcement priority in the criminal justice system. Like other laws of similar status, unless there is an unrelenting and harsh willingness to pursue abuse, violations will ordinarily be tolerated. The worst thing to me about my experience in Holland was the casual, seemingly indifferent attitude toward abuse. I think that would happen everywhere.

Why would it be hard to precisely write, and then enforce, the law? The Dutch speak about the requirement of "unbearable" suffering, but admit that such a term is just about indefinable, a highly subjective matter admitting of no objective standards. A requirement for outside opinion is nice, but it is easy to find complaisant colleagues. A requirement that a medical condition be "terminal" will run aground on the notorious difficulties of knowing when an illness is actually terminal.

Apart from those technical problems there is a more profound worry. I see no way, even in principle, to write or enforce a meaningful law that can guarantee effective procedural safeguards. The reason is obvious yet almost always overlooked. The euthanasia transaction will ordinarily take place within the boundaries of the private and confidential doctor-patient relationship. No one can possibly know what takes place in that context unless the doctor chooses to reveal it. In Holland, less than 10 percent of the physicians report their acts of euthanasia and do so with almost complete legal impunity. There is no reason why the situation should be any better elsewhere. Doctors will have their own reasons for keeping euthanasia secret, and some patients will have no less a motive for wanting it concealed.

I would mention, finally, that the moral logic of the motives for euthanasia contain within them the ingredients of abuse. The two standard motives for euthanasia and assisted suicide are said to be our right of self-determination, and our claim upon the mercy of others, especially doctors, to relieve our suffering. These two motives are typically spliced together and presented as a single justification. Yet if they are considered independently—and there is no inherent reason why they must be linked—they reveal serious problems. It is said that a competent, adult person should have a right to euthanasia for the relief of suffering. But why must the person be suffering? Does not that stipulation already compromise the principle of self-determination? How can self-determination have any limits? Whatever the person's motives may be, why are they not sufficient?

Consider next the person who is suffering but not competent, who is perhaps demented or mentally retarded. The standard argument would deny euthanasia to that person. But why? If a person is suffering but not competent, then it would seem grossly unfair to deny relief solely on the grounds of incompetence. Are the incompetent less entitled to relief from suffering than the competent? Will it only be affluent, middle-class people, mentally fit and savvy about working the medical system, who can qualify? Do the incompetent suffer less because of their incompetence?

> Callahan presents us with a slippery slope argument based on the value of both beneficence ("Medical staff should not prolong suffering") and autonomy ("I should be able to end my life if I have decisional capacity"). If we accept autonomy as our justification for euthanasia, but only if the person has good rational reasons like unbearable suffering, what do we do with those who lack autonomy but are suffering? If autonomy is not a factor, doesn't our value of patient beneficence mean that we should still consider euthanasia?

Considered from these angles, there are no good moral reasons to limit euthanasia once the principle of taking life for that purpose has been legitimated. If we really believe in self-determination, then any competent person should have a right to be killed by a doctor for any reason that suits him. If we believe in the relief of suffering, then it seems cruel and capricious to deny it to the incompetent. There is, in short, no reasonable or logical stopping point once the turn has been made down the road to euthanasia which could soon turn into a convenient and commodious expressway.

Euthanasia and Medical Practice

A fourth kind of argument one often hears both in the Netherlands and in this country is that euthanasia and assisted suicide are perfectly compatible with the aims of medicine. I would note at the very outset that a physician who participates in another person's suicide already abuses medicine. Apart from depression (the main statistical cause of suicide), people commit suicide because they find life empty, oppressive, or meaningless. Their judgment is a judgment about the value of continued life, not only about health (even if they are sick). Are doctors now to be given the right to make judgments about the kinds of life worth living and to give their blessing to suicide for those they judge wanting? What conceivable competence, technical or moral, could doctors claim to play such a role? Are we to medicalize suicide, turning judgments about its worth and value into one more clinical issue? Yes, those are rhetorical questions.

Yet they bring us to the core of the problem of euthanasia and medicine. The great temptation of modern medicine, not always resisted, is to move beyond the promotion and preservation of health into the boundless realm of general human happiness and wellbeing. The root problem of illness and mortality is both medical and philosophical or religious. "Why must I die?" can be asked as a technical, biological question or as a question about the meaning of life. When medicine tries to respond to the latter, which it is always under pressure to do, it moves beyond its proper role.

It is not medicine's place to lift from us the burden of that suffering which turns on the meaning we assign to the decay of the body and its eventual death. It is not medicine's place to determine when lives are not worth living or when the burden of life is too great to be borne. Doctors have no conceivable way of evaluating such claims on the part of patients, and they should have no right to act in response to them. Medicine should try to relieve human suffering, but only that suffering which is brought on by illness and dying as biological phenomena, not that suffering which comes from anguish or despair at the human condition.

Doctors ought to relieve those forms of suffering that medically accompany serious illness and the threat of death. They should relieve pain, do what they can to allay anxiety and uncertainty, and be a comforting presence. As sensitive human beings, doctors should be prepared to respond to patients who ask why they must die, or die in pain. But here the doctor and the patient are at the same level. The doctor may have no better an answer to those old questions than anyone else; and certainly no special insight from his training as a physician. It would be terrible for physicians to forget this, and to think that in a swift, lethal injection, medicine has found its own answer to the riddle of life. It would be a false answer, given by the wrong people. It would be no less a false answer for patients. They should neither ask medicine to put its own vocation at risk to serve their private interests, nor think that the answer to suffering is to be killed by another. The problem is precisely that, too often in human history, killing has seemed the quick, efficient way to put aside that which burdens us. It rarely helps, and too often simply adds to one evil still another. That is what I believe euthanasia would accomplish. It is self-determination run amok.

Reading 5.3: J. McMahan, "Killing, Letting Die, and Withdrawing Aid"

Philosopher Jeff McMahan (b. 1954) lays out a case for when withdrawing aid like removing a ventilator is killing and when it is letting die. In doing so, he engages in some extensive casuistry (see Chapter 2) to argue for how we can know when an action or inaction is morally wrong or morally permissible.

Introduction

... One of the aims of this article is to contribute to the identification of the empirical criteria governing the use of the concepts of killing and letting die. I will not attempt a comprehensive analysis of the concepts but will limit the inquiry to certain problematic cases—namely, cases involving the removal or withdrawal of life-supporting aid or protection.[1] The analysis of these cases will, however, shed light on the criteria for distinguishing killing and letting die in other cases as well.

My overall aims in the article are partly constructive and partly skeptical. I hope to advance our understanding of the nature of the distinction between killing and letting die. This, I believe, will enable us to defend the moral relevance of the distinction against certain objections—in particular, objections that claim that the distinction fails to coincide with commonsense moral intuitions. Yet I will suggest that, as we get clearer about the nature of the distinction and the sources of its intuitive appeal, it may seem that the intuitions it supports are not so well grounded as one could wish.

In the above paragraph, McMahan lays out his thesis. Can you figure out why his aim is both constructive and skeptical? What is he skeptical about?

Withdrawing Aid

In this section, McMahan uses several hypothetical cases to argue against the idea that the distinction between killing and letting die is the same as between act and omission or even doing and allowing. His target is an argument by moral philosopher Philippa Foot (1920–2010). He concludes that Foot's analysis of killing and letting die needs some work.

Let us assume, as I have suggested, that the distinction between killing and letting die exemplifies the broader distinction between doing and allowing. How should the broader distinction be analyzed? Perhaps the most influential analysis is the one advanced by Philippa Foot. Focusing specifically on doing harm and allowing harm to occur, Foot contends that the relevant distinction is between, on the one hand, initiating a threatening sequence of events or keeping it going and, on the other hand, allowing a threatening sequence that is already in train to continue.[2] She then distinguishes further between two ways of allowing an existing sequence to continue, one of which involves "forbearing to prevent" the sequence from continuing while the other involves "the removal of some obstacle which is, as it were, holding back a train of events."[3]

Two points about Foot's analysis should be noted. First, Foot's distinction does not coincide with the distinction between action and inaction, or that between action and omission. She notes that "the first kind of allowing requires an omission, but there is no other general correlation between omission and allowing, commission and bringing about or doing."[4] This, I believe, is right—at least as regards the claim that there is no correlation between allowing and inaction. Consider the following example.

> *The Aborted Rescue.*—Two persons are in the water when one begins to drown. The other attempts to haul the drowning man to shore but the latter, in a panic, begins to claw and encumber his rescuer in a way that threatens to drown him as well. To extricate himself from this peril, the erstwhile rescuer has to push the drowning man off and swim away from him while the drowning man goes under.

The erstwhile rescuer clearly does not kill the other man when he leaves him to drown. He merely lets him die, or fails to save him (for there was some possibility that, had he continued to try, he might have succeeded in saving him). Yet in order to allow the drowning man to die, the erstwhile rescuer had to do something—namely, actively prevent the drowning man from trying to save himself at his rescuer's expense.[5]

The second noteworthy point is that Foot believes that the distinction between killing and letting die exemplifies her broader distinction only imperfectly. For she believes that there are certain cases in which one kills by allowing a threatening sequence to continue. The example she cites is:

> The Involuntary Donor.—One has been involuntarily hooked up to a patient with a normally fatal disease who can survive only if he continues to draw life-support from one's body for a number of months. If one removes the tubes connecting one's body to his, he will die. One removes the tubes.[6]

Since what the agent does in this case is to withdraw a barrier that stands in the way of the patient's death, Foot's distinction implies that this is a case of allowing harm to occur. Thus she describes it as a "refusal to save a life."[7] Yet she also says that the agent who removes the tubes kills the patient who is thereby removed from his source of life-support. But this, she writes, shows only "that the use of 'kill' is not important: what matters is that the fatal sequence resulting in death [i.e., the disease] is not initiated but is rather allowed to take its course."

Since, however, this is a case in which, according to Foot's own distinction, the agent allows the patient to die, Foot here commits herself to the position that the agent both kills the patient and allows him to die—indeed, that the agent kills the patient by allowing him to die. I believe that this is a mistake. To refuse to save a life is not normally to kill. The exceptions are cases in which the act of killing has the death of the victim as a delayed effect which the agent could prevent during the period between the performance of the act and the occurrence of the effect ...

How, then, is the relevant distinction to be drawn? Is Foot's analysis the right one? I believe that it too is defective and that ... it is undermined by cases involving the active withdrawal of aid or protection from a threat. Consider:

> Respirator.—A person is stricken with an ailment that would normally be fatal but is given mechanical life-support to sustain him until the condition can be cured. While the patient is on a respirator, his enemy surreptitiously enters the hospital and turns the machine off. The patient dies.[8]

Since the agent in this case simply removes a barrier that is, as it were, holding death at bay, his action falls on the negative side of Foot's distinction. It counts as allowing harm to occur rather than doing harm. If we believe, with Foot, that her distinction marks an intuitively morally important difference, then I think that we must conclude that it misclassifies this case. If we believe, as I have suggested we should, that the distinction between killing and letting die exemplifies the broad distinction that she is trying to capture and derives its moral significance from that broader distinction, then Foot's distinction classifies Respirator as a case of letting a patient die and suggests that there is a presumption that the agent's action is less objectionable than it would be in an otherwise comparable case involving killing. But it is more natural to describe this as a case of killing; and we certainly evaluate it as such.[9]

Another case of this sort is:

> *Burning Building.*—A person trapped atop a high building that is on fire leaps off. Seeing this, a firefighter quickly stations a self-standing net underneath and then dashes off to assist with other work. The imperiled person's enemy is, however, also present and, seeing his opportunity, swiftly removes the net so that the person hits the ground and dies.

Here too Foot's distinction implies that the agent merely allows his enemy to die by removing a barrier to a threat. Yet again it seems more natural to describe this as a case of doing harm rather than allowing harm to occur—of killing rather than letting die—and we certainly evaluate it as such.

It is significant that the cases that resist assimilation into the categories established by [Foot's distinction] are all cases involving the active withdrawal of aid or protection against a threat. Foot's distinction locates all such cases on the negative side of the divide, classing them as instances of allowing harm to occur or, in cases in which the harm is death, as instances of letting die (provided, of course, that I am right that the distinction between killing and letting die exemplifies the broader distinction). Yet at least some of these cases seem to belong on the positive side; they are cases of killing rather than letting die....

Other writers have, moreover, thought that they should be classed as instances of doing harm rather than allowing harm to occur, or as cases of killing rather than letting die. Frances Myrna Kamm, for example, explicitly claims that "a case in which one removes a barrier to the cause of death [is] a killing, not a letting die."[10]

A review of the cases we have considered so far should convince us that all of these views are mistaken. For some cases of withdrawing aid or protection are cases of killing, while others are cases of letting die. As we have just noted, the agent's withdrawal of the patient's lifesupport mechanism in Respirator seems a clear instance of killing, as does the agent's removal of the protective net in Burning Building. By contrast, the rescuer's withdrawing his aid to the drowning man in the Aborted Rescue is uncontroversially an instance of letting die. And, though this may seem less obvious, disconnecting oneself from the patient for whom one has been involuntarily providing life-support is also best understood as allowing the dependent patient to die of the disease from the effects of which one has been protecting him (albeit involuntarily).

> Pay close attention to this next section, where McMahan offers his explanation as to why our intuitions sometimes see withdrawal of aid as killing and immoral and sometimes as letting die and morally acceptable. He reasons that if we are the ones who initiated the aid and then remove it, then it "feels" more like letting die than killing. We just cancel out the aid we render. However, if we do not initiate the aid, then removing it feels more like killing, not "letting die." Further, this intuition can be refined even further, when the intervention we initiated is self-sustaining rather than ongoing. It is a subtle point, but, if you agree, it can have profound implications about withdrawing or removing life-sustaining treatment.

What is the basis of our classing some of these cases as killings and others as instances of letting die? One suggestion is that whether an act of withdrawing aid or protection counts as killing or letting die depends on whether the barrier to death that one removes is a barrier that one has oneself provided. Thus it might be argued that, in general, if one withdraws a barrier that protects a person from death, one's action counts as letting the person die if the barrier is one that one has oneself interposed or provided, whereas it counts as killing if the barrier was not interposed or provided by oneself.[11] If, in other words, one temporarily intervenes to block a threat and then withdraws, one simply allows the threat to continue, thereby allowing its victim to die. Withdrawing one's own previous aid or protection simply nullifies one's initial intervention: the net effect is tantamount to nonintervention (apart from any benefit that the initial intervention may have provided). But to remove a barrier that exists independently of anything one has done is totally unlike nonintervention. While in many cases it may be infelicitous to characterize action of this sort as creating a threat, since the threat already exists but is blocked, it is relevantly like the creation of a new threat in that the victim would have been entirely safe independently of any intervention by oneself.

I believe that this suggestion is on the right track. It gives what seem to be the right descriptions in the Aborted Rescue, Involuntary Donor, Respirator, and Burning Building cases. Nevertheless, it is, as it stands, too crude. For consider:

> *The Pipe Sealer.*—An earthquake cracks a pipe at a factory, releasing poisonous chemicals into the water supply. Before a dangerous amount is released, a worker seals the pipe. But a year later he returns and removes the seal. As a result, numerous people die from drinking contaminated water.[12]

In this case, the worker removes a barrier or protection against a threat that he himself has provided. Yet clearly, he does not merely allow the victims to die but instead kills them. Thus the suggested ground for distinguishing between cases involving the withdrawal of aid or protection must be refined.

It seems that what makes the pipe sealer's action an instance of killing is that, although he removes a protection that he himself has provided, the barrier that he has created was both complete and self-sustaining, requiring no further contribution from him in order to keep the threat at bay. Indeed, because the barrier he interposed was operative, complete, and self-sustaining, it may seem appropriate in this case to say that the threat was not merely blocked but eliminated.

If so, his action in removing the barrier he interposed may be said to have created a new threat rather than merely unblocking or releasing an existing threat. In this respect, his action is analogous to that of a person who rescues a drowning man from the water but then throws him back—a clear case of killing, in contrast to the action of a person who merely abandons an attempt at rescue, as in the Aborted Rescue.

Now contrast the case of the Pipe Sealer with a variant of the classic tale of the little Dutch boy.

> *The Dutch Boy.*—A little Dutch boy, seeing that the dike is beginning to crack, valiantly sticks his finger in the crack to prevent the dike from breaking and flooding the town. He waits patiently but after many hours, no one has come along who can help. Eventually succumbing to boredom and hunger, the boy withdraws his finger and

leaves. Within minutes the dike bursts and a flood engulfs the town, killing many.

Whereas it seems clear that the pipe sealer causes rather than merely allows the poisonous chemicals to be released into the water supply, it is equally clear that the Dutch boy merely allows rather than causes the town to be flooded. Thus, while the pipe sealer kills the victims of the poison, the Dutch boy merely lets the inhabitants of the town die, or allows them to be killed. Yet both remove or withdraw a barrier that they themselves have provided.

The difference seems to be that, while the barrier provided by the pipe sealer is complete and self-sustaining, the protection provided by the Dutch boy is, when withdrawn, still in progress and requires further and indeed continuous contributions from the boy to be sustained. This suggests that the original proposal should be refined in the following way: when an agent withdraws aid or protection from a lethal threat that he has not himself provided, or when he withdraws aid or protection that he has provided but which was complete and self-sustaining, his action counts as killing; but when an agent withdraws aid or protection that he himself has provided but which requires further contributions from him to be effective, then his action counts as letting the victim die.

This way of distinguishing between different instances of withdrawing aid or protection appears to follow our general sense of linguistic propriety in classifying instances of doing and allowing rather than merely following our moral intuitions about the different examples. Thus, the pipe sealer does not allow the poisons to escape but instead releases them, whereas the Dutch boy does not cause the flood but merely allows it to occur. The same descriptions would be appropriate even if each's action were expected to have good consequences rather than bad. Yet this proposal yields the intuitively correct classifications of all of the cases so far considered. In Respirator and Burning Building, each agent removes a barrier that was provided by someone else and each seems intuitively to be guilty of killing. In Pipe Sealer, the agent removes a barrier that he himself has provided but which was complete and self-sustaining; he too seems to be guilty of killing. But in the cases of the Aborted Rescue, the Involuntary Donor, and the Dutch Boy, each agent withdraws aid or protection that he has himself provided but which is in progress and requires more from the agent to be finally effective. In these cases, it seems clear that the agents merely allow people to die and are not guilty of killing.

Operative and As-Yet-Inoperative Aid

> In true philosopher fashion, McMahan is now going to consider slightly different versions of some of his original cases (Burning Building, Dutch Boy) in order to tease out another distinction in our intuitions. We distinguish, intuitively, between aid that is already operating before we get there (e.g., a patient already on respirator) and aid that is yet inoperative (e.g., we must decide whether to give a patient on a ventilator a hole in the throat for a breathing tube—because they will be on a ventilator for the long term). Do not assume that McMahan thinks there is something morally compelling about our intuitions. He is only trying to explain why it seems to make a difference in our intuitions. Later he will question whether our intuitions really should follow these distinctions.

... [I]f aid or protection against a lethal threat is both operative and self-sustaining, withdrawing it appears to count as killing irrespective of whether the person who withdraws it is also the person who provided it. But, when aid that is as-yet-inoperative is withdrawn, it seems to make a difference to whether this counts as killing or letting die whether the person who withdraws it is also the person who provided it. Thus compare Burning Building with:

> *Burning Building 2.*—A person trapped atop a high building that is on fire leaps off. Seeing this, a firefighter quickly stations a self-standing net underneath. But he then immediately notices that two other persons have jumped from a window several yards away. He therefore repositions the net so that it catches the two. The first jumper then hits the ground and dies.

In this case, it seems absurd to say that the firefighter kills the one; rather, he merely allows him to die....

In cases in which aid is operative but ongoing rather than self-sustaining, it is less clear that it matters whether the person who withdraws the aid also provided it, but there is some support for the claim that it does. Consider:

> *The Involuntary Donor 2.*—The same as Involuntary Donor except that it is a person who wanders in off the street who removes the tubes so that the patient dies....

> *The Dutch Boy 2.*—The same as Dutch Boy except that it is the Dutch boy's father, annoyed because his son is late for dinner, who yanks the boy's finger out of the dike.

In both of these cases the agent who terminates the aid or protection is not the person who has been providing it. And in both it seems natural to say that the agent kills the victims rather than merely allowing them to die.

It seems, therefore, that various factors are relevant in determining whether an instance of withdrawing aid or protection from a threat counts as killing or letting die. Among these are whether the person who terminates the aid or protection is the person who has provided it, whether the aid or protection is self-sustaining or requires more from the agent, and whether the aid or protection is operative or as yet inoperative. Thus matters are already quite complex. In the next section, I will introduce further complications.

Problem Cases

…

> *Burning Building 3.*—A person trapped atop a high building that is on fire leaps off. Seeing this, a firefighter quickly stations a self-standing net underneath and then dashes off to assist with other work. A second firefighter sees that two other persons have also jumped from an adjacent window. He therefore moves the net over to catch the two, with the consequence that the first jumper hits the ground and dies.

> *The Involuntary Donor 3.*—The same as in Involuntary Donor except that it is a doctor acting at the donor's request who removes the tubes connecting the donor to the dependent patient.

These cases appear to be counterexamples to my proposed way of distinguishing among cases of withdrawing aid. In Burning Building 3, the agent withdraws a self-sustaining though as-yet-inoperative barrier that someone else has provided. So my proposed distinction should classify it as a case of killing; but intuitively we regard it as a case of letting die. It is hard to believe that the firefighter in Burning Building 3 kills the falling person while the firefighter in Burning Building 2 merely lets him die, especially if this alleged difference is thought to make a moral difference.

In Involuntary Donor 3, the agent terminates operative aid that is being provided by someone else (the donor). Hence my proposal should classify it as a case of killing; yet it too may seem to be a case of letting die. Again, it is hard to believe that the doctor in Involuntary Donor 3 kills the patient while the donor in Involuntary Donor merely allows him to die, especially if this alleged difference is thought to make a moral difference.

Perhaps one could try to defend my proposal by claiming that these two most recent cases are in fact cases of killing that we are mistakenly disposed to regard as instances of letting die because we believe that what the agent does in each case is permissible in the same way that it would be if it were done by the person who provided the aid that is terminated (as is the case in Burning Building 2 and Involuntary Donor). I think, however, that this is the wrong response. These cases show that my proposal requires further refinements....

Suppose the second firefighter in Burning Building 3 is accused of killing the first jumper. His accuser might argue as follows: "You didn't let him die; for he was quite safe independently of you. It is not as if you were saving him but then withdrew to save the other two instead. Rather, you killed him in order to be able to save the other two." It seems to me that the firefighter could appropriately respond, "It's not true that the jumper would have been safe if not for me. If it looked as if he would be safe, that is because we, the team of firefighters, were there in our role as firefighters. When the first firefighter placed the net under the first jumper, he was fulfilling the requirements of his role. When I moved the net, I was fulfilling the requirements of the same role. It makes no difference which individual does what when they are all acting in a role-based capacity. If I had moved the net out of malice, then of course I could be accused of killing—not because my action would have been wrong (though it would have been) but because I would then have been acting in my capacity as a private individual and not in the role of a firefighter." This seems a cogent reply.

Involuntary Donor 3 requires a different response. To understand why this is a case of letting die rather than killing, we must distinguish between the decision to withdraw aid and the execution of that decision. What is important, in determining whether an act of terminating aid or protection counts as killing or letting die, is who decides to terminate it, not who physically implements the decision. In Involuntary Donor 3, it is the person who has been providing the aid who decides to terminate it. And it is this fact, together with the fact that the aid was in progress rather than self-sustaining, that makes this a case of letting die. When the doctor removes the tubes, he acts as an agent whose principal is the donor herself. His action thus counts as action by proxy, or vicarious action, on behalf of the donor.

These two refinements should be read back into the earlier claim that it makes a difference, in cases of withdrawing aid, whether the person who withdraws the aid is also the person who provided it. We see now that this was only a crude approximation to the truth. Doubtless there are other subtle refinements that are necessary but which I have overlooked.

There is one further matter that should be addressed in this section. I have argued that the removal of aid or protection that is both operative and self-sustaining counts as killing irrespective of whether the person who terminates it is also the person who provided it, but that the termination of aid or protection that is operative but not self-sustaining, in that it requires more from the agent, counts as letting die if the person who terminates it is also the agent who has provided it.[13] Thus the question whether aid that an agent has provided is self-sustaining or whether it requires more from the agent is a critical question; yet the relevant notions here are vague, and this can lead to uncertainties about how certain cases should be classified.

Return to the case I have called Respirator. In this case, the agent terminates life-supporting aid that he has had no part in providing. Hence, his action counts as killing. This seems intuitively right; and it would seem right even if the agent did not have a discreditable motive but intended his act as an instance of euthanasia—that is, an act intended to benefit the person who dies. Now consider:

> Respirator 2.—A person is stricken with an ailment that would normally be fatal but is given mechanical life-support to sustain him. Eventually, however, the doctor who ordered that the patient should receive life-support concludes that the patient will never regain consciousness and so turns the respirator off.

Many people regard this as a case in which the doctor lets the patient die.[14] And the fact that the doctor was himself responsible for providing the aid he discontinues supports this assessment. Other people, however, have doubts and suspect that the act of turning off or disconnecting a life-support machine must always count as killing.

Perhaps this uncertainty derives from a lack of clarity about whether or not a life-support machine counts as a self-sustaining form of aid. Clearly the provision of a life-support machine does not require continuous intervention and effort in the way that hauling a drowning man to shore or keeping one's finger in the dike does. Compared to these forms of aid or protection, the provision of a life-support mechanism seems a relatively self-sustaining form of aid—hence the temptation to call its withdrawal, even by its provider, an act of killing. Yet a life-support machine requires monitoring and maintenance, and keeping it functioning draws continuously on the provider's resources and exacts opportunity costs from him. In these respects it falls far short of being self-sustaining in the way that, for example, the pipe sealer's patch is; hence the temptation to call its withdrawal by its provider an instance of letting die. (Note that it seems appropriate to describe what the doctor does in Respirator 2 as discontinuing the patient's life-support—implying that he—the doctor—would otherwise be continuing it. It would, by contrast, be inappropriate to describe what the agent does in Respirator in this way.) If I am right that whether the withdrawal of operative aid or protection by its provider counts as killing or letting die depends on whether the aid is self-sustaining, then it should not be surprising that vagueness as to what kinds of aid count as self-sustaining should lead to the sorts of taxonomical and moral uncertainties that surround cases involving the termination of mechanical life-support....

> One takeaway from McMahan's examples is that our intuitions about cases may operate on distinctions and biases we are not even aware we have. Did you find that once McMahan explained why we tend to think what the pipe sealer did was a kind of killing and not just letting die, this was what was really making you think the pipe sealer is liable for the deaths because of his actions? What does this say about the value of intuitions in your own decision making?

It is, perhaps, surprising that what most people have taken to be simple, basic distinctions (doing and allowing, killing and letting die) should turn out to be complex and multifaceted. This confusion is, I think, readily explicable. Our intuitions about killing and letting die are indeed based on considerations that are relatively simple, as I will suggest in the final section. But, because of the unruly complexity of reality, it is often difficult to determine what these considerations imply about the classification of a particular case. Thus, while there are clear paradigm cases of killing and letting die in which the relevant considerations appear in relatively pure forms, there are also numerous gray areas in which these same considerations are more difficult to discern or interpret. We have, nevertheless, somehow evolved inexplicit rules for the classification even of most of the cases in the gray areas. But, because the function of these rules is to sort a welter of diverse and heterogeneous cases into two apparently simple categories, the rules are necessarily intricate, involving distinctions that are subtle and nuanced....

General Reflections

I have argued that certain cases of withdrawing aid or protection count as acts of killing while others count as instances of letting die. This does not, however, imply that all instances of withdrawing aid that let the victim die must be morally just like other instances of letting die, if other things are equal. It is possible, for example, that letting a person die by actively withdrawing aid in progress is generally more objectionable than letting a person die by simply failing to intervene at all to arrest a sequence of events by which he is threatened. We may feel that letting a person die by withdrawing aid in progress is more like killing than simple nonintervention is (perhaps because withdrawing aid may involve action, or because releasing a threat that has been blocked is more like initiating a threat than simply failing to block a threat is).

Similarly, killing by withdrawing aid or protection may seem generally less objectionable, and perhaps more like letting die, than killing by initiating a lethal threat, other things being equal. There are certainly precedents for drawing a moral distinction in this way between different ways of killing. It has been plausibly suggested, for example, that we distinguish morally between killing via the creation of a lethal threat where none previously existed and killing via the redistribution or redirection of a preexisting threat, holding that the latter is less objectionable than the former, other things being equal.[15] Some have, moreover, sought to explain the plausibility of this distinction between ways of killing in a way that resembles standard explanations of why letting die is in general less bad than killing.[16] And just as killing via redistributing a threat may be less bad than killing via the creation of a threat because the former has more in common with letting die than the latter, so killing via withdrawing aid may be less bad than killing via the creation of a threat for much the same reason.

These claims are, of course, speculative; and limitations of space preclude a thorough defense of them here. But they suggest a conclusion that I believe to be true. This is that, because the distinction between killing and letting die is not a simple distinction, but is, as I noted earlier, based on a variety of subfactors, it is not the case that all instances of killing differ morally from all instances of letting die in exactly the same way, at least with respect to the difference that is marked by the distinction between killing and letting die. Instead, rather than distinguishing two simple and opposed categories, the distinction between killing and letting die marks a rough division along a spectrum of cases....

The paragraph above is a very important one. McMahan's argument, if correct, expands Rachels's thesis about killing and letting die. What counts as killing and what counts as letting die are not simply a matter of action vs. inaction or act vs. omission. Nor is it as simple as all killing is morally worse than all instances of "letting die." In the last section, McMahan suggests that, if he is correct, maybe we should question whether the killing/letting die distinction is as morally useful when talking about whether someone who kills/lets die is morally responsible, as previously thought.

It is also important to note that there are, in commonsense morality, numerous factors that may affect the moral status of a course of conduct that has lethal consequences other than the distinction between killing and letting die. The most commonly noted among these further considerations is whether a person's death is an intended effect of an agent's action; but there are others as well.... The recognition of these facts may also help to explain how it can be that in certain comparisons the difference between killing and letting die may seem to make no intuitive difference....

Conclusion

... In short, the fundamental intuitive difference between killing and letting die is that in cases of killing we assign primary causal responsibility for a person's death to an agent's intervention in the person's life, whereas, in cases of letting die, primary responsibility for the death is attributed to factors other than any intervention by the agent....

Suppose that this is right—that our tendency to distinguish morally between killing and letting die as well as our tendency to distinguish morally within the two categories themselves both reflect a concern with the form and degree of an agent's causal responsibility for a person's death. We should ask whether these considerations are really sufficiently important to support the full moral significance that we attribute to the distinction.

Our aversion to being causally implicated in the death of an innocent person shows up in contexts in which its rationality is open to question. It influences us, for example, in cases in which killing an innocent person would not be worse for that person....

The aversion further manifests itself in cases in which one kills an innocent person but in which one cannot be held responsible or blamable for doing so. Again, a case of Bernard Williams's illustrates this point.[17] If a person who is driving carefully and alertly runs into a small child who has darted unexpectedly from behind a parked car, we expect the driver to feel an agonizing form of regret that other passengers in the car will not feel, even though the driver is not at fault because there was nothing that he or she could have been expected to do to avoid the accident....

When we reflect on these cases, we may find that our intuitive responses, while deeply ingrained and difficult to repudiate, nevertheless strike us as primitive or atavistic impulses that critical moral thinking might enable us to rise above. On reflection, the importance we intuitively attribute to mere causal responsibility for a death may seem excessive. Similarly, the significance that we attribute to differences in the form and degree of causal responsibility for a death when we distinguish between killing and letting die may also seem excessive....

Notes

1. I will use the terms 'withdrawal' and 'removal' interchangeably. Later, however ... I will draw a distinction that might be articulated by distinguishing between withdrawing and removing [see n. 11 below].

2. Philippa Foot, "The Problem of Abortion and the Doctrine of Double Effect" in her *Virtues and Vices* (Oxford: Basil Blackwell, 1978), p. 26. Also see her "Morality, Action, and Outcome," in *Morality and Objectivity*, ed. Ted Honderich (London: Routledge & Kegan Paul, 1985), p. 24, and "Killing and Letting Die," in *Abortion: Moral and Legal Perspectives*, ed. Jay L. Garfield and Patricia Hennessey (Amherst: University of Massachusetts Press, 1984), pp. 178–80.

3. Foot, "The Problem of Abortion and the Doctrine of Double Effect," p. 26.

4. Ibid.

5. See the similar case presented by H. M. Malm in her "Killing, Letting Die, and Simple Conflicts," *Philosophy and Public Affairs* 18 (1989): 254–55.

6. This is the well-known case introduced by Judith Thomson as an analogue of abortion in "A Defense of Abortion," *Philosophy and Public Affairs* 1 (1971): 47–66. Foot's reference to it is on pp. 184–85 of "Killing and Letting Die."

7. Foot, "Killing and Letting Die," p. 184.

8. Compare Shelly Kagan, *The Limits of Morality* (Oxford: Oxford University Press, 1989), p. 101.

9. In fairness to Foot, it should be noted that she focuses (in "The Problem of Abortion and the Doctrine of Double Effect") her initial discussion on the contrast between doing and allowing in the first of her two senses—i.e., allowing as "forbearing to prevent." Respirator, however, is a case involving allowing in her second sense of allowing as "enabling." Thus, if her claims about the contrast between doing and allowing were restricted to comparisons between doing and allowing in the first sense, Respirator as a counterexample might miss its target. But in the later paper ("Killing and Letting Die," p. 185), she contends that the agent's action in Involuntary Donor is "completely different" from normal instances of killing since "the fatal sequence resulting in death is not initiated but is rather allowed to take its course." Since Involuntary Donor is a case involving enabling rather than forbearing to prevent, this passage shows that she intends her claims about the contrast between doing and allowing to apply to both forms of allowing.

10. Frances Myrna Kamm, "Harming, Not Aiding, and Positive Rights," *Philosophy and Public Affairs* 15 (1986): 310, n. 5.

11. One might articulate this suggestion by drawing a distinction between withdrawing and removing. Withdrawing might be understood as a subspecies of removing in that removing aid, protection, or, more generally, a barrier counts as an instance of withdrawing only if the agent who removes the aid, protection, or barrier is also the agent who provided it. Given this understanding of the terms, the suggestion in the text is that, while withdrawing life-supporting aid or protection counts as letting die, all other instances of removing life-supporting aid or protection count as killing. I have not adopted

this use of the terms in the text because the dictionary recognizes a sense of withdrawing such that one can withdraw what one has not oneself provided.

12. I owe this case, and the objection it raises, to Heidi Malm.

13. Here and elsewhere one should read in the refinements suggested above.

14. See, e.g., George P. Fletcher, "Prolonging Life: Some Legal Considerations," *Washington Law Review* 42 (1967): 999–1016, reprinted in Bonnie Steinbock, ed., *Killing and Letting Die* (Englewood Cliffs, NJ: Prentice-Hall, 1980), p. 50. Others have objected to this classification of Respirator 2 on the ground that it is "structurally similar" to Respirator, which seems a clear case of killing. Shelly Kagan, e.g., suggests that the similarity challenges the idea that the intuitive difference between the two cases can be explained by appealing to the claim that one is a case of killing and the other a case of letting die (*The Limits of Morality*, p. 101). Also see Christopher Boorse and Roy A. Sorensen, "Ducking Harm," *Journal of Philosophy* 85 (1988): 126.

15. See, e.g., Judith Thomson, "The Trolley Problem," in her *Rights, Restitution, and Risk*, ed. William Parent (Cambridge, MA: Harvard University Press, 1986).

16. Eric Mack, e.g., argues that "when generally perilous and inevitably injurious forces confront a person such that, no matter how that person acts, some nonaggressor(s) will be injured, the antecedent perilous forces bear the predominant causal responsibility for the subsequent injuries" ("Three Ways to Kill Innocent Bystanders," *Social Philosophy and Policy* 3 [1985]: p. 17). In other words, responsibility for the harm is traced, as it is in cases in which one fails to arrest a harmful sequence, to the preexisting sequence of events rather than to the agent.

17. Bernard Williams, "Moral Luck," in his *Moral Luck* (Cambridge: Cambridge University Press, 1981), p. 28.

<hr>

ETHICS COMMITTEE

<hr>

A Chilly Reception[*]

Martha Kinder is an 85-year-old female who suffered a heart attack at home in rural North Carolina. She was brought into the Emergency Room at 4:30 a.m. by ambulance when she was found by a neighbor. By the time paramedics arrived she was unconscious and unresponsive. The standard wisdom is that with a heart attack, time is at issue. Because Martha was in such a remote setting, the paramedics began therapeutic hypothermia to preserve both her heart tissue and brain tissue.[†] In essence, emergency medical providers lower the patient's body temperature through cold IV fluids and ice packs. In order to prevent shivering during this process the patient is given both a sedative (making the patient unconscious) and paralytic medications, which render the patient unable to move or breathe on their own. A breathing tube is inserted and the patient is given artificial respiration until paramedics transport her to the ER.

Shortly after arriving at the ER, the patient's daughter (a local attorney), who serves as her medical decision maker, protests that her mother has a do not

<hr>

[*] This case study is adapted from J.K. Miles and Jeri Conboy, "Warm and Dead? (Therapeutic Hypothermia)," *Hastings Center Report* 45, no. 5 (2015): 9–10.

[†] Because of dilemmas like the one in this case study and extensive medical research, therapeutic hypothermia has now fallen into disuse. However, I include this true story (with patient details changed) because I think it illustrates problems with Callahan's claim that "passive euthanasia" can be distinguished by the cause of death being "the underlying illness."

resuscitate order that explicitly states she did not want extraordinary measures and demands that the breathing tube and any other measures be withdrawn and her mother be allowed to die.

Once medical staff initiate therapeutic hypothermia, it takes up to six hours to completely reverse the process. If the vent (breathing tube) is removed before the paralytic drug has time to wear off, the patient will not have a natural death but rather will essentially "stop breathing" immediately.

As one nurse in the ER says, "Might as well put a pillow over her face. It's the same thing." The attending physician agrees and states he will not engage in "active euthanasia." He considers therapeutic hypothermia analogous to surgery, where all do not resuscitate orders are ignored until the patient is out of surgery. Support medical staff and the doctor on duty do not want to stop the therapy until it can be reversed naturally (6–8 hours) at which point the staff would then stop all "extraordinary measures." This will mean that the staff will have to continue giving CPR in the interval since the therapeutic hypothermia can cause cardiac arrest.

The patient's daughter claims that she understands the implications but would rather have a "moment" of "not breathing" rather than all of this intervention. "Mom said she never wanted to have a machine breathe for her." She wants the vent removed immediately so that her mother can die with dignity according to her explicitly stated wishes.

As a group, discuss the following: Would removing the breathing tube without waiting for the paralytic medications to wear off be killing or letting die? Is this morally significant, given our discussions? Which principles are in conflict here? There do not seem to be any other options. Should the staff agree to remove the breathing vent or should they simply wait until the therapeutic hypothermia process wears off and then honor the patient's wishes?

CHAPTER 6

Dilemmas with Scarce Medical Resources

Was the Drug Lottery Fair?

Some have called state lotteries a progressive tax on the poor, since poor people are more likely to spend hundreds, even thousands, on lottery tickets without realizing that their chances of winning the big jackpot are alarmingly low. Many poor people will spend hundreds of dollars a year without considering the odds. Some will play the lottery only when the jackpot is enormous. Others will play only when it is small, reasoning that fewer people playing means greater odds. In a state lottery, the odds are the same whether the pot is large or small. Officials choose numbers at random. If you are aiming to win, it is not rational to play the lottery.

What about a lottery for a new drug, where the odds are based on how many people apply? Would it be rational to play? In 1994, Berlex Pharmaceuticals offered such a lottery, and 67,000 multiple sclerosis (MS) patients decided to take their chances. In 1994, no MS drugs on the market actually treated the disease. They only managed the symptoms. Then came Betaseron, a genetically engineered drug. Berlex knew that there would not be enough of the drug to go around, given the 300,000 people in 1994 with Relapsing/Remitting MS (RRMS), the kind of MS flare-ups that in clinical trials Betaseron reduced by a staggering 30 per cent.

Berlex officials said, "We talked to patient groups and doctors and distribution experts and the lottery seemed the fairest way." Doctors certified that each candidate had RRMS and was early enough in the disease progression that they could walk unassisted. They advertised the lottery with the National Multiple Sclerosis Society in order to keep the process completely transparent. They turned down senators and congressional representatives who wanted a better spot in line.

When asked about the risks, many patients were aware of them but hopeful: "I know I'm taking a chance with a new drug, but what else is there?" A doctor interviewed was less optimistic: "I'm hopeful about Betaseron but we don't really know if, in two years, it will look as good." Another said, "I'm fascinated and a little bit discouraged that people with chronic diseases will try almost anything." A large number of the doctors surveyed thought it would be wrong to offer Betaseron to patients when there was no proven effectiveness, especially since there was not enough to go around.[*]

WHAT'S AT STAKE?

"Who gets what, how much, and when?" are the central questions of distributive justice. The list of principles in Chapter 2 mentions a few of these. These principles obtain when there are not enough resources to go around—what economists call "conditions of scarcity." It is important to note that in a medical setting just about everything is a scarce resource, not just equipment and medicines but personnel too. Nursing staff are often just as much a scarce resource as beds in the Intensive Care Unit.

Patient Perspective:
Understanding that almost every medical resource is a scarce resource is important not just for those who must decide how to distribute the scarce resources. It is also important for those who request and receive them. Patients, like doctors, can get tunnel vision. The attitude is understandable: "I'm paying for this. I expect my doctor or nurse to stay with me as long as I need them too." Patients can violate the principle of justice just like providers if they monopolize time or resources, unaware that they could deprive other patients of the scarce resource of physician time.

---

[*] Quotes taken from "Experimental Drug is Prize in a Highly Unusual Lottery," *New York Times*, Jan. 7, 1994, A1.

Distributing Scarce Resources: Fairness vs. Equality

The principle of contribution states that those who bear the most burden of contributing to the community should receive the first or most of the resources. For example, if a community's taxes paid for a new dialysis treatment center, then locals should receive first priority over people from outside the area. The principle of need, however, says that those who need the resources most deserve to get them first. If there are only two viable kidneys, then only those with the most acute kidney failure should get them, not the people who paid the local taxes.

Both of these are principles of fairness, but neither necessarily leads to equal distribution. Fairness and equality are not the same thing. Some distributions can be fair without being equal, as when acute patients receive care first or those with a greater chance to live take priority when providers cannot save everyone. Likewise, equal distribution may not always be fair, such as when all 67,000 MS sufferers had an equal chance to get Betaseron, even though some were suffering more than others.

Now consider what a North Texas hospital system proposed. There were only about 80 ICU beds for a system that served over four million people, so the hospital would have to implement triage protocols. What about vaccination status? Normally, vaccination status would not be a factor, but COVID-19 was something unprecedented. There was a vast difference in the survival rate of moderate to severe COVID between those vaccinated and those not vaccinated. With this in mind, administrators circulated a memo to their medical staff indicating that vaccination status could be used as a factor in triage. When it was reported in the news, the hospital called it a "homework assignment."

In a pandemic, standard practice dictates that health workers get any new vaccine first, mainly because their health ensures the health of others but also because the principle of justice holds that those who contribute the most by treating others get the first doses. What is the best way to distribute vaccines? Given that the principles of need and contribution were taken care of, most public-health officials decide on a first-come, first-served (FCFS) principle of justice. People lined up around the block and waited hours in some cases to get the vaccine. Was this a fair distribution? Maybe not, considering that the working poor might not be able to get off work to stand in line. Would a lottery have been fairer, since everyone would have had an equal chance at the scarce vaccine?

First-come, first-served and random selection like the lottery are both thought to be based on the principle of equality. However, assuming that FCFS is just as equal as a random lottery is problematic, but FCFS is easier to implement. It is familiar to everyone and requires few resources to distribute. A lottery is complicated and requires more administration. FCFS is also easy to monitor, as most people will not tolerate someone breaking in line. Lotteries can be manipulated.

Increasing the Supply of Scarce Resources: Nudging vs. Payment

There are two ways to deal with the problem of scarce resources: we can limit the demand using a selection criterion like a lottery, or we can increase supply. We have covered the principles for distribution of scarce resources. What about the morality of trying to increase the supply of scarce resources rather than limit the demand? No surprise: moral problems loom here as well.

When it comes to the problem of scarce medical resources, by far the best-known issue is the problem of suitable organs for transplant. There are three ways most often proposed for increasing the supply of scarce organs: we can increase supply by making it easier to donate; we can make organ donation mandatory; or we might incentivize providing organs to the transplant network by paying organ providers or their families.

Is it ethical to assume that all viable organs are, by default, the property of the state to be distributed to those that need them? Family members who do not want viable organs harvested would have to have a compelling reason (and likely a court order) to prevent the harvesting. The problem with this should be apparent if you have been paying attention in this book: it would be coercive. It is a kind of eminent domain, except instead of seizing land to build an airport, the state would seize viable organs. We couldn't even call this a "donation."

A less extreme way to encourage donation is to "nudge" people toward donation by playing on their natural preference for the status quo. We have data indicating that 95 per cent of US citizens support organ donation, but only 54 per cent opt in to be a donor by signing the donor designation on their driver's license.

We know from social psychology that this is explained partly by the status quo bias. If the status quo is that I am not an organ donor unless I opt in, then I am likely not to bother. Some ethicists argue that we should change the status quo in favor of organ donation by requiring people to "opt out" of organ donation instead of the current opt-in approach. Medical providers would then assume that all patients are organ donors unless the patient or other authorized medical decision maker specifically made a request to opt out as a donor. The status quo would be donation. The current "opt-in" system still requires medical providers to get consent at the time of death from family members, who can reject the request even if the driver's license indicates the donor was "opt-in."

The other option to increase supply is to pay for organs. This is far more controversial than nudging people to opt in for donation. It is no surprise that arguments in favor of organ sales hinge primarily on autonomy. I own my body and what I own I can sell:

1. If I own anything, I own my body.
2. My kidney is part of my body.
3. Therefore, I own my kidney.
4. But what is owned can be sold.
5. Therefore: I should be able to sell a kidney to someone who needs one.

This self-ownership argument is a familiar one. It is used to justify abortion, legalized prostitution, and the right for people to engage in risky work for higher pay (oil rig workers, combat pay for soldiers, etc.). If a person has the right to "sell" their body doing dangerous work and is lauded for their bravery, why do we object to someone selling an organ, since the risk is the same for both donating a kidney and selling one? Proponents of organ sales point out that everyone *except* the donor (and the recipient) is paid. The doctors, nurses, and staff do not have a duty to donate their time or labor. Why think differently for the person providing the kidney? Notice that this argument says nothing about whether organ donation is better or worse at increasing the supply of organs. Organ sales and organ donations could occur at the same time. Proponents argue that organ sales are morally permissible even if organ donation is praiseworthy or "above and beyond the call of duty."

Still, someone might object that the market is the problem, not the individual sale. There is no such thing as a harmless market, the objection goes. Some things should not be for sale because the act of selling and buying sullies the process. A similar argument can be made about paying research participants. One response to this sort of objection is to concede that no one condones what goes on in black-market organ sales, where the ultra-rich prey on the poor and only the rich get the benefit. Are legal organ markets like this? One example we have of a functioning legal market in organs is in Iran. There, only Iranian citizens can sell or buy. The government matches sellers and buyers (private sales are illegal) and pays for the surgery, and sellers get discounted health care for a year after surgery. The government sets a price of US$4,600. However, even with all this regulation, illegal side payments (sometimes thousands of dollars) do occur, and there is a thriving black market for organs in Iran. There is, however, no substantial shortage of kidneys there; in the United States, the average wait time for a kidney is three-and-a-half years.

There is one other substantial objection to organ sales: it could discourage donation. The assumption here is that regardless of utility (the benefit to society as a whole), donation is morally preferable to organ sales. If this is true, then what happens to organ donation if we legalize organ sales? Some argue that organ sales will "crowd out" organ donation. It is an empirical question whether organ donations would be lower if organ sales were an option in a country like the United States. We just do not have the data.

In another sense, it is, not surprisingly, a moral question. An action that is not required but praiseworthy is *supererogatory* in ethics. Is donation supererogatory or a duty? If donation is a duty, then why is there such an emphasis on the gift of donation? If it is supererogatory, above and beyond duty, then why is not it permissible to pay those who don't want to go above and beyond?

WHAT'S THE DEBATE?

Reading 6.1: Leslie P. Scheunemann and Douglas B. White, "The Ethics and Reality of Rationing in Medicine"

The article begins with a conflict in medicine. Medical providers are reluctant to admit that rationing occurs because of their commitment to beneficence and justice. No one likes having to deny some patients resources. No one likes choosing between patients. However, one element stands as the stark reality in the title of this article: No one wants to admit that rationing occurs to cut costs. Money is a repugnant justification for rationing.

Health-care reform has remained a controversial sociopolitical issue for the last 2 decades. Part of the controversy at the policy level arises from the question of whether health-care reform will involve rationing medical care. This topic raises fears about unfair treatment of individuals,[1] which have been inflamed by assertions that rationing devalues human life.[2]

Physicians have struggled with the controversy surrounding rationing.[3,4] Some deny that rationing occurs and contend that their professional obligations require them not to participate in rationing.[5-7] Others admit to rationing[8,9] and see just allocation of medical care as part of physicians' ethical duties.[10] Intensivists share this ambivalence. In a recent survey, only 60% vouched that they provide "every patient all beneficial therapies without regard to costs."[11]

To be thoughtful participants in the social debate about rationing in medicine, physicians must be well informed. The purpose of this article is to address the following topics: (1) the inevitability of rationing of social goods, including medical care; (2) types of rationing; (3) ethical principles and procedures for fair allocation; and (4) whether rationing ICU care to those near the end of life would result in substantial cost savings.

What Is Rationing?

Although rationing has been defined in slightly different ways by different groups, most definitions cluster around one central idea: denying a potentially beneficial treatment to a patient on the grounds of scarcity.[12] The focus on potentially beneficial treatments is appropriate because virtually no treatment in medicine offers certain benefit for an individual patient and because a central point of controversy is whether the potential benefit is large enough or likely enough to occur in order to justify the expense. In this document, we use the terms "rationing" and "resource allocation" synonymously, although we acknowledge that the emotional valence of the two terms is clearly different.

> The authors make a distinction between cost-cutting and rationing. What is the distinctive feature of rationing and why does it seem more moral?

It is also important to note that not all efforts to control health-care costs involve rationing. For example, choosing a less expensive treatment over a more-expensive one does not entail rationing if both are equally effective, because selecting the less costly of the two does not result in the patient being denied a potentially beneficial treatment.[12] In addition, strategies focused on reducing administrative costs and waste in health care (e.g., reducing duplicative testing and administrative inefficiencies) are generally not rationing because they do not entail denying patients potentially beneficial care.

Rationing Is Unavoidable

In many industrialized countries, social goods—including health care, education, defense, infrastructure, environmental protection, and public health—draw funding from a common pool. Although need for such social goods is limitless, the resources available to supply them are limited.[6,13–15] Inevitably, difficult choices must be made to allocate finite resources in a way that achieves a reasonable balance across the range of important social goods. Attempting to meet all health-care needs would likely overwhelm our capacity to supply basic elements of other social goods, such as public safety, education, and defense. Therefore, some degree of rationing of health care is necessary for the overall well-being of society.

Rationing decisions pervade daily practice in ICUs.[5,12,16] For example, it is common to transfer a patient out of an ICU when she might still derive some small degree of benefit from ongoing monitoring; such transfers accommodate the needs of sicker patients in the face of a finite number of ICU beds. Physicians in ICUs also routinely ration their time.[12] They must decide which patients to see first and how much time to spend with each. Physicians also must balance the needs of patients against their nonprofessional obligations, such as responsibilities to their families. It is undoubtedly true that physicians cannot provide every potential benefit to every critically ill patient. Therefore, the reality of practice in ICUs is that patients are routinely denied some potential benefit—however small—through implicit rationing decisions made by physicians at the bedside.

The Appropriateness of Rationing Is Context Specific

The necessity of some rationing in medicine does not mean that all such rationing is ethically justifiable, and a justifiable rationing decision in one health-care system may not be similarly justifiable in another. One example is the rules in many health systems requiring less expensive, less beneficial drugs to be first-line choices over more expensive, more beneficial drugs. This type of rationing is relatively easy to justify in single-payer systems (e.g., the government-sponsored health-care plans in Canada and many European countries), in which savings are reinvested in programs to improve the health of the population. Such rationing decisions are harder to justify in a for-profit health system with wasteful administrative mechanisms and in which most profits are passed on to employees and shareholders rather than invested in improving the quality of care for patients.

> Do you agree with the last sentence? Does it seem simplistic to say that single-payer systems are efficient and for-profit health systems are "wasteful administrative mechanisms"?

Levels and Transparency of Rationing

Rationing can occur at multiple levels. The clearest conceptual distinction exists between "macroallocation" and "microallocation" decisions.[17,18] Macroallocation occurs at the societal level and includes decisions about how to allocate funds across a range of public goods. For example, macroallocation decisions determine how a particular society's public funds are allocated across social goods, such as defense, education, infrastructure, public health, and health care. Microallocation decisions involve bedside decisions about whether an individual patient will or will not receive a scarce medical resource. Although conceptually distinct, macroallocation decisions and microallocation decisions are related. For example, restrictive macroallocation decisions regarding healthcare funding will create more situations in which individual patients must be denied potentially beneficial treatments.

Perhaps the most straightforward examples of the rationing in medicine occur when there is an absolute scarcity of a medical resource, such as organs for transplantation....

Rationing also occurs because of general fiscal scarcity rather than an absolute scarcity of a particular medical resource. For example, in the early 1990s, Oregon had to cope with escalating medical expenditures for Medicaid recipients in the face of budget deficits. The resulting Oregon Health Plan concurrently set a firm annual health-care budget and expanded the Medicaid eligibility criteria to include all below the federal poverty level.[23,24] The initial macroallocation decision balanced state health-care spending against competing social goods, such as education, infrastructure, and prisons.[24] The second macroallocation traded providing a larger range of health-care services to less than one-half the state's poor for providing a basic level of health care to all Oregonians living in poverty.[23,25,26] Oregon covered services according to a published priority list until projected expenditures exhausted the budget; there was not publicly funded coverage for the remaining services.[23-26] This entailed denying beneficial therapies to some patients (microallocation).

Both the UNOS [United Network for Organ Sharing] strategy for organ allocation and the Oregon Health Plan are examples of explicit rationing; these rationing decisions arise from stated principles and rules. In contrast, implicit rationing occurs without formally stated rules or principles. The 46 million uninsured in the United States are an example of implicit rationing at the macro level.[27,28] Intensivists' decisions about how much time to spend with each patient are also examples of implicit rationing because they are generally not based on publicly disclosed reasons. In general, implicit rationing raises more concerns about fairness than explicit rationing because the basis of the decisions is not disclosed and because unspoken and illegitimate biases may exert undue influence on the decisions....

A survey of US intensivists suggests that many believe that they do not ration.[11] These results may reflect a lack of understanding of what rationing is or may reflect a symbolic belief about what physicians should do. In either case, the lack of insight about the inevitability of rationing in ICUs is problematic, because it suggests that many intensivists are not well positioned to be informed participants in the social conversation about how best to make the difficult decisions regarding competing social goods.

What Principles Could Guide Rationing?

A substantial barrier to moving from implicit to explicit approaches to rationing health care is the failure to specify what principle(s) should guide allocation. Many principles could form the basis of rationing decisions in health care, each of which represents a different interpretation of distributive justice. For example, the following have been proposed as valid material principles of distributive justice: (1) to each person an equal share, (2) to each according to need, (3) to each according to effort, (4) to each according to free market conditions, (5) to each so as to maximize overall usefulness.[22] A more comprehensive description of the principles—and how they might be combined into multiprinciple allocation strategies—can be found elsewhere.[22,33,34]

A foundational debate about distributive justice is how to navigate the conflicting impulses to maximize efficiency (making decisions so as to produce the most good with the least expenditure), equity (treating individuals equally), and prioritarian conceptions of justice (favoring the worst off). Therefore, we briefly discuss three approaches to allocating scarce resources grounded in these radically different philosophical notions of justice: utilitarianism, egalitarianism, and prioritarianism. We also introduce the "rule of rescue."

To Each to Maximize Overall Quality-Adjusted Life Years: Utilitarianism

In general terms, utilitarianism seeks to maximize overall benefits at the societal level. There are numerous approaches to quantifying benefits related to health care. Many health economists advocate use of the quality-adjusted life years (QALYs) as the best metric.[35] Rationing by QALYs involves two steps: selecting outcome measures that adjust life-years for quality, and then allocating so as to maximize QALYs....

Rationing by maximizing QALYs has limitations. First, there are important unanswered questions regarding the best methods to quantify quality of life.[23,33] For example, a person who has over time adapted to using a wheelchair may rate her quality of life the same as someone who is ambulatory, whereas someone recently confined to a wheelchair might rate her quality of life lower....

Discounting lower quality of life may also systematically disadvantage those with chronic illness compared with those with good health; such practice opposes a commonly held moral intuition that it is important to help the worst off, or at least not to enable their poor health to be a self-fulfilling prophesy ...

To Each an Equal Opportunity: Egalitarianism

Egalitarianism emphasizes the equal moral status of individuals by trying to provide equal opportunity to have the basic goods in life.[22] A straightforward example of an egalitarian approach to rationing is a lottery to determine priority for receiving a scarce resource.[18,33] Many citizens have strong moral intuitions toward egalitarian allocation strategies, even when they come at the expense of utility maximization.[42] For example, if there were an insufficient supply of ICU beds for the number of patients in need, an egalitarian might advocate for a lottery to randomly select which patients would be admitted. Lotteries require little knowledge about recipients, can occur rapidly, and resist corruption.[33] On the other hand, lotteries—and egalitarian principles of justice in general—are insensitive to factors that are also intuitively important to many, such as patients' need and likelihood of deriving benefit from treatment.[33]

First-come, first-served strategies to allocate scarce resources appear to be egalitarian, but often are not.[18,33] Existing guidelines support allocating ICU beds in this way,[43,44] and prior to 2005 waiting time was the primary criterion for allocating lungs for transplantation.[19] However, time on the waitlist for organ transplantation is not "random" in two ways. First, it favors those with diseases who are well enough to wait the longest.[19] Second, those with power, knowledge, and connections often have the social resources to more quickly secure a position in the queue compared with those who have poor health-care access.[18,33]

To Each to Favor the Worst Off: Prioritarianism

In general terms, prioritarianism attempts to help those who are considered the worst off by giving them priority in situations in which all cannot receive a particular resource.[33] For example, a prioritarian might preferentially allocate medical resources to the young over the old because the young have had the least chance to live through life's stages.[33,34] This "life cycle principle"—which is one example of a prioritarian allocation strategy—has been advocated as a way to allocate scarce organs for transplantation and mechanical ventilators during an influenza pandemic.[34,45] The justification for this principle does not rely on considerations of one's intrinsic worth or social usefulness. Rather, the goal is to give all individuals equal opportunity to live a normal life span. When used alone to guide allocation decisions, the life cycle principle ignores prognostic differences among individuals. This type of objection points to the possibility that multiprinciple allocation strategies may better account for the complex moral considerations at play in such decisions compared with single-principle allocation strategies.[34]

The Rule of Rescue

The rule of rescue describes a powerful psychologic impulse to attempt to save those facing death, no matter how expensive or how small the chance of benefit. The philosopher Albert Jonsen coined the term and describes it as "the moral response to the imminence of death [which] demands that we rescue the doomed."[46] In many ways, the impulse underlying the rule of rescue is an admirable human response to suffering. However, it also can lead to decisions that confound priority setting meant to maximize population-level outcomes. When Oregon refused to cover a potentially lifesaving bone marrow transplantation for 7-year-old Coby Howard, there was tremendous public outrage and negative media coverage, which likely arose as a consequence of not satisfying the psychologic impulse to rescue identifiable persons facing death.[47] The emotional costs of rationing ICU care would likely be similarly high because it would lead to the loss of identifiable lives.

Conflicts between Efficiency, Equity, and the Rule of Rescue

The deep moral tensions between efficiency, equity, and responding to those facing death should not be underestimated. In surveys of physicians, citizens, and economists about how to balance such trade-offs, people generally prioritize treatment that can be made available to everyone, but this view is tempered by impulses to maximize usefulness[34,45,46] and to rescue those in need.[42,48–52] Finding an acceptable balance between these competing ethical goals remains a serious challenge for the development of explicit rationing policies.

> In the section below, the authors present four characteristics of fair allocation. If you have read Chapter 2, how many of the principles from that chapter can you identify in these characteristics?

Fair Processes of Rationing

In morally pluralistic societies, reasonable people may be unable to agree about which principles should guide rationing. When such conflicts arise concerning high-stakes outcomes, using fair processes to make decisions acquires special ethical importance.[14,53] Daniels and Sabin[14] and Daniels[53] have proposed four characteristics of fair processes related to allocation: oversight by a legitimate institution, transparent decision making, reasoning according to information and principles that all can accept as relevant, and procedures for appealing and revising individual decisions.[14,53] A fifth aspect of procedural fairness is meaningful public engagement.[54] This step is important to identify unanticipated needs and values and to obtain public support.[54,55] ...

> In this next section the authors argue that fair distribution of scarce resources will always be at odds with our individual cognitive biases toward the rule of rescue and our deep-seated fear of moral responsibility when it results in death.

Will Fair Processes Fail for Tragic Choices?

Although public engagement and transparency seem indispensable for ethical priority setting in medicine, critics have argued that the emotionally and morally difficult choices raised by the rationing of life-saving medical therapies may prove resistant to rational debate. In their book *Tragic Choices*, Calabresi and Bobbitt[18] argue that society is unlikely to be able to produce a durable, acceptable solution to the issue of scarcity in medicine because the consequences of denying these treatments to individual patients are intolerable.

They argue that individuals collectively attempt to deny moral responsibility for their role in choices—no matter how ethical or necessary—that consign individuals to death. This denial involves creating the illusion that the suffering arises out of nature rather than from conscious choices. For example, the safety standards in the mining industry do not create the safest possible environment for coal miners; doing so would be prohibitively expensive and threaten the market competitiveness of mining companies. However, when there is a mine accident and identifiable miners are trapped, nothing is spared to save them. This response supports the illusion that the mining accident was not preventable and that all was done to safeguard the lives at stake, while ignoring the initial decision that allowed people to work in conditions with a certain level of risk.

Two repeating processes characterize tragic choices. First, society iteratively remakes macro- and micro-allocation decisions to make human suffering appear as infrequent and random as possible. Second, society chooses ostensibly non-controversial values to justify rationing decisions until the inherent conflict with basic values is exposed. For example, when hemodialysis was first developed as a life-saving therapy for patients with renal failure, demand outstripped supply, and the Seattle Dialysis Committee was formed to determine who would receive dialysis.[57] This panel made decisions that entailed refusing treatment to patients who died as a result. An exposé of the committee's decisions was published in LIFE magazine,[58] which generated a national public firestorm. The public's distaste for allowing identifiable patients to die partly led Congress to authorize universal coverage for hemodialysis. In doing so, society was able to better tolerate the (still unresolved) societal question of how to allocate scarce medical resources because the proposed solution minimized the number of identifiable lives lost. In the last decade, the debate has reemerged in a predictable way, now focused on controlling spending while ensuring a minimum acceptable level of basic care for all. It is not yet clear whether the next iteration of health care reform will produce substantive changes rather than changes that appease our consciences but leave unaddressed the inevitability of tragic choices....

References

1. Holtz-Eakin D. All's not fair in health reform bills. *The Boston Globe*. December 10, 2009. http://www.boston.com/bostonglobe/editorial_opinion/oped/articles/2009/12/10/alls_not_fair_in_health_reform_bills. Accessed December 28, 2010.
2. Singer P. Why we must ration healthcare. *The New York Times*. July 15, 2009. www.nytimes.com/2009/07/19/magazine/19healthcare-t.html. Accessed December 28, 2010.
3. Levinsky NG. The doctor's master. *N Engl J Med*. 1984;311(24):1573–75.
4. Strech D, Persad G, Marckmann G, Danis M. Are physicians willing to ration health care? Conflicting findings in a systematic review of survey research. *Health Policy*. 2009;90(2–3):113–24.
5. Strech D, Synofzik M, Marckmann G. How physicians allocate scarce resources at the bedside: a systematic review of qualitative studies. *J Med Philos*. 2008;33(1):80–99.
6. Sulmasy DP. Physicians, cost control, and ethics. *Ann Intern Med*. 1992;116(11):920–26.
7. Angell M. The doctor as double agent. *Kennedy Inst Ethics J*. 1993;3(3):279–86.
8. Hurst SA, Slowther AM, Forde R, et al. Prevalence and determinants of physician bedside rationing: data from Europe. *J Gen Intern Med*. 2006;21(11):1138–43.
9. Sinuff T, Kahnamoui K, Cook DJ, Luce JM, Levy MM. Values Ethics and Rationing in Critical Care Task Force Rationing critical care beds: a systematic review. *Crit Care Med*. 2004;32(7):1588–97.

10. Cooke M. Cost consciousness in patient care—what is medical education's responsibility? *N Engl J Med.* 2010;362(14):1253–55.

11. Ward NS, Teno JM, Curtis JR, Rubenfeld GD, Levy MM. Perceptions of cost constraints, resource limitations, and rationing in United States intensive care units: results of a national survey. *Crit Care Med.* 2008;36(2):471–76.

12. Truog RD, Brock DW, Cook DJ, et al. for the Task Force on Values, Ethics, and Rationing in Critical Care (VERICC). Rationing in the intensive care unit. *Crit Care Med.* 2006;34(4):958–63.

13. Veatch RM. Physicians and cost containment: the ethical conflict. *Jurimetrics.* 1990;30(4):461–82.

14. Daniels N, Sabin J. Limits to health care: fair procedures, democratic deliberation, and the legitimacy problem for insurers. *Philos Public Aff.* 1997;26(4):303–50.

15. King D, Maynard A. Public opinion and rationing in the United Kingdom. *Health Policy.* 1999;50(1–2):39–53.

16. Halpern NA. Can the costs of critical care be controlled? *Curr Opin Crit Care.* 2009;15(6):591–96.

17. Skowronski GA. Bed rationing and allocation in the intensive care unit. *Curr Opin Crit Care.* 2001;7(6):480–84.

18. Calabresi G, Bobbitt P. *Tragic Choices: The Conflicts Society Confronts in the Allocation of Tragically Scarce Resources.* New York, NY: W.W. Norton & Company; 1978.

19. Egan TM, Kotloff RM. Pro/Con debate: lung allocation should be based on medical urgency and transplant survival and not on waiting time. *Chest.* 2005;128(1):407–15.

...

22. Childress J, Beauchamp T. *Principles of Biomedical Ethics.* New York, NY: Oxford University Press; 2009.

23. Hadorn D. The Oregon priority-setting exercise: quality of life and public policy. *Hastings Cent Rep.* 1991;21(3):11–16.

24. Kitzhaber J, Gibson M. The crisis in health care—The Oregon Health Plan as a strategy for change. *Stanford Law & Policy Review.* 1991;3:64–72.

25. Oberlander J, Marmor T, Jacobs L. Rationing medical care: rhetoric and reality in the Oregon Health Plan. *CMAJ.* 2001;164(11):1583–87.

26. Jacobs L, Marmor T, Oberlander J. The Oregon Health Plan and the political paradox of rationing: what advocates and critics have claimed and what Oregon did. *J Health Polit Policy Law.* 1999;24(1):161–80.

27. Feldman R. The cost of rationing medical care by insurance coverage and by waiting. *Health Econ.* 1994;3(6):361–72.

28. Kennedy J, Morgan S. Health care access in three nations: Canada, insured America, and uninsured America. *Int J Health Serv.* 2006;36(4):697–717.

...

33. Persad G, Wertheimer A, Emanuel EJ. Principles for allocation of scarce medical interventions. *Lancet.* 2009;373(9661):423–31.

34. White DB, Katz MH, Luce JM, Lo B. Who should receive life support during a public health emergency? Using ethical principles to improve allocation decisions. *Ann Intern Med.* 2009;150(2):132–38.

35. Neumann PJ, Weinstein MC. Legislating against use of cost-effectiveness information. *N Engl J Med.* 2010;363(16):1495–97.

...

42. Ubel PA, Baron J, Nash B, Asch DA. Are preferences for equity over efficiency in health care allocation "all or nothing"? *Med Care.* 2000;38(4):366–73.

43. American Thoracic Society. Fair allocation of intensive care unit resources. *Am J Respir Crit Care Med.* 1997;156(4 pt 1):1282–1301.

44. Guidelines for intensive care unit admission, discharge, and triage. Task Force of the American College of Critical Care Medicine, Society of Critical Care Medicine. *Crit Care Med.* 1999;27(3):633–38.

45. Emanuel EJ, Wertheimer A. Public health. Who should get influenza vaccine when not all can? *Science.* 2006;312(5775):854–55.

46. Jonsen AR. Bentham in a box: technology assessment and health care allocation. *Law Med Health Care.* 1986;14(3–4):172–74.

47. Egan T. Rebuffed by Oregon, patients take their life-or-death cases public. *New York Times.* May 1, 1988. http://www.nytimes.com/1988/05/01/us/rebuffed-by-oregon-patients-take-their-life-or-death-cases-public.html?scp=1&sq=may%201%201988%20coby%20oregon&st=cse. Accessed November 6, 2010.

48. Ubel PA, DeKay ML, Baron J, Asch DA. Cost-effectiveness analysis in a setting of budget con-straints—is it equitable? *N Engl J Med.* 1996;334(18):1174–77.

49. Perneger TV, Martin DP, Bovier PA. Physicians' attitudes toward health care rationing. *Med Decis Making.* 2002;22(1):65–70.

50. Ubel PA, Loewenstein G, Scanlon D, Kamlet M. Individual utilities are inconsistent with rationing choices: a partial explanation of why Oregon's cost-effectiveness list failed. *Med Decis Making.* 1996;16(2):108–16.

51. Ubel PA, Loewenstein G. The efficacy and equity of retransplantation: an experimental survey of public attitudes. *Health Policy.* 1995;34(2):145–51.

52. Ubel PA. How stable are people's preferences for giving priority to severely ill patients? *Soc Sci Med.* 1999;49(7):895–903.

53. Daniels N. Accountability for reasonableness. BMJ. 2000;321(7272):1300–01.

54. Baum NM, Jacobson PD, Goold SD. "Listen to the people": public deliberation about social dis-tancing measures in a pandemic. *Am J Bioeth.* 2009;9(11):4–14.

55. Danis M, Ginsburg M, Goold S. Experience in the United States with public deliberation about health insurance benefits using the small group decision exercise, CHAT. *J Ambul Care Manage.* 2010;33(3):205–14.

...

57. Rescher N. The allocation of exotic medical lifesaving therapy. *Ethics.* 1969;79(3):173–86.

58. Alexander S. They decide who lives, who dies. LIFE. November 19, 1962;53(19):102–25.

...

Reading 6.2: George Annas, "The Prostitute, the Playboy, and the Poet: Rationing Schemes for Organ Transplantation"

George Annas (b. 1945) considers four methods for rationing organ transplants. He rejects a market-based approach outright and presents a program for incorporating the best of the other three.

In the public debate about the availability of heart and liver transplants, the issue of rationing on a massive scale has been credibly raised for the first time in United States medical care. In an era of scarce resources, the eventual arrival of such a discussion was, of course, inevitable.[1] Unless we decide to ban heart and liver transplantation, or make them available to everyone, some rationing scheme must be used to choose among potential transplant candidates. The debate has existed throughout the history of medical ethics. Traditionally it has been stated as a choice between saving one of two patients, both of whom require the immediate assistance of the only available physician to survive.

National attention was focused on decisions regarding the rationing of kidney dialysis machines when they were first used on a limited basis in the late 1960s. As one commentator described the debate within the medical profession:

"Shall machines or organs go to the sickest, or to the ones with the most promise of recovery; on a first-come, first served basis; to the most 'valuable' patient (based on wealth, education, position, what?); to the one with the most dependents; to women and children first; to those who can pay; to whom? Or should lots be cast, impersonally and uncritically?"[2]

In Seattle, Washington, an anonymous screening committee was set up to pick who among competing candidates would receive the life-saving technology. One lay member of the screening committee is quoted as saying:

The choices were hard ... I remember voting against a young woman who was a known prostitute. I found I couldn't vote for her, rather than another candidate, a young wife and mother. I also voted against a young man who, until he learned he had renal failure, had been a ne'er do-well, a real playboy. He promised he would reform his character, go back to school, and so on, if only he were selected for treatment. But I felt I'd lived long enough to know that a person like that won't really do what he was promising at the time.[3]

When the biases and selection criteria of the committee were made public, there was a general negative reaction against this type of arbitrary device. Two experts reacted to the "numbing accounts of how close to the surface lie the prejudices and mindless clichés that pollute the committee's deliberations," by concluding that the committee was "measuring persons in accordance with its own middle-class values." The committee process, they noted, ruled out "creative nonconformists" and made the Pacific Northwest "no place for a Henry David Thoreau with bad kidneys."[4]

To avoid having to make such explicit, arbitrary, "social worth" determinations, the Congress, in 1972, enacted legislation that provided federal funds for virtually all kidney dialysis and kidney transplantation procedures in the United States.[5] This decision, however, simply served to postpone the time when identical decisions will have to be made about candidates for heart and liver transplantation in a society that does not provide sufficient financial and medical resources to provide all "suitable" candidates with the operation.

There are four major approaches to rationing scarce medical resources: the market approach; the selection committee approach; the lottery approach; and the "customary" approach.[6]

The Market Approach

The market approach would provide an organ to everyone who could pay for it with their own funds or private insurance. It puts a very high value on individual rights, and a very low value on equality and fairness. It has properly been criticized on a number of bases, including that the transplant technologies have been developed and are supported with public funds, that medical resources used for transplantation will not be available for higher priority care, and that financial success alone is an insufficient justification for demanding a medical procedure. Most telling is its complete lack of concern for fairness and equity.[7]

A "bake sale" or charity approach that requires the less financially fortunate to make public appeals for funding is demeaning to the individuals involved, and to society as a whole. Rationing by financial ability says we do not believe in equality, but believe that a price can and should be placed on human life and that it should be paid by the individual whose life is at stake. Neither belief is tolerable in a society in which income is inequitably distributed.

The Committee Selection Process

The Seattle Selection Committee is a model of the committee process. Ethics Committees set up in some hospitals to decide whether or not certain handicapped newborn infants should be given medical care may represent another.[8] These committees have developed because it was seen as unworkable or unwise to explicitly set forth the criteria on which selection decisions would be made. But only two results are possible, as Professor Guido Calabrezi has pointed out: either a pattern of decision-making will develop or it will not. If a pattern does develop (e.g., in Seattle, the imposition of middle-class values), then it can be articulated and those decision "rules" codified and used directly, without resort to the committee. If a pattern does not develop, the committee is vulnerable to the charge that it is acting arbitrarily, or dishonestly, and therefore cannot be permitted to continue to make such important decisions.[9]

In the end, public designation of a committee to make selection decisions on vague criteria will fail because it too closely involves the state and all members of society in explicitly preferring specific individuals over others, and in devaluing the interests those others have in living. It thus directly undermines, as surely as the market system does, society's view of equality and the value of human life.

The Lottery Approach

> This paragraph illustrates the important distinction between equality and fairness. Lotteries are equal, Annas claims, but not fair.

The lottery approach is the ultimate equalizer which puts equality ahead of every other value. This makes it extremely attractive, since all comers have an equal chance at selection regardless of race, color, creed, or financial status. On the other hand, it offends our notions of efficiency and fairness since it makes no distinctions among such things as the strength of the desires of the candidates, their potential survival, and their quality of life. In this sense it is a mindless method of trying to solve society's dilemma which is caused by its unwillingness or inability to spend enough resources to make a lottery unnecessary. By making this macro spending decision evident to all, it also undermines society's view of the pricelessness of human life. A firstcome, first-served system is a type of natural lottery since referral to a transplant program is generally random in time. Nonetheless, higher income groups have quicker access to referral networks and thus have an inherent advantage over the poor in a strict first-come, first-served system.[10,11]

The Customary Approach

Society has traditionally attempted to avoid explicitly recognizing that we are making a choice not to save individual lives because it is too expensive to do so. As long as such decisions are not explicitly acknowledged, they can be tolerated by society. For example, until recently there was said to be a general understanding among general practitioners in Britain that individuals over age 55 suffering from endstage kidney disease not be referred for dialysis or transplant. In 1984, however, this unwritten practice became highly publicized, with figures that showed a rate of new cases of end-stage kidney disease treated in Britain at 40 per million (versus the US figure of 80 per million) resulting in 1500–3000 "unnecessary deaths" annually.[12] This has, predictably, led to movements to enlarge the National Health Service budget to expand dialysis services to meet this need, a more socially acceptable solution than permitting the now publicly recognized situation to continue.

In the US, the customary approach permits individual physicians to select their patients on the basis of medical criteria or clinical suitability. This, however, contains much hidden social worth criteria. For example, one criterion, common in the transplant literature, requires an individual to have sufficient family support for successful aftercare. This discriminates against individuals without families and those who have become alienated from their families. The criterion may be relevant, but it is hardly medical.

Annas makes a strong claim here that the availability of family support in deciding who gets an organ is relevant but not medical. Is there reason to question this? Studies have shown that continuity of aftercare is a key factor in recovery.

Similar observations can be made about medical criteria that include IQ, mental illness, criminal records, employment, indigency, alcoholism, drug addiction, or geographical location. Age is perhaps more difficult, since it may be impressionistically related to outcome. But it is not medically logical to assume that an individual who is 49 years old is necessarily a better medical candidate for a transplant than one who is 50 years old. Unless specific examination of the characteristics of older persons that make them less desirable candidates is undertaken, such a cut off is arbitrary, and thus devalues the lives of older citizens. The same can be said of blanket exclusions of alcoholics and drug addicts.

In short, the customary approach has one great advantage for society and one great disadvantage: it gives us the illusion that we do not have to make choices; but the cost is mass deception, and when this deception is uncovered, we must deal with it either by universal entitlement or by choosing another method of patient selection.

A Combination of Approaches

A socially acceptable approach must be fair, efficient, and reflective of important social values. The most important values at stake in organ transplantation are fairness itself, equity in the sense of equality, and the value of life. To promote efficiency, it is important that no one receive a transplant unless they want one and are likely to obtain significant benefit from it in the sense of years of life at a reasonable level of functioning.

Accordingly, it is appropriate for there to be an initial screening process that is based exclusively on medical criteria designed to measure the probability of a successful transplant, i.e., one in which the patient survives for at least a number of years and is rehabilitated. There is room in medical criteria for social worth judgments, but there is probably no way to avoid this complete-ly. For example, it has been noted that "in many respects social and medical criteria are inextricably intertwined" and that therefore medical criteria might "exclude the poor and disadvantaged because health and socioeconomic status are highly interdependent."[13] Roger Evans gives an example. In the End Stage Renal Disease Program, "those of lower socioeconomic status are likely to have multiple comorbid health conditions such as diabetes, hepatitis, and hyperten-sion" making them both less desirable candidates and more expensive to treat.[13]

> Annas makes an important point here. Most everyone will agree that who gets which organ should avoid racism, sexism, and judgments about peo-ple's lifestyles in order to be fair. It is very difficult, however, to separate medical and non-medical criteria.

To prevent the gulf between the haves and have-nots from widening, we must make every reasonable attempt to develop medical criteria that are objective and independent of social worth categories. One minimal way to approach this is to require that medical screening be reviewed and approved by an ethics committee with significant public representation, filed with a public agency, and made readily available to the public for comment. In the event that more than one hospital in a state or region is offering a particular transplant service, it would be most fair and efficient for the individual hospitals to perform the initial medical screening themselves (based on the uniform, objective criteria), but to have all subsequent non-medical selection done by a method approved by a single selection committee composed of representatives of all hospitals engaged in the particular transplant procedure, as well as significant representation of the public at large.

As this implies, after the medical screening is performed, there may be more acceptable candidates in the "pool" than there are organs or surgical teams to go around. Selection among waiting candidates will then be necessary. This situation occurs now in kidney transplantation, but since the organ matching is much more sophisticated than in hearts and livers (permitting much more precise matching of organ and recipient), and since dialysis permits individuals to wait almost indefinitely for an organ without risking death, the situations are not close enough to permit use of the same matching criteria. On the other hand, to the extent that organs are specifically tissue- and size-matched and fairly distributed to the best-matched candidate, the organ distribution system itself will resemble a natural lottery.

When a pool of acceptable candidates is developed, a decision about who gets the next available, suitable organ must be made. We must choose between using a conscious, value-laden, social worth selection criterion (including a committee to make the actual choice), or some type of random device. In view of the unacceptability and arbitrariness of social worth criteria being applied, implicitly or explicitly, by committee, this method is neither viable nor proper. On the other hand, strict adherence to a lottery might create a situation where an individual who has only a one-in-four chance of living five years with a transplant (but who could survive another six months without one) would get an organ before an individual who could survive as long or longer, but who will die within days or hours if he or she is not immediately transplanted. Accordingly, the most reasonable approach seems to be to allocate organs on a first-come, first-served basis to members of the pool but permit individuals to "jump" the queue if the second level selection committee believes they are in immediate danger of death (but still have a reasonable prospect for long-term survival with a transplant) and the person who would otherwise get the organ can survive long enough to be reasonably assured that he or she will be able to get another organ.

The first-come, first-served method of basic selection (after a medical screen) seems the preferred method because it most closely approximates the randomness of a straight lottery without the obviousness of making equity the only promoted value. Some unfairness is introduced by the fact that the more wealthy and medically astute will likely get into the pool first, and thus be ahead in line, but this advantage should decrease sharply as public awareness of the system grows. The possibility of unfairness is also inherent in permitting individuals to jump the queue, but some flexibility needs to be retained in the system to permit it to respond to reasonable contingencies.

We will have to face the fact that should the resources devoted to organ transplantation be limited (as they are now and are likely to be in the future), at some point it is likely that significant numbers of individuals will die in the pool waiting for a transplant. Three things can be done to avoid this: 1) medical criteria can be made stricter, perhaps by adding a more rigorous notion of "quality" of life to longevity and prospects for rehabilitation; 2) resources devoted to transplantation and organ procurement can be increased; or 3) individuals can be persuaded not to attempt to join the pool.

Of these three options, only the third has the promise of both conserving resources and promoting autonomy. While most persons medically eligible for a transplant would probably want one, some would not—at least if they understood all that was involved, including the need for a lifetime commitment to daily immunosuppression medications, and periodic medical monitoring for rejection symptoms. Accordingly, it makes public policy sense to publicize the risks and side effects of transplantation, and to require careful explanations of the procedure be given to prospective patients before they undergo medical screening. It is likely that by the time patients come to the transplant center they have made up their minds and would do almost anything to get the transplant. Nonetheless, if there are patients who, when confronted with all the facts, would voluntarily elect not to proceed, we enhance both their own freedom and the efficiency and cost-effectiveness of the transplantation system by screening them out as early as possible.

Conclusion

Choices among patients that seem to condemn some to death and give others an opportunity to survive will always be tragic. Society has developed a number of mechanisms to make such decisions more acceptable by camouflaging them. In an era of scarce resources and conscious cost containment, such mechanisms will become public, and they will be usable only if they are fair and efficient. If they are not so perceived, we will shift from one mechanism to another in an effort to continue the illusion that tragic choices really don't have to be made, and that we can simultaneously move toward equity of access, quality of services, and cost containment without any challenges to our values. Along with the prostitute, the playboy, and the poet, we all need to be involved in the development of an access model to extreme and expensive medical technologies with which we can live.

Notes

1. Calabresi G, Bobbitt P: *Tragic Choices*. New York: Norton, 1978.
2. Fletcher J: Our shameful waste of human tissue. *In:* Cutler DR (ed): *The Religious Situation*. Boston: Beacon Press, 1969; 223–52.
3. Quoted in Fox R, Swazey J: *The Courage to Fail*. Chicago: Univ of Chicago Press, 1974; 232.
4. Sanders & Dukeminier: Medical advance and legal lag: hemodialysis and kidney transplantation. *UCLA L Rev* 1968; 15:357.
5. Rettig RA: The policy debate on patient care financing for victims of end stage renal disease. *Law & Contemporary Problems* 1976; 40:1.
6. Calabresi G, Bobbitt P: *Tragic Choices*. New York: Norton, 1978.
7. President's Commission for the Study of Ethical Problems in Medicine: *Securing Access to Health Care*. VS Govt Printing Office, 1983; 25.
8. Annas GJ: Ethics committees on neonatal care: substantive protection or procedural diversion? *Am J Public Health* 1984; 74:843–45.
9. Calabresi G, Bobbitt P: *Tragic Choices*. New York: Norton, 1978.
10. Bayer R: Justice and health care in an era of cost containment: allocating scarce medical resources. *Soc Responsibility* 1984; 9:37–52.
11. Annas GJ: Allocation of artificial hearts in the year 2002: *Minerva v National Health Agency*. *Am J Law Med* 1977; 3:59–76.
12. Commentary: UK's poor record in treatment of renal failure. *Lancet* July 7, 1984; 53.
13. Evans R: Health care technology and the inevitability of resource allocation and rationing decisions, Part II. *JAMA* 1983; 249:2208, 2217.

Reading 6.3: Ezekiel J. Emanuel et al., "Fair Allocation of Scarce Medical Resources in the Time of COVID-19"

Writing early on in the COVID crisis, Emanuel and colleagues argue that in a pandemic, concerns about scarcity require that we alter normal ethical guidelines for allocation so that providers maximize benefit to those most likely to survive.

COVID-19 is officially a pandemic. It is a novel infection with serious clinical manifestations, including death, and it has reached at least 124 countries and territories. Although the ultimate course and impact of COVID-19 are uncertain, it is not merely possible but likely that the disease will produce enough severe illness to overwhelm health care infrastructure. Emerging viral pandemics "can place extraordinary and sustained demands on public health and health systems and on providers of essential community services."[1] Such demands will create the need to ration medical equipment and interventions.

Rationing is already here. In the United States, perhaps the earliest example was the near-immediate recognition that there were not enough high-filtration N-95 masks for health care workers, prompting contingency guidance on how to re-use masks designed for single use.[2] Physicians in Italy have proposed directing crucial resources such as intensive care beds and ventilators to patients who can benefit most from treatment.[3,4] Daegu, South Korea—home to most of that country's COVID-19 cases—faced a hospital bed shortage, with some patients dying at home while awaiting admission.[5] In the United Kingdom, protective gear requirements for health workers have been downgraded, causing condemnation among providers.[6] The rapidly growing imbalance between supply and demand for medical resources in many countries presents an inherently normative question: How can medical resources be allocated fairly during a COVID-19 pandemic?

Health Impacts of Moderate-to-Severe Pandemics

In 2005, the U.S. Department of Health and Human Services (HHS) developed a Pandemic Influenza Plan that modeled the potential health care impact of moderate and severe influenza pandemics. The plan was updated after the 2009 H1N1 outbreak and most recently in 2017.[1] It suggests that a moderate pandemic will infect about 64 million Americans, with about 800,000 (1.25%) requiring hospitalization and 160,000 (0.25%) requiring beds in the intensive care unit (ICU)....[1] A severe pandemic would dramatically increase these demands ...

In what follows, Emanuel et al. describe the anticipated shortages of medical supplies, specifically ventilators. They also point out that one of the greatest shortages might be skilled medical staff.

Health System Capacity

Even a conservative estimate shows that the health needs created by the coronavirus pandemic go well beyond the capacity of U.S. hospitals.[9] ...Other estimates of ICU bed capacity, which try to account for purported undercounting in the American Hospital Association data, show a total of 85,000 adult ICU beds of all types.[13]

There are approximately 62,000 full-featured ventilators (the type needed to adequately treat the most severe complications of COVID-19) available in the United States.[14] Approximately 10,000 to 20,000 more are estimated to be on call in our Strategic National Stockpile,[15] and 98,000 ventilators that are not full-featured but can provide basic function in an emergency during crisis standards of care also exist.[14] Supply limitations constrain the rapid production of more ventilators; manufacturers are unsure of how many they can make in the next year.[16] However, in the COVID-19 pandemic, the limiting factor for ventilator use will most likely not be ventilators but healthy respiratory therapists and trained critical care staff to operate them safely over three shifts every day. In 2018, community hospitals employed about 76,000 full-time respiratory therapists,[12] and there are about 512,000 critical care nurses—of which ICU nurses are a subset.[17] California law requires one respiratory therapist for every four ventilated patients; thus, this number of respiratory therapists could care for a maximum of 100,000 patients daily (25,000 respiratory therapists per shift).

Given these numbers—and unless the epidemic curve of infected individuals is flattened over a very long period of time—the COVID-19 pandemic is likely to cause a shortage of hospital beds, ICU beds, and ventilators. It is also likely to affect the availability of the medical workforce, since doctors and nurses are already becoming ill or quarantined.[18] Even in a moderate pandemic, hospital beds and ventilators are likely to be scarce in geographic areas with large outbreaks, such as Seattle, or in rural and smaller hospitals that have much less space, staff, and supplies than large academic medical centers.

Diagnostic, therapeutic, and preventive interventions will also be scarce. Pharmaceuticals like chloroquine, remdesivir, and favipiravir are currently undergoing clinical trials, and other experimental treatments are at earlier stages of study.[19-21] ...

> Now the authors move from the empirical to the normative. Can you spot where they appeal to the principles of utility and equality as well as Rawls's difference principle (priority to the worst-off patients) in order to make their argument?

Ethical Values for Rationing Health Resources in a Pandemic

Previous proposals for allocation of resources in pandemics and other settings of absolute scarcity, including our own prior research and analysis, converge on four fundamental values: maximizing the benefits produced by scarce resources, treating people equally, promoting and rewarding instrumental value, and giving priority to the worst off.[24-29] Consensus exists that an individual person's wealth should not determine who lives or dies.[24-33] Although medical treatment in the United States outside pandemic contexts is often restricted to those able to pay, no proposal endorses ability-to-pay allocation in a pandemic.[24-33]

Each of these four values can be operationalized in various ways (Table 2). Maximization of benefits can be understood as saving the most individual lives or as saving the most life-years by giving priority to patients likely to survive longest after treatment.[24,26,28,29] Treating people equally could be attempted by random selection, such as a lottery, or by a first-come, first-served allocation.[24,28] Instrumental value could be promoted by giving priority to those who can save others, or rewarded by giving priority to those who have saved others in the past.[24,29] And priority to the worst off could be understood as giving priority either to the sickest or to younger people who will have lived the shortest lives if they die untreated.[24,28-30]

The proposals for allocation discussed above also recognize that all these ethical values and ways to operationalize them are compelling. No single value is sufficient alone to determine which patients should receive scarce resources.[24-33] Hence, fair allocation requires a multivalue ethical framework that can be adapted, depending on the resource and context in question.[24-33]

TABLE 2

Ethical Values to Guide Rationing of Absolutely Scarce Health Care Resources in a COVID-19 Pandemic.

Ethical Values and Guiding Principles	Application to COVID-19 Pandemic
Maximize benefits	
Save the most lives	Receives the highest priority
Save the most life-years—maximize prognosis	Receives the highest priority
Treat people equally	
First-come, first-served	Should not be used
Random selection	Used for selecting among patients with similar prognosis
Promote and reward instrumental value (benefit to others)	
Retrospective—priority to those who have made relevant contributions	Gives priority to research participants and health care workers when other factors such as maximizing benefits are equal
Prospective—priority to those who are likely to make relevant contributions	Gives priority to health care workers
Give priority to the worst off	
Sickest first	Used when it aligns with maximizing benefits
Youngest first	Used when it aligns with maximizing benefits such as preventing spread of the virus

The authors take a pluralistic approach, arguing for the priority of some principles (overall utility) over other principles (treating equally). This pluralistic weighing of principles yields a series of policy recommendations.

Who Gets Health Resources in a COVID-19 Pandemic?

These ethical values—maximizing benefits, treating equally, promoting and rewarding instrumental value, and giving priority to the worst off—yield six specific recommendations for allocating medical resources in the COVID-19 pandemic: maximize benefits; prioritize health workers; do not allocate on a first-come, first-served basis; be responsive to evidence; recognize research participation; and apply the same principles to all COVID-19 and non–COVID-19 patients.

Recommendation 1: In the context of a pandemic, the value of maximizing benefits is most important.[3,26,28,29,31-33] This value reflects the importance of responsible stewardship of resources: it is difficult to justify asking health care workers and the public to take risks and make sacrifices if the promise that their efforts will save and lengthen lives is illusory.[29] Priority for limited resources should aim both at saving the most lives and at maximizing improvements in individuals' post-treatment length of life. Saving more lives and more years of life is a consensus value across expert reports.[26,28,29] It is consistent both with utilitarian ethical perspectives that emphasize population outcomes and with non-utilitarian views that emphasize the paramount value of each human life.[34] There are many reasonable ways of balancing saving more lives against saving more years of life;[30] whatever balance between lives and life-years is chosen must be applied consistently.

Limited time and information in a COVID-19 pandemic make it justifiable to give priority to maximizing the number of patients that survive treatment with a reasonable life expectancy and to regard maximizing improvements in length of life as a subordinate aim. The latter becomes relevant only in comparing patients whose likelihood of survival is similar. Limited time and information during an emergency also counsel against incorporating patients' future quality of life, and quality-adjusted life-years, into benefit maximization. Doing so would require time-consuming collection of information and would present ethical and legal problems.[28,34] However, encouraging all patients, especially those facing the prospect of intensive care, to document in an advance care directive what future quality of life they would regard as acceptable and when they would refuse ventilators or other life-sustaining interventions can be appropriate.

Operationalizing the value of maximizing benefits means that people who are sick but could recover if treated are given priority over those who are unlikely to recover even if treated and those who are likely to recover without treatment. Because young, severely ill patients will often comprise many of those who are sick but could recover with treatment, this operationalization also has the effect of giving priority to those who are worst off in the sense of being at risk of dying young and not having a full life.[25,29,30]

This is an interesting argument. Emanuel and his colleagues argue that maximizing benefits for the people who are likely to survive (versus those most sick) actually does give priority to the worst off, but only if we define "worst off" as those who are at risk of dying young and not living a full life. Do you agree with this definition of the worst off? Why or why not? In the next section the authors consider the conflict between first-come, first-served and maximizing utility for the critical rationing of ventilators, arguing that it is ethical to withdraw treatment from a patient with a poor prognosis to use this ventilator on another patient.

Because maximizing benefits is paramount in a pandemic, we believe that removing a patient from a ventilator or an ICU bed to provide it to others in need is also justifiable and that patients should be made aware of this possibility at admission.[3,28,29,33,35] Undoubtedly, withdrawing ventilators or ICU support from patients who arrived earlier to save those with better prognosis will be extremely psychologically traumatic for clinicians—and some clinicians might refuse to do so. However, many guidelines agree that the decision to withdraw a scarce resource to save others is not an act of killing and does not require the patient's consent.[26,28,29,33,35] We agree with these guidelines that it is the ethical thing to do.[26] Initially allocating beds and ventilators according to the value of maximizing benefits could help reduce the need for withdrawal.

In Recommendation 2, the authors confirm the principle of priority for first responders. What normative reason do they give?

Recommendation 2: Critical COVID-19 interventions—testing, PPE, ICU beds, ventilators, therapeutics, and vaccines—should go first to front-line health care workers and others who care for ill patients and who keep critical infrastructure operating, particularly workers who face a high risk of infection and whose training makes them difficult to replace.[27] These workers should be given priority not because they are somehow more worthy, but because of their instrumental value: they are essential to pandemic response.[27,28] If physicians and nurses are incapacitated, all patients—not just those with COVID-19—will suffer greater mortality and years of life lost. Whether health workers who need ventilators will be able to return to work is uncertain, but giving them priority for ventilators recognizes their assumption of the high-risk work of saving others, and it may also discourage absenteeism.[28,36] Priority for critical workers must not be abused by prioritizing wealthy or famous persons or the politically powerful above first responders and medical staff—as has already happened for testing.[37] Such abuses will undermine trust in the allocation framework.

Recommendation 3: For patients with similar prognoses, equality should be invoked and operationalized through random allocation, such as a lottery, rather than a first-come, first-served allocation process. First-come, first-served is used for such resources as transplantable kidneys, where scarcity is long-standing and patients can survive without the scarce resource. Conversely, treatments for coronavirus address urgent need, meaning that a first-come, first-served approach would unfairly benefit patients living nearer to health facilities. And first-come, first-served medication or vaccine distribution would encourage crowding and even violence during a period when social distancing is paramount. Finally, first-come, first-served approaches mean that people who happen to get sick later on, perhaps because of their strict adherence to recommended public health measures, are excluded from treatment, worsening outcomes without improving fairness.[33] In the face of time pressure and limited information, random selection is also preferable to trying to make finer-grained prognostic judgments within a group of roughly similar patients.

Recommendation 4: Prioritization guidelines should differ by intervention and should respond to changing scientific evidence. For instance, younger patients should not be prioritized for COVID-19 vaccines, which prevent disease rather than cure it, or for experimental post- or pre-exposure prophylaxis. COVID-19 outcomes have been significantly worse in older persons and those with chronic conditions.[8] Invoking the value of maximizing saving lives justifies giving older persons priority for vaccines immediately after health care workers and first responders. If the vaccine supply is insufficient for patients in the highest risk categories—those over 60 years of age or with coexisting conditions—then equality supports using random selection, such as a lottery, for vaccine allocation.[24,28] Invoking instrumental value justifies prioritizing younger patients for vaccines only if epidemiologic modeling shows that this would be the best way to reduce viral spread and the risk to others.

Epidemiologic modeling is even more relevant in setting priorities for coronavirus testing. Federal guidance currently gives priority to health care workers and older patients,[22] but reserving some tests for public health surveillance (as some states are doing) could improve knowledge about COVID-19 transmission and help researchers target other treatments to maximize benefits.[39]

Conversely, ICU beds and ventilators are curative rather than preventive. Patients who need them face life-threatening conditions. Maximizing benefits requires consideration of prognosis—how long the patient is likely to live if treated—which may mean giving priority to younger patients and those with fewer coexisting conditions. This is consistent with the Italian guidelines that potentially assign a higher priority for intensive care access to younger patients with severe illness than to elderly patients.[3,4] Determining the benefit-maximizing allocation of antivirals and other experimental treatments, which are likely to be most effective in patients who are seriously but not critically ill, will depend on scientific evidence. These treatments may produce the most benefit if preferentially allocated to patients who would fare badly on ventilation.

> Do you agree with the authors that our ethical obligations differ whether the scarce resource is preventative (e.g., vaccines) or curative (e.g., ventilators)? If so, is this sort of common-sense intuition dependent on the principle of maximizing benefits, or could you make this case in other ways? In Recommendation 5, the authors argue for the principle of contribution, giving priority to those who participate in research, but only among those with the same level of expected outcome.

Recommendation 5: People who participate in research to prove the safety and effectiveness of vaccines and therapeutics should receive some priority for COVID-19 interventions. Their assumption of risk during their participation in research helps future patients, and they should be rewarded for that contribution. These rewards will also encourage other patients to participate in clinical trials. Research participation, however, should serve only as a tiebreaker among patients with similar prognoses.

Recommendation 6: There should be no difference in allocating scarce resources between patients with COVID-19 and those with other medical conditions. If the COVID-19 pandemic leads to absolute scarcity, that scarcity will affect all patients, including those with heart failure, cancer, and other serious and life-threatening conditions requiring prompt medical attention. Fair allocation of resources that prioritizes the value of maximizing benefits applies across all patients who need resources. For example, a doctor with an allergy who goes into anaphylactic shock and needs life-saving intubation and ventilator support should receive priority over COVID-19 patients who are not front-line health care workers....

Conclusions

Governments and policy makers must do all they can to prevent the scarcity of medical resources. However, if resources do become scarce, we believe the six recommendations we delineate should be used to develop guidelines that can be applied fairly and consistently across cases. Such guidelines can ensure that individual doctors are never tasked with deciding unaided which patients receive life-saving care and which do not. Instead, we believe guidelines should be provided at a higher level of authority, both to alleviate physician burden and to ensure equal treatment. The described recommendations could shape the development of these guidelines.

References

1. Pandemic influenza plan: 2017 update. Washington, DC: Department of Health and Human Services, 2017 (https://www.cdc.gov/flu/pandemic-resources/pdf/pan-flu-report-2017v2.pdf).

2. Strategies for optimizing the supply of N95 respirators. Atlanta: Centers for Disease Control and Prevention, 2020 (https://www.cdc.gov/coronavirus/2019-ncov/hcp/respirators-strategy/ index.html).

3. Vergano M, Bertolini G, Giannini A, et al. Clinical Ethics Recommendations for the Allocation of Intensive Care Treatments, in Exceptional, Resource-Limited Circumstances. Italian Society of Anesthesia, Analgesia, Resuscitation, and Intensive Care (SIAARTI). March 16, 2020 (http://www.siaarti.it/SiteAssets/News/COVID19%20-%20documenti%20SIAARTI/SIAARTI%20-%20Covid-19%20-%20Clinical%20Ethics%20Reccomendations.pdf).

4. Mounk Y. The extraordinary decisions facing Italian doctors. *Atlantic*. March 11, 2020 (https://www.theatlantic.com/ideas/archive/2020/03/who-gets-hospital-bed/607807/).

5. Kuhn A. How a South Korean city is changing tactics to tamp down its COVID-19 surge. *NPR*. March 10, 2020 (https://www.npr.org/sections/goatsandsoda/2020/03/10/812865169/how-a-south-korean-city-is-changing-tactics-to-tamp-down-its-covid-19-surge).

6. Campbell D, Busby M. 'Not fit for purpose': UK medics condemn Covid-19 protection. *The Guardian*. March 16, 2020 (https://www.theguardian.com/society/2020/mar/16/not-fit-for-purpose-uk-medics-condemn-covid-19-protection).

...

8. Wu Z, McGoogan JM. Characteristics of and important lessons from the coronavirus disease 2019 (COVID-19) outbreak in China: summary of a report of 72 314 cases from the Chinese Center for Disease Control and Prevention. *JAMA* 2020 February 24 (Epub ahead of print).

9. Ferguson NM, Laydon D, Nedjati-Gilani G, et al. Impact of non-pharmaceutical interventions (NPIs) to reduce COVID-19 mortality and healthcare demand. London: Imperial College London, March 16, 2020 (https://www.imperial.ac.uk/media/imperial-college/medicine/sph/ide/gida-fellowships/Imperial-College-COVID19-NPI-modelling-16-03-2020.pdf).

...

12. AHA annual survey database. Chicago: American Hospital Association, 2018.

13. Sanger-Katz M, Kliff S, Parlapiano A. These places could run out of hospital beds as coronavirus spreads. *New York Times*. March 17, 2020 (https://www.nytimes.com/interactive/2020/03/17/upshot/hospital-bed-shortages-coronavirus.html).

14. Rubinson L, Vaughn F, Nelson S, et al. Mechanical ventilators in US acute care hospitals. *Disaster Med Public Health Prep* 2010;4:199–206.

15. Jacobs A, Fink S. How prepared is the U.S. for a coronavirus outbreak? *New York Times*. February 29, 2020 (https://www.nytimes.com/2020/02/29/health/coronavirus-preparation-united-states.html).

16. Cohn J. How to get more ventilators and what to do if we can't. *Huffington Post*. March 17, 2020 (https://www.huffpost.com/entry/coronavirus-ventilators-supply-manufacture_n_5e6dc4f7c5b6747ef11e8134).

17. Critical care statistics. Mount Prospect, IL: Society of Critical Care Medicine (https://www.sccm.org/Communications/ Critical-Care-Statistics).

18. Gold J. Surging health care worker quarantines raise concerns as coronavirus spreads. *Kaiser Health News*. March 9, 2020 (https://khn.org/news/surging-health-care-worker-quarantines-raise-concerns-as-coronavirus-spreads/).

19. Casadevall A, Pirofski LA. The convalescent sera option for containing COVID-19. *J Clin Invest* 2020 March 13 (Epub ahead of print).

20. Zimmer C. Hundreds of scientists scramble to find a coronavirus treatment. *New York Times*. March 17, 2020 (https://www.nytimes.com/2020/03/17/science/coronavirus-treatment.html).

21. Harrison C. Coronavirus puts drug repurposing on the fast track. *Nat Biotechnol* 2020 February 27 (Epub ahead of print).

22. Devlin H, Sample I. Hopes rise over experimental drug's effectiveness against coronavirus. *The Guardian*. March 10, 2020 (https://www.theguardian.com/world/2020/mar/10/hopes-rise-over-experimental-drugs-effectiveness-against-coronavirus).

...

24. Persad G, Wertheimer A, Emanuel EJ. Principles for allocation of scarce medical interventions. *Lancet* 2009;373:423–31.

25. Emanuel EJ, Wertheimer A. Public health: who should get influenza vaccine when not all can? *Science* 2006;312:854–55.

26. Biddison LD, Berkowitz KA, Courtney B, et al. Ethical considerations: care of the critically ill and injured during pandemics and disasters: CHEST consensus statement. *Chest* 2014;146:4 Suppl:e145S-e155S.

27. Interim updated planning guidance on allocating and targeting pandemic influenza vaccine during an influenza pandemic. Atlanta: Centers for Disease Control and Prevention, 2018 (https://www.cdc.gov/flu/pandemic-resources/national-strategy/ planning-guidance/index.html).

28. Rosenbaum SJ, Bayer R, Bernheim RG, et al. Ethical considerations for decision making regarding allocation of mechanical ventilators during a severe influenza pandemic or other public health emergency. Atlanta: Centers for Disease Control and Prevention, 2011 (https://www.cdc.gov/od/science/integrity/phethics/docs/Vent_Document_Final_Version.pdf).

29. Zucker H, Adler K, Berens D, et al. Ventilator allocation guidelines. Albany: New York State Department of Health Task Force on Life and the Law, November 2015 (https://www.health.ny.gov/regulations/task_force/reports_publications/docs/ventilator_guidelines.pdf).

30. Christian MD, Sprung CL, King MA, et al. Triage: care of the critically ill and injured during pandemics and disasters: CHEST consensus statement. *Chest* 2014;146:4 Suppl:e61S–e74S.

31. Responding to pandemic influenza—the ethical framework for policy and planning. London: UK Department of Health, 2007 (https://webarchive.nationalarchives.gov.uk/20130105020420/http://www.dh.gov.uk/prod_consum_dh/groups/dh_digitalassets/@dh/@en/documents/digitalasset/dh_080729.pdf).

32. Toner E, Waldhorn R. What US hospitals should do now to prepare for a COVID-19 pandemic. Baltimore: Johns Hopkins University Center for Health Security, 2020 (http://www.centerforhealthsecurity.org/cbn/2020/cbnreport-02272020.html).

33. Influenza pandemic—providing critical care. North Sydney, Australia: Ministry of Health, NSW, 2010 (https://www1.health.nsw.gov.au/pds/ActivePDSDocuments/PD2010_028.pdf).

34. Kerstein SJ. Dignity, disability, and lifespan. *J Appl Philos* 2017;34:635–50.

35. Hick JL, Hanfling D, Wynia MK, Pavia AT. Duty to plan: health care, crisis standards of care, and novel coronavirus SARS-CoV-2. *NAM Perspectives*. March 5, 2020 (https://nam.edu/duty-to-plan-health-care-crisis-standards-of-care-and-novel-coronavirus-sars-cov-2/).

36. Irvin CB, Cindrich L, Patterson W, Southall A. Survey of hospital healthcare personnel response during a potential avian influenza pandemic: will they come to work? *Prehosp Disaster Med* 2008;23:328–35.

37. Biesecker M, Smith MR, Reynolds T. Celebrities get virus tests, raising concerns of inequality. *Associated Press* March 19, 2020 (https://apnews.com/b8dcd1b369001d5a70eccdb1f75ea4bd).

...

39. COVID-19 sentinel surveillance. Honolulu: State of Hawaii Department of Health, 2020 (https://health.hawaii.gov/docd/covid-19-sentinel-surveillance/).

Reading 6.4: Lynette Reid, "Triage of Critical Care Resources in COVID-19: A Stronger Role for Justice"

Lynette Reid offers a rebuttal to Emanuel et al.'s maximizing argument. She says that medical providers must resist the urge to jettison values like social justice in conditions of absolute scarcity; in fact, maximizing benefits may reinforce existing injustice.

Introduction

Some ethicists assert that there is a consensus in favour of maximising medical outcomes in emergency triage of absolutely scarce resources.[1,2] Debate turns to the kind or kinds of outcome maximisation that should be adopted, for example, lives or life years,[1,2] and to whether the same principle also licenses resource reallocation.[3] Equity considerations may be integrated into triage[1] but only if they do not interfere with the goal of maximising outcomes.[a]

Should it be a commonplace? Should it apply to our response to critical care triage in the current severe acute respiratory syndrome-related coronavirus 2 (SARS-CoV-2) pandemic?

Weaknesses in Arguments for Maximising Medical Outcomes

Decades ago, we could contrast the ethics of clinical care, with its focus on the good of a patient to whom the physician owes a special duty of care, against emergency triage and public health ethics, with their prioritisation of outcomes.[2] Clinical practice is now shaped by considerations of "good value" care, and the gap between clinical and triage ethics is less categorical. In other allocation processes, we balance maximising medical outcomes with various values. In health technology assessment, some form of values pluralism is reflected in multidimensional decision-making in many jurisdictions.[4,5] In organ allocation, despite the absolute scarcity of a life-saving resource, need still plays a strong role and equity considerations are taken into account.[6] Public health ethics, contrary to the claim of White and Lo,[2] is informed by values beyond utilitarianism,[7-11] such as social justice and legitimacy in public policy. The latter is particularly important when we are at odds in our fundamental moral commitments about values like justice and outcome maximisation.

Triage of critical care resources in the SARS-CoV-2 pandemic shares some features with emergency triage and other features with resource allocation decisions in routine care. The situation is unprecedented, and we face momentary, absolute resource scarcity. However, the current situation is also going to be a prolonged one. Public health has engaged the entire population in an outbreak response that fundamentally alters our day-to-day lives. That broader public health response takes into account values beyond outcome maximisation. A few countries (New Zealand, Vietnam[12] and some countries of Sub-Saharan Africa[13]) have maximised lives saved by immediately implementing containment. The goal of most countries has been to keep the outbreak within expanded critical care capacity. Many countries are reopening despite ongoing community transmission.

Furthermore, the pandemic and our public health response expose disadvantaged groups to risks that raise justice concerns. Consider two persons. One is a middle-aged person in good health with a life expectancy in their mid-80s, who can work from home with full salary and no threat to housing security. Their home is spacious, well ventilated with little pollution, and they enjoy access to green space. They can pay to have necessities delivered. If they must have some contact with the public, they can afford measures to avoid household transmission.

The second person is the same age but of lower socioeconomic status and works in precarious employment that cannot be done from home. They have either been designated essential or they cannot leave work because they have no resources to sustain unemployment. Their housing is crowded, with poor ventilation and no green space; the pandemic increases their housing insecurity. They cannot afford temporary shelter apart from their family; the whole family faces a substantial risk of household transmission. Government financial assistance may provide some relief, but it also saddles them with debt after the pandemic. They rely on public transit to get to and from work and for essential shopping. In many countries, they are disproportionately immigrants or members of racialised minorities and/or immigrant groups.[14,15] They are exposed to a greater risk of contracting COVID-19[14,16] for the very reasons that they are at greater risk of chronic health conditions that may lower their likelihood of responding favourably to intensive care unit (ICU) or organ support in the case of severe COVID-19.[17]

In the current pandemic, maximising outcomes in critical care triage may compound the injustices of the social determinants of health and have negative implications for equity of racialised groups.[18,19] Concern with these inequities is at least consistent with public health ethics, if not also core to public health ethics. Decades of work in resource allocation about balancing equity and efficiency should be brought to bear on critical care resource triage in a pandemic.[b]

Equity versus Efficiency in Resource Allocation

The goal of maximising outcomes in the specific form of maximising lives saved seems highly morally plausible until one considers the unacceptable results of its pursuit at all costs. Decades of research into public attitudes and of ethical debate[20-24] have explored three forms of justice in tension with outcome maximisation.

I will label these forms of justice concerns as follows: the *egalitarian* concern to give everyone a chance, connected to a fundamental sense of human equality,[25,26] the *non-discrimination* concern to protect those at risk of discrimination and the *social justice* concern to address unjust health detriments, whether relating to natural (e.g., ability or age) or social (e.g., socioeconomic status or racialised identity) categories. I will also refer to *procedural justice* concerns and *domain-specific fairness*[27] for the distribution of a good.[c]

> Reid highlights the fact of pluralism by arguing that maximizing outcomes competes with maximizing equality in the form of non-discrimination and social justice. She then discusses balancing these against utility. She argues that during crises we may be tempted to ignore the magnitude of differences between expected patient outcomes.

Surveys of public and professional attitudes in the 1990s suggest that some persons are committed to maximising outcomes and other persons are committed to maximising equality by, for example, granting *more* livers in organ allocation to those less likely to benefit in order to improve equality of outcomes. This latter commitment is consistent with our approach to disabilities in many realms, and a positive argument for abandoning it in pandemic response, if there is one, must be made. Many people can be described as "balancers" who prefer distributions that give weight to both equity and efficiency.[22-24,28,29] The metaphor of "balancing" as I use it here captures the idea that we resolve moral dilemmas by developing approaches that take into consideration multiple values: each value retains metaphorical weight, even when it does not dominate. When we cannot do as much good as we should in some dimension, we have responsibilities to limit and mitigate the harm this causes.

In balancing conflicting values, risk and uncertainty come into play, specifically epistemic uncertainty, risk of bias and the moral irrelevance of small differences in risk. For example, in allocation dilemma research, balancers were willing to sacrifice equal chances for all in order to save a greater number of persons, but only where the difference in probability of benefit was substantial and where epistemic warrant for categorising individuals was good. In the process of balancing competing, important moral claims that could not all be maximised, they wanted decisive rather than marginal considerations to tip the scale.

Balancing considerations can also reflect an *egalitarian* concern that persons deserve an equal opportunity or deserve not to have their chance taken away because it is smaller than another's. That is, a balancer might readily agree to prioritise saving the most lives if the choice is between a person who has a 10% chance of survival and a person who has a 90% chance of survival. Where the differences are smaller, it is plausible to reason that the differences in survival probability between two persons do not justify a categorical difference in treatment: for example, a person with a 45% and one with a 55% chance of survival both deserve an equal chance at their marginally different possibility of benefiting from access to ICU.

We may have reasons to be more or less sensitive to the size of difference in probability to benefit as it relates to concerns of discrimination, fundamental human equality or social justice. An epistemic metaconsideration that has long led people to adopt random selection (by lottery[d] or by using time as a natural, but imperfect, randomiser in a wait list or first-come, first-served situation) is that it is both difficult and time consuming to categorise persons in fair ways. This is particularly difficult to accomplish under emergency conditions or conditions of competing resource claims. When considerations of procedural justice and the possibility of appeal come into play, the supposed efficiencies of acting to save the greatest number by applying defensible categories in a fair way may be lost.

Contrary to the argument of Emanuel *et al*,[1] balancing competing values in resolving ethical dilemmas does not render "illusory" our commitment to values that we compromise. Compromise across deeply held, diverse moral values is essential to the legitimacy of pandemic policy.

Three Ways to Take Equity into Account in Triage

Avoid bias and discrimination

In this approach, medical criteria should be designed solely to maximise outcomes. Bias would be detrimental to those subject to triage, and would also interfere with outcome maximisation.

Insofar as social injustice occurs because of bias and discrimination, non-discrimination also addresses some social justice concerns. However, it does not address all of them: the consistent application of criteria that exclude people with health detriments that are due to the social determinants of health compounds existing health injustices. Neither does non-discrimination address the egalitarian or epistemic balancing concern that differences in probabilities must be substantial in order to dissuade us from treating everyone equally or from attending to social justice. These are not reasons to reject unbiased application of medical criteria, of course, but reasons to think that this solution is an incomplete response to concerns of justice.

Note that some concerns about discrimination are not about irrelevant criteria or inconsistent application of relevant criteria, but about a predetermined idea of persons against whom it is impermissible to discriminate. As Johnson points out,[18] no one has proposed prioritising women over men for ICU admission, even where there has been evidence that men with COVID-19 are less likely to survive. The grounds for this (in balancing considerations or in social justice concerns) must be made transparent and consistent with other groups for whom discrimination is a threat.

Another disadvantage is that consistent application of outcome-maximising criteria creates a relatively homogenous treatment pool, such that poor prognosis becomes a self-fulfilling prophecy. As people with certain conditions are excluded from ICU, the opportunity for healthcare providers to refine their management of persons with these conditions is lost, along with the opportunity to improve outcomes.

We should modify critical care resource triage on the basis of considerations of justice, even at the cost of saving fewer lives

In this section, I review several possible balancing solutions that reflect a willingness to sacrifice outcome maximisation for justice considerations.

One way to give weight to social justice considerations is to refuse outcome-maximising criteria that further structural inequalities. That is, outcome-maximising criteria could be adopted only where they are neutral in distribution among categories relevant to justice, such as socioeconomic status, gender and racialised groups. Triage protocols based on life expectancy or chronic multimorbidities may fail this test in relation to concerns about health inequities, as would the use of quality-adjusted life years in relation to disabled persons. If no such criteria can be found, then we can move to random allocation by lottery or time.

Another balancing approach would be to allow outcome maximisation to outweigh social justice considerations and fundamental egalitarian concerns, but only where the distinctions we apply make a substantial difference and the categories are homogeneous enough to warrant discrimination among individuals. Note that the differences in odds of surviving critical care between groups are not 9–1.[e] Preliminary UK data on critical care survival suggest differences of 10–14 percentage points between risk categories (including adjacent age categories).[17]

A third approach would be to use justice considerations to limit our choice of which outcome-maximising principle or principles to use. Some candidates are lives, life years, quality of life and fair innings. Adopting several outcome-maximising principles at the same time would further compound health inequities. For example, given a 10-to-30-year difference in life expectancy for persons of different socioeconomic status and different chronic disease patterns,[30] including life years saved or quality-of-life considerations in addition to probability of survival-to-discharge in critical care triage, would doubly advantage persons who already enjoy a considerable health advantage. We should instead choose whichever single outcome-maximising principle is least detrimental to social justice and to egalitarian opportunity. Since saving the most lives limits each person's claim to a maximum of one, it is theoretically more egalitarian than saving the most life years, a principle that allows one person's claim to outweigh another person's by much more.

Another approach would be to place the most weight on pure egalitarian concerns in order to give everyone the same opportunity to have their existing chance, within a reasonable range of chances. This could be operationalised through randomisation by lottery or time. The same approach could be chosen on the basis of epistemic considerations: in circumstances where judgments of individual probabilities are uncertain, risks of bias are high and/or categorical differences in possibility of benefit are small, it may be preferable to turn to random allocation.

Social justice considerations should play a role in how we operationalise random allocation. Using time to randomise (by wait lists or first-come, first-served) is more publicly acceptable than using a lottery, but it is an imperfect randomiser.[f] Healthier persons of higher socioeconomic status are likely to be more successful in seeking care and navigating systems than disadvantaged persons, and will have more alternatives for care. It is feasible for healthcare systems and providers to make judgments about, for example, delayed care seeking, the availability of care alternatives, the burden of returning for reassessment or a limited accessibility for follow-up care. Such an approach would also tie our response to health inequities closely to dimensions in which healthcare providers and systems can support disadvantaged patients. Non-critical care resources can be called on to assist in improving outcome potential, for example, by addressing gaps in postdischarge care or supporting home care to delay or prevent admissions.[19]

We should modify how we pursue the goal of saving the greatest number in order to also achieve equitable outcomes

A solution that maximises both equity and efficiency without sacrificing either would be ideal. One way to address the limitations in the "avoid bias and discrimination" approach discussed above has been proposed by Schmidt[31] and is permitted by Emanuel et al:[1] among those who meet the chosen threshold of likelihood to survive ICU and organ support, we could prioritise disadvantaged persons. We would then (in theory) save the same number of lives but save more lives of disadvantaged persons. This would be a form of affirmative action in medical resource allocation. Proponents point out that we may be able to save even more lives of the disadvantaged than we would on the balancing solutions canvassed above. However, this proposal faces two normative challenges from quite different perspectives.

First, if we take this approach, we will fail to remedy social injustice. If we select healthy disadvantaged persons, ones whose health is not detrimentally affected by the social determinants of health, then we will not interfere with the way that maximising outcomes compounds the health inequities caused by socioeconomic or racialised inequalities. We will save only those disadvantaged persons who have escaped the health effects of their disadvantage. This can be described as awarding resources to those who share a feature that is proxy for health injustice but is not itself health injustice.

Second, this approach violates competing principles of domain-specific fair distribution. If we take an affirmative action approach, we attract the objection that access to medical care should be based on medical, not social, criteria.[g] We would also face feasibility challenges that support concerns about domain-specific fairness, even if we reject the controversial idea that appropriate allocation principles flow from the nature of what is being allocated. These include the preparation of healthcare providers and healthcare systems to discern the categories of social disadvantage in question.[h] Data on race and ethnicity but not class are routinely collected in some health systems, such as in the USA, and not in others, such as Canada. These data are collected for monitoring health system performance and enabling epidemiological surveillance. They are unlikely to have the accuracy sufficient to inform life and death decisions for individuals. Consider the use of postal codes to support judgments of socioeconomic status based on neighbourhood income, which would privilege gentrifiers. If the role of racial, ethnic or socioeconomic markers in affirmative action were known, they would be subject to manipulation. Asking healthcare providers to distribute resources based on social inequities may increase rather than mitigate vulnerability to discrimination. Expecting people to triage against their own class identities may not be feasible. Addressing procedural justice concerns would readily swamp the efficiency gains that the proposal otherwise promises.

Furthermore, the proposal would achieve its goal only where triage protocols are categorical, such that there is a group above a threshold chance of benefit but still too large for the available resources, and further selection to maximise outcomes is not possible. (If further outcome maximising is possible using a scalar approach, but that has been rejected, then the proposal no longer demonstrates true outcome maximising.[2]) Empirically, this group must contain enough disadvantaged persons such that preferentially selecting these persons will address the fundamental concerns of social justice raised by medical criteria that are designed to maximise outcomes.

Proponents of affirmative action argue that it could achieve even greater benefits for those worse off than could the balancing solutions I have proposed in the previous section, such that rejecting outcome maximisation and affirmative action would constitute levelling down for the disadvantaged themselves. The argument is that admitting all of the disadvantaged persons who have escaped the health detriments associated with disadvantage could result in admitting more disadvantaged persons than would be admitted under a lottery that includes a broader group of both advantaged and disadvantaged persons who are on average less likely to survive.

However, my normative critique of outcome-maximising affirmative action would still apply under this so-called levelling down scenario. On this proposal, we select those who have not experienced the health detriments of the social determinants of health. This achieves, at best, an ambiguous case of levelling up. Its application in disability cases, for example, involves playing the interests of the "healthy disabled" against those whose disabilities imply greater health detriments or shorter life expectancy. Insofar as it does this, it weakens the claim that those with greater health vulnerabilities or shorter life expectancy should see the persons who are preferentially selected as levelling up for a group with which they identify.

Because only those with fewer health detriments are treated, the problem of the self-fulfilling prophecy still applies. And like the "avoid bias and discrimination" approach, it does not address the egalitarian sense that differences in probabilities of survival must be substantial to override a fundamental commitment to human equality.

Conclusion

In this paper, I have challenged the claim that there is a consensus in a pandemic emergency triage of scarce critical care resources that the value of maximising outcomes should dominate. My argument draws on work in resource allocation and organ allocation, where balancing multiple criteria is common. I focus on concerns of justice, specifically fundamental egalitarian concerns, social justice concerns and non-discrimination concerns. In addition to arguing that maximising outcomes is detrimental to egalitarian and social justice concerns, I have also described balancing considerations that should come into play. In resolving dilemmas, competing values retain their weight even when they do not dominate. They can set standards for evidence and limit the lengths to which we are prepared to go to maximise the value we think is more important. They establish responsibilities to support those of us who are harmed by our failure to live up to values that matter to us, in order to mitigate or compensate for these harms.

In addition to these general considerations in favour of balancing justice and outcomes in emergency triage, there are considerations specific to the current SARS-CoV-2 pandemic that favour triage rules informed by solidarity with those experiencing health detriments arising from social determinants of health and compounded by racialisation. Furthermore, it is not clear what in the current pandemic warrants abandoning existing societal commitments to inclusion for disabled persons. This pandemic has required, and will continue to require, an enormously disruptive societal response with substantially inequitable effects. We should broaden our focus beyond which form or forms of maximising outcomes are appropriate in a pandemic response. We need to consider mitigating the health inequities of a global pandemic, in critical care resource allocation and beyond.

Notes

a. Every ICU admission involves a judgment of need and a judgment of potential to benefit. Even the most extreme outcome maximising triage proposal can be described as a modification of needs-based ICU admission, to be applied only where there are too many patients of equal need. My discussion is about triage protocols adopted when existing standards for ICU admission and the surge in demand for critical care resources present the healthcare system with a shortage.

b. Note that the hospital triage process is not the only priority-setting question in pandemic response. We raise justice concerns when we prioritise hospital admission (assigning risk to caregivers and families in the community), balance tertiary-care surge-capacity preparation with continuing care sector preparedness and community public health response (testing and tracing for outbreak control), and decide which services are necessary and which characterised as elective can be safely postponed. We also ration personal protective equipment and will likely ration vaccines when they become available but are not yet plentiful. The broader public health response raises substantial justice questions that are beyond the scope of this paper. Many of these other prioritisation questions will affect far more people than the subject of this paper.

c. The interpretation and specification of each of these forms of justice are controversial, but they are still legitimate concerns in public policy.

d. Broome articulates the classic moral case for random selection, distinct from the argument for its use as a tie breaker in uncertainty.[32]

e. The extensive literature on the imperative to save the greatest number (SGN), following Taurek's provocative arguments,[33] focuses on saving 1 versus ≥2 lives, not saving 4 versus 5 lives, and Taurek himself argued against SGN on the grounds of partiality, not justice. The deontologist or contractualist who advocates matching procedures for settling these cases might construe all tradeoffs, ultimately, as ≥2/1 cases—the leftover after matching. I think this reveals that the contractualist/deontological matching process is a poor representation of equity concerns.

f. Thanks to Jeff Kirby for pressing this question in response to an earlier draft.

g. Sen characterises this as a "procedural" objection to achieving health equity by discrimination.[34] I have discussed this as a social justice concern. Affirmative action in education can be justified by the argument that students of low socioeconomic status have abilities that are not adequately reflected in prior performance: they will succeed once given the chance. This rationale would not be available in medical affirmative action. A rationale that will stand up in law is necessary for an affirmative action approach.

h. Compare my proposal above for mitigating social justice concerns with wait lists, where the healthcare system is not asked to make global judgments of relative disadvantage, but to identify and address barriers more proximal to healthcare.

References

1. Emanuel EJ, Persad G, Upshur R, et al. Fair allocation of scarce medical resources in the time of COVID-19. *N Engl J Med* 2020;382(21):2049–55. doi:10.1056/NEJMsb2005114 pmid:http://www.ncbi.nlm.nih.gov/pubmed/32202722

2. White DB, Lo B. A framework for rationing ventilators and critical care beds during the COVID-19 pandemic. *JAMA* 2020;323(18):1773–4. doi:10.1001/jama.2020.5046 pmid:http://www.ncbi.nlm.nih.gov/pubmed/32219367

3. Peterson A, Largent EA, Karlawish J. Ethics of reallocating ventilators in the covid-19 pandemic. *BMJ* 2020;369:m1828. doi:10.1136/bmj.m1828 pmid:http://www.ncbi.nlm.nih.gov/pubmed/32398225

4. NICE. *Social value judgments: principles for the development of NICE guidance.* 2nd Edn, 2008.

5. Kristensen FB, Lampe K, Wild C, et al. The HTA Core Model®—10 Years of Developing an International Framework to Share Multidimensional Value Assessment. *Value Health* 2017;20(2):244–50. doi:10.1016/j.jval.2016.12.010 pmid:http://www.ncbi.nlm.nih.gov/pubmed/28237203

6. Stegall MD, Stock PG, Andreoni K, et al. Why do we have the kidney allocation system we have today? a history of the 2014 kidney allocation system. *Hum Immunol* 2017;78(1):4–8. doi:10.1016/j.humimm.2016.08.008 pmid:http://www.ncbi.nlm.nih.gov/pubmed/27554430

7. Selgelid MJ. A moderate pluralist approach to public health policy and ethics. *Public Health Ethics* 2009;2:195–205. doi:10.1093/phe/php018

8. Grill K, Dawson A. Ethical frameworks in public health decision-making: defending a value-based and pluralist approach. *Health Care Anal* 2017;25(4):291–307. doi:10.1007/s10728-015-0299-6 pmid:http://www.ncbi.nlm.nih.gov/pubmed/26170178

9. Kirby J. Enhancing the Fairness of pandemic critical care triage. *J Med Ethics* 2010;36(12):758–61. doi:10.1136/jme.2010.035501 pmid:http://www.ncbi.nlm.nih.gov/pubmed/20940175

10. Munthe C. The goals of public health: an integrated, multidimensional model. *Public Health Ethics* 2008;1:39–52. doi:10.1093/phe/phn006

11. Powers M, Faden R. *Social justice: the moral foundations of public health and health policy.* New York: Oxford University Press, 2008: 248.

12. Klingler-Vidra R, Tran B-L. Vietnam has reported no coronavirus deaths—how? the conversation, 2020. Available: https://theconversation.com/vietnam-has-reported-no-coronavirus-deaths-how-136646 [Accessed 25 May 2020].

13. Moore J. What African nations are teaching the West about fighting the coronavirus, 2020. Available: https://www.newyorker.com/news/news-desk/what-african-nations-are-teaching-the-west-about-fighting-the-coronavirus [Accessed 20 May 2020].

14. Bhala N, Curry G, Martineau AR, et al. Sharpening the global focus on ethnicity and race in the time of COVID-19. *The Lancet* 2020;395(10238):1673–6. doi:10.1016/S0140-6736(20)31102-8

15. Yancy CW. COVID-19 and African Americans. *JAMA* 2020;323(19):1891–2. doi:10.1001/jama.2020.6548

16. Office for national statistics. deaths involving COVID-19 by local area and socioeconomic deprivation: deaths occurring between 1 March and 17 April 2020, 2020. Available: https://www.ons.gov.uk/peoplepopulationandcommunity/birthsdeathsandmarriages/deaths/bulletins/deathsinvolvingcovid19bylocalareasanddeprivation/deathsoccurringbetween1marchand17april [Accessed 20 May 2020].

17. Intensive Care National Audit & Research Centre. ICNARC report on COVID-19 in critical care, 2020. Available: https://www.icnarc.org/DataServices/Attachments/Download/b8c18e7d-e791-ea11-9125-00505601089b [Accessed 20 May 2020].

18. Johnson LSM. Prioritizing justice in ventilator allocation, 2020. Available: https://blogs.bmj.com/medical-ethics/2020/04/15/prioritizing-justice-in-ventilator-allocation/ [Accessed 20 May 2020].

19. Sederstrom NO. Unblinded: systematic racism, institutional oppression, and colorblindness, 2020. Available: http://www.bioethics.net/2020/05/unblinded-systematic-racism-institutional-oppression-and-colorblindness/ [Accessed 20 May 2020].

20. Wagstaff A. QALYs and the equity-efficiency trade-off. *J Health Econ* 1991;10(1):21–41. doi:10.1016/0167-6296(91)90015-F pmid:http://www.ncbi.nlm.nih.gov/pubmed/10113661

21. Nord E. The QALY—a measure of social value rather than individual utility? *Health Econ* 1994;3(2):89–93. doi:10.1002/hec.4730030205 pmid:http://www.ncbi.nlm.nih.gov/pubmed/8044215

22. Ubel PA, DeKay ML, Baron J, et al. Cost-effectiveness analysis in a setting of budget constraints—is it equitable? *N Engl J Med* 1996;334(18):1174–7. doi:10.1056/NEJM199605023341807 pmid:http://www.ncbi.nlm.nih.gov/pubmed/8602185

23. Nord E, Pinto JL, Richardson J, et al. Incorporating societal concerns for fairness in numerical valuations of health programmes. *Health Econ* 1999;8(1):25–39. doi:10.1002/(SICI)1099-1050(199902)8:1<25::AID-HEC398>3.0.CO;2-H pmid:http://www.ncbi.nlm.nih.gov/pubmed/10082141

24. Ubel PA, Loewenstein G. Distributing scarce livers: the moral Reasoning of the general public. *Soc Sci Med* 1996;42(7):1049–55. doi:10.1016/0277-9536(95)00216-2 pmid:http://www.ncbi.nlm.nih.gov/pubmed/8730910

25. Broome J. Fairness versus doing the most good. *Hastings Cent Rep* 1994;24(4):36–9. doi:10.2307/3562844 pmid:http://www.ncbi.nlm.nih.gov/pubmed/7960705

26. Fairness BJ. *Proceedings of the Aristotelian Society.* 91, 1990: 87–101.

27. Walzer M. *Spheres of justice: a defense of pluralism and equality.* New York: Basic Books, 2008.

28. Ubel PA, Baron J, Nash B, et al. Are preferences for equity over efficiency in health care allocation "all or nothing"? *Med Care* 2000;38(4):366–73. doi:10.1097/00005650-200004000-00003 pmid:http://www.ncbi.nlm.nih.gov/pubmed/10752968

29. Neuberger J, Ubel PA. Finding a place for public preferences in liver allocation decisions. *Transplantation* 2000;70(10):1411–3. doi:10.1097/00007890-200011270-00001 pmid:http://www.ncbi.nlm.nih.gov/pubmed/11118080

30. Marmot M. *The health gap: the challenge of an unequal world.* London: Bloomsbury Publishing, 2015.

31. Schmidt H. The way we ration ventilators is biased, 2020. Available: https://www.nytimes.com/2020/04/15/opinion/covid-ventilator-rationing-blacks.html [Accessed 20 May 2020].

32. Broome J. Selecting people randomly. *Ethics* 1984;95(1):38–55. doi:10.1086/292596 pmid:http://www.ncbi.nlm.nih.gov/pubmed/11651785

33. Taurek JM. Should the numbers count? *Philos Public Aff* 1977;6(4):293–316. pmid:http://www.ncbi.nlm.nih.gov/pubmed/11662404

34. Sen A. Why health equity? *Health Econ* 2002;11(8):659–66. doi:10.1002/hec.762. pmid:http://www.ncbi.nlm.nih.gov/pubmed/12457367

ETHICS COMMITTEE

Ira Harker Needs a Kidney*

60-year-old Ira Harker needs a liver transplant badly. There is no question that on the PELD/MELD criteria that determine how badly someone needs a liver transplant, Ira's numbers were right up there with anyone on the list for hospital transplant in his area. If Ira does not get a liver transplant in the next three months, he could die. He got to the point where he needs a liver lobe so badly because of prolonged alcohol abuse. The only transplant center within driving distance of his home is County Hospital. According to the UNOS (United Network for Organ Sharing) guidelines that County must follow, decisions about transplant eligibility must be based on medical criteria and consider all ethical principles. The ethics committee at County meets to consider adding Ira to its transplant list. One committee member asks how long Mr. Harker has been sober, since to be eligible, no candidates for a liver transplant should drink alcohol. Harker just received his one-year chip from Alcoholics Anonymous and reports that he hasn't drunk alcohol (except for one three-day relapse) in two years. He is otherwise in average health for a 60-year-old man.

Here are some other facts brought up in the committee:

- The five-year survival rate of sober patients is 63%—equal to or above the next five patients on the current list waiting for a liver transplant.

- There is no statistical evidence that alcoholics are more likely than non-alcoholics to drink after their transplant.

- Some studies suggest that alcoholics and non-alcoholics consume similar amounts of alcohol following their transplants.

> As a committee, decide if Ira Harker should be listed as a transplant candidate.

---

* This case study is based on Vanessa Williamson, "The Liver Transplant Dilemma: The Alcoholic Medicaid Patient" [3 Rich. J.L. & Pub. Int. 94 (1998)]. I've altered some information and added some details.

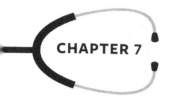

CHAPTER 7

Dilemmas in Genetic and Reproductive Technology

OPENING GAMBIT

Screening for the Breast Cancer Gene

Mrs. Hockney and her husband sat in the office of the fertility clinic, hands desperately clasped together. Dr. Randall wanted to talk to them about their options. The Hockneys came to the clinic because Mr. Hockney had a family history that included Tay-Sachs disease, a debilitating childhood illness. Children with Tay-Sachs rarely make it to age five. Dr. Randall's clinic offered the Hockneys a way to prevent passing Tay-Sachs to their children using in vitro fertilization and preimplantation genetic diagnosis (PGD) to identify which embryos would have the genetic markers for Tay-Sachs and implant only the ones that did not.

It was Mrs. Hockney's other request, however, that had Dr. Randall over an ethical barrel: "Can we also screen for the BRCA mutation?" The BRCA mutation Mrs. Hockney referred to can increase the chance of developing certain kinds of cancer. Women with a BRCA-1 gene mutation, for example, are five times more likely to get breast cancer, according to some studies. The clinic had a standing policy, however, that prevented such screenings. The clinic would screen for debilitating childhood diseases like Tay-Sachs but not adult-onset diseases. Screening for genetic markers that did not guarantee disease, like the BRCA mutation, was an ongoing debate among the partners at the clinic.

"You realize that a BRCA mutation doesn't guarantee a child will get breast cancer? She could go her whole life without getting it. Many women never get it. And we would be destroying embryos that might develop perfectly healthy babies," Dr. Randall explained.

Mrs. Hockney was not dissuaded. "I understand, but my mom and Greg's sister both went through breast cancer nightmares. I want to stop it from spreading in this family. I don't want any female embryos implanted that have that mutation." Dr. Randal sighed. "So you want us to screen for the sex of the embryos and then test for the BRCA mutation?" Mrs. Hockney smiled. "You can do that? Oh, we would really like a girl. Let's just implant those embryos." Dr. Randall rubbed her temples, feeling a headache coming on.

WHAT'S AT STAKE?

Some of the most perplexing and debilitating diseases are genetic ones. Unlike viruses and bacterial infections, which can be passed from one person to another by contact, genetic disorders can be just as harmful but are passed by reproduction. This means it is possible to stop genetic diseases by altering reproduction. For instance, Tay-Sachs disease is a debilitating genetic disorder that runs in certain ethnic populations: Ashkenazi (European) Jews, Québécois, and Cajuns. Theoretically, if we could prevent carriers of these diseases from passing on the bad gene traits, we could wipe out these diseases in much the same way we wiped out polio by a concerted national vaccination program. However, this would require people to voluntarily alter their reproductive choices. No easy thing.

Because of the horrors of diseases like Tay-Sachs, Jewish communities have set up programs to do this very thing. The Dor Yeshorim (Hebrew for "Generation of the Righteous") has a program where Jewish high schools have mass screenings.

From the Dor Yeshorim website

During mass/school screening events (or private appointments), blood is drawn for testing and each participant receives a nine-digit identification number. Blood samples are sent for intensive DNA analysis and results entered into a centralized database. Individuals seeking a partner in marriage have unlimited, 24-hour access to the Dor Yeshorim automated hotline, where they are asked to enter both parties' ID number and day and month of birth. Within a few business hours, a trained specialist returns the call and informs both parties whether they are compatible. Couples found to be incompatible are offered guidance and assistance.

Source: https://doryeshorim.org/faq/.

If programs like the Dor Yeshorim are successful at preventing births with debilitating diseases, such programs are not only permissible but perhaps mandatory, provided there are precautions for privacy and safety. Here we have a clash between autonomy on the one hand, and beneficence and non-maleficence on the other. Eradicating genetic disease like Tay-Sachs is certainly beneficial, and preventing the conception of babies who will die by the time they are five years old from neuro-muscular failure is certainly consistent with non-maleficence. Doing so would require couples to go childless if one of them is a carrier.

There is also the worry that such centralized regulation will lead to a kind of manipulation of the gene pool. This is a familiar kind of slippery slope argument. Consider the following argument:

1. If it is permissible to prevent certain genetic diseases on the basis that it is better for the child and the population, then people who are born with genetic diseases would not have been born if such programs were in place.
2. It would have been better if those people had never been born.
3. To say it would be better if someone had never been born because of their handicap disrespects handicapped people.
4. Conclusion: Preventing genetic diseases on the basis of utility (the greater good of society) disrespects every handicapped person.

This is one reason that disability advocacy groups often oppose measures to prevent births of those with genetic diseases. Today it is Tay-Sachs, they say; tomorrow it is Down's syndrome or brittle-bone disease.

Defenders of this sort of testing point out that there is a very big difference between Tay-Sachs and Down's syndrome. Tay-Sachs is fatal, while those with Down's syndrome can live happy, fruitful lives. It is wrong, they say, to throw the baby out with the bathwater. If Tay-Sachs can be prevented by genetic screening, as in the Dor Yeshorim program, and no one's privacy is violated, then there is no reason not to screen. We have a moral duty to prevent this harm if possible. Genetic screening can identify carriers of genetic defects that would be passed on to a child by couples, who then choose not to conceive. But what about couples who choose to conceive and later find out that one of them is a carrier of a debilitating, fatal, genetic disease?

Huntington's Disease (HD) is a genetic disorder of the number of chromosomes: a chromosome copying error. When cells divide, they copy DNA traits, but with HD some genes replicate more than necessary. The higher the number of replication errors, the worse the HD symptoms. HD is a debilitating neurological and physical disease whose sufferers develop symptoms of dementia and muscle deterioration. Depending on how high the number of replications, these symptoms can show up early in life or even up into middle age. Because it is a DNA replication problem, there is no cure. Couples where one partner has HD find themselves with a choice: they can choose not to reproduce at all in order to prevent harm to a future child who may or may not develop a high replication number, or they can select embryos that have the lowest chance of developing HD. This latter option requires in vitro fertilization (IVF) and something called pre-implantation genetic diagnosis (PGD)

In vitro is Latin for "in glass" and refers to fertilization taking place outside of the womb in a glass container. Nearly all IVF procedures create more embryos than will be implanted safely. Therefore, IVF involves a choice of which embryos fertility technicians will implant. This provides an opportunity for selecting embryos based on the principles of beneficence and non-maleficence. PGD screens embryos for implantation by taking samples of DNA. Fertility specialists can now screen for up to thirty different genetic abnormalities. For instance, if an embryo has a high replication error number for HD it can be frozen or discarded, and replaced with embryos with low replication errors. Likewise, embryos that have the genetic marker for Tay-Sachs can be selected out in favor of embryos that do not have the marker. PGD can achieve the same results as the Dor Yeshorim project without couples worrying if they are compatible and without stigmatizing an ethic group.

Are there any problems with IVF and PGD? Some studies show that IVF increases the chances of birth defects and miscarriages. This is one reason that PGD is often offered in conjunction with IVF because PGD gives fertility specialists ways to select embryos that will have a greater chance of coming to term without birth defects. But once we go down the road of selecting embryos to screen out traits like Tay-Sachs, why would we stop there? If our duty is to non-maleficence (the duty to not harm a baby by causing it to be born with a birth defect), then surely this duty would extend to every single genetic abnormality we could screen for. Why not screen for as many as we can?

Julian Savulescu (b. 1963) argues that our duty is not just to prevent harm (non-maleficence) but also to provide the greatest life possible for the future child (beneficence). This would include not just *screening out* diseases but also *selecting for* positive traits like intelligence and physical health. This is not science fiction. Humans have mapped the genome, and to the extent that our intelligence and physical fitness are genetic, we are not far from being able to make these sorts of selections.

But, morally, should we? If our duty is to beneficence, then it would seem that yes, we should. If our duty is only to non-maleficence, then it would seem that this sort of selection for traits would be less important. If we could identify genetic markers for obesity and arthritis, wouldn't our commitment to non-maleficence oblige us to screen embryos to prevent these physical defects in future children? You might think the reasons we should not start selecting for genetic traits have to do with diversity and respect for those who have disabilities. National disability groups have expressed grave concerns about PGD because it treats future persons who might come from genetic abnormalities as somehow defective. These groups argue that this kind of selection says, in effect, "It would be better if these kinds of people were never born."

We have a four-way clash of principles here: non-maleficence (screen out genetic diseases that harm) and beneficence (choose the embryos that will have the best chance at the best life), and the principles of justice (do not treat genetic disabilities as defective) and respect (those born with disabilities are ends in themselves, not a means to some end).

Notice, however, that the reasons for not discriminating against genetic diseases and for *not* selecting the best embryos actually make permissible selecting embryos *for* genetic diseases. Sharon Duchesneau and Candy McCullough made headlines not because they wanted to have a child together but because they chose a sperm donor who had five generations of deafness. Both Sharon and Candy were deaf, and they wanted a deaf child. They were doing with artificial insemination what couples using PGD do, namely increasing the chances of having a child with a particular genetic trait. Now, notice that the reasons for *not* allowing genetic screening for positive traits (justice and respect for the disabled) seem to argue *for* allowing PGD to select for some genetic defect, provided the disability is not painful or terminal. Deafness and dwarfism are two such traits.

As philosopher Jeff McMahan has pointed out, if we say to couples, "You can't select for positive traits because it would be unjust and disrespects diversity," then we would have to allow couples to intentionally create genetic disabilities by selecting embryos for implantation because this would increase diversity, show respect for the differently abled, and increase equality. McMahan's argument forces us into a dilemma: either we allow people to select for positive

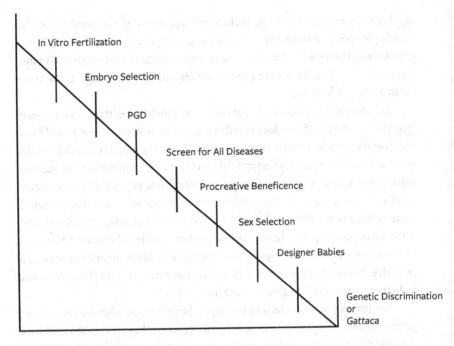

FIGURE 7.1

traits and against genetic disorders or we accept selection for disabilities on the grounds of justice and respect for diversity.*

By now you may be thinking, "This sort of selection starts to sound more like 'design' than prevention." We have discussed slippery slopes before, but not all slippery slopes are faulty reasoning. Here we have what may be a genuine slippery slope argument, where starting with embryo selection and PGD leads to further reproductive choices, none of which seems too objectionable until we realize that we have gone from preventing disease to designing a baby (see Figure 7.1).

At the bottom of this slippery slope is wholesale genetic discrimination, something that is graphically portrayed in the science-fiction movie *Gattaca*, where the main character is barred from jobs and opportunities based not on his race or gender but on genetic imperfection.

Here is an argument that illustrates the moral reasoning that would lead, partially, down this slippery slope:

---

* Jeff McMahan, "Causing Disabled People to Exist and Causing People to Be Disabled," *Ethics* 116, no. 1 (2005): 77–99.

1. In IVF, selection of embryos is inevitable, since more embryos are created than can be implanted.
2. If selection is inevitable, there seem to be reasons to select based on criteria that are not just arbitrary (i.e., we should not simply choose at random).
3. If selection should be non-arbitrary, then it should be based on moral criteria (all things being equal, our reasons for selecting *this* embryo rather than *that* one should be based on, or at least consistent with, moral reasons).
4. Moral criteria for selection are often (typically?) based on avoiding harmful diseases and physical defects.
5. If selecting embryos is based on the principle of non-maleficence (causing no harm), then it is also moral to make a selection on the basis of positive traits, such as intelligence, good looks, and athleticism, since they make the future person better off.
6. Conclusion: It is moral to select for positive traits if we engage in IVF.

One way to avoid this slippery slope is, of course, not to get on it in the first place. Many people argue that IVF itself is immoral because of how it treats embryos. If embryos have the same moral status as persons, then any discrimination of persons is immoral. The response to this is that some genetic diseases like Tay-Sachs or Huntington's are so bad that we have a duty to prevent that level of suffering if we can. We can do that only with IVF and PGD, or by not reproducing.

This does not mean that we have to go any further than screening out for these few childhood incurable diseases. We could stop the slippery slope by saying, "This far and no further!" The moral quandary, however, is this: What are our moral reasons for saying we will screen for these few diseases because they are so harmful, but not for any other diseases? And if we screen for harmful diseases, why not for positive traits? We need a good reason to say, "This far and no further."

And this is not even the cutting edge of genetic and reproductive technology. Two new technologies actually take designing to a new level. CRISPRCas9 is a technology that can turn genes on and off using chemical transmitters. Dr. Jiankui He, a researcher in China, took a break from the university where he worked to put in time at a family fertility clinic. The project was designed to study couples where one partner had HIV and the other did not. Dr. He used CRISPRCas9 to alter one couple's embryos so that the children would have a resistance to HIV by turning off a gene known to be associated with HIV called the CCR-5 gene. Dr. He claims that the first genetically edited human children, twins, were born healthy.

The medical community was considerably upset that Dr. He had done this without proper precautions and oversight. There did seem to be concerns that fall within the ethical principles of research (see Chapter 4). For instance, the editing seems to have been successful only at turning off the CCR-5 gene in one of the twins. However, both twins were brought to term. Lulu and Nana, as they were nicknamed, represent a major escalation toward gene-edited children, and the scientific community has reacted with caution and concern. Francis Collins, leader of the Human Genome Project and discoverer of many genetic diseases, said, "This work represents a deeply disturbing willingness by Dr. He and his team to flaunt [*sic*] international ethical norms. The project was largely carried out in secret, the medical necessity for inactivation of CCR5 in these infants is utterly unconvincing, the informed consent process appears highly questionable, and the possibility of damaging off-target effects has not been satisfactorily explored."*

The second major technological breakthrough that has caused ethical concerns is the advent of three-parent babies. Mitochondrial (mtDNA) disease is a rare but potentially destructive genetic disease that can affect all major organs including the heart, lungs, and kidneys. Defective mitochondria (the engines that power cells) are debilitating, and there is no cure. However, researchers in Great Britain have successfully transplanted healthy mitochondria into embryos. These embryos do not develop mitochondrial disease because cell replication proceeds with healthy mitochondria. There is the worry, however, that the children in these circumstances technically have DNA from three parents. Mitochondrial replacement challenges our views on reproductive technology as well as our intuitions about who gets to be counted as parents. Is parentage a social construction or a biological fact?

This is not a trivial question. A great number of duties and responsibilities come with parentage, including financial ones. Legally, it matters who is considered a parent. We have good evidence that what makes us who we are genetically (our traits, our characteristics) are found in the nuclear DNA, not the mitochondrial DNA, but this has not stopped ethical concerns about the social conventions of maternity and worries about the long-term effects of mitochondrial replacement.

You might think, "Three-parent babies aren't really all that new, are they?" Since the advent of artificial insemination, children have been born with three parents thanks to surrogacy. But surrogacy itself as an institution has challenged traditional norms regarding parentage. As ethicist Elizabeth Anderson (b. 1959) has argued, biological/genetic ties have been the traditional

---

* "Statement on Claim of First Gene-Edited Babies by Chinese Researcher," National Institutes of Health, Nov. 28, 2018, https://www.nih.gov/about-nih/who-we-are/nih-director/statements/statement-claim-first-gene-edited-babies-chinese-researcher.

norm we have adopted to ensure that children are cared for even if their parents do not want the responsibility.* Surrogacy challenges this norm because it makes labor (the labor of the surrogate) into a commodity, thus straining the ties between parent and child. However, for couples who cannot have children and cannot adopt, surrogacy remains a viable alternative to traditional birth. What both of these examples of new reproductive technology show is that the link between biological processes and ethical norms is not easy to establish or maintain in a society.

WHAT'S THE DEBATE?

Reading 7.1: Julian Savulescu, "Procreative Beneficence: Why We Should Select the Best Children"

Julian Savulescu argues that if we use pre-implantation genetic diagnosis (PGD), we have a moral duty to select those embryos that have the best chance for the best life, and this includes selecting for non-disease traits such as intelligence.

...

Introduction

Imagine you are having in vitro fertilisation (IVF) and you produce four embryos. One is to be implanted. You are told that there is a genetic test for predisposition to scoring well on IQ tests (let's call this intelligence). If an embryo has gene subtypes (alleles) A, B there is a greater than 50% chance it will score more than 140 if given an ordinary education and upbringing. If it has subtypes C, D there is a much lower chance it will score over 140. Would you test the four embryos for these gene subtypes and use this information in selecting which embryo to implant?

Many people believe intelligence is a purely social construct and so it is unlikely to have a significant genetic cause. Others believe there are different sorts of intelligence, such as verbal intelligence, mathematical intelligence, musical ability and no such thing as general intelligence. Time will tell. There are several genetic research programs currently in place which seek to elucidate the genetic contribution to intelligence. This paper pertains to any results of this

---

* Elizabeth S. Anderson, "Is Women's Labor a Commodity?" *Philosophy & Public Affairs* 19, no. 1 (1990): 71–92.

research even if it only describes a weak probabilistic relation between genes and intelligence, or a particular kind of intelligence.

Many people believe that research into the genetic contribution to intelligence should not be performed, and that if genetic tests which predict intelligence, or a range of intelligence, are ever developed, they should not be employed in reproductive decision-making. I will argue that we have a moral obligation to test for genetic contribution to non-disease states such as intelligence and to use this information in reproductive decision-making.

Imagine now you are invited to play the Wheel of Fortune. A giant wheel exists with marks on it from 0-$1,000,000, in $100 increments. The wheel is spun in a secret room. It stops randomly on an amount. That amount is put into Box A. The wheel is spun again. The amount which comes up is put into Box B. You can choose Box A or B. You are also told that, in addition to the sum already put in the boxes, if you choose B, a dice will be thrown and you will lose $100 if it comes up 6.

Which box should you choose?

The rational answer is Box A. Choosing genes for non-disease states is like playing the Wheel of Fortune. You should use all the available information and choose the option most likely to bring about the best outcome.

Procreative Beneficence: The Moral Obligation to Have the Best Children

I will argue for a principle which I call Procreative Beneficence:

> couples (or single reproducers) should select the child, of the possible children they could have, who is expected to have the best life, or at least as good a life as the others, based on the relevant, available information.

I will argue that Procreative Beneficence implies couples should employ genetic tests for non-disease traits in selecting which child to bring into existence and that we should allow selection for non-disease genes in some cases even if this maintains or increases social inequality.

By "should" in "should choose," I mean "have good reason to." I will understand morality to require us to do what we have most reason to do. In the absence of some other reason for action, a person who has good reason to have the best child is morally required to have the best child....

DEFINITIONS

A disease gene is a gene which causes a genetic disorder (e.g., cystic fibrosis) or predisposes to the development of disease (e.g. the genetic contribution to cancer or dementia). A non-disease gene is a gene which causes or predisposes to some physical or psychological state of the person which is not itself a disease state, e.g. height, intelligence, character (not in the sub-normal range).

SELECTION

It is currently possible to select from a range of possible children we could have. This is most frequently done by employing fetal selection through prenatal testing and termination of pregnancy. Selection of embryos is now possible by employing in vitro fertilization and preimplantation genetic diagnosis (PGD). There are currently no genetic tests available for non-disease states except sex. However, if such tests become available in the future, both PGD and prenatal testing could be used to select offspring on the basis of non-disease genes. Selection of sex by PGD is now undertaken in Sydney, Australia.[1] PGD will also lower the threshold for couples to engage in selection since it has fewer psychological sequelae than prenatal testing and abortion.

In the future, it may be possible to select gametes according to their genetic characteristics. This is currently possible for sex, where methods have been developed to sort X and Y bearing sperm.[2]

BEHAVIOURAL GENETICS

Behavioural Genetics is a branch of genetics which seeks to understand the contribution of genes to complex behaviour. The scope of behavioural genetics is illustrated in Table 1.

An Argument for Procreative Beneficence

Consider the *Simple Case of Selection for Disease Genes*. A couple is having IVF in an attempt to have a child. It produces two embryos. A battery of tests for common diseases is performed. Embryo A has no abnormalities on the tests performed. Embryo B has no abnormalities on the tests performed except its genetic profile reveals it has a predisposition to developing asthma. Which embryo should be implanted?

Embryo B has nothing to be said in its favour over A and something against it. Embryo A should (on pain of irrationality) be implanted. This is like choosing Box A in the Wheel of Fortune analogy.

TABLE 1
Behavioural Genetics

Aggression and criminal behaviour
Alcoholism
Anxiety and Anxiety disorders
Attention Deficit Hyperactivity Disorder (ADHD)
Antisocial personality disorder
Bipolar disorder
Homosexuality
Maternal Behaviour
Memory and intelligence
Neuroticism
Novelty Seeking
Schizophrenia
Substance Addiction

Why shouldn't we select the embryo with a predisposition to asthma? What is relevant about asthma is that it reduces quality of life. Attacks cause severe breathlessness and in extreme cases, death. Steroids may be required to treat it. These are among the most dangerous drugs which exist if taken long term. Asthma can be lifelong and require lifelong drug treatment. Ultimately it can leave the sufferer wheelchair bound with chronic obstructive airways disease. The morally relevant property of "asthma" is that it is a state which reduces the well-being a person experiences.

PARFITIAN DEFENCE OF VOLUNTARY PROCREATIVE
BENEFICENCE IN THE SIMPLE CASE

The following example, after Parfit,[3] supports Procreative Beneficence. A woman has rubella. If she conceives now, she will have a blind and deaf child. If she waits three months, she will conceive another different but healthy child. She should choose to wait until her rubella is passed.

Or consider the Nuclear Accident. A poor country does not have enough power to provide power to its citizens during an extremely cold winter. The government decides to open an old and unsafe nuclear reactor. Ample light and heating are then available. Citizens stay up later, and enjoy their lives much more. Several months later, the nuclear reactor melts down and large amounts of radiation are released into the environment. The only effect is that a large number of children are subsequently born with predispositions to early childhood malignancy.

The supply of heating and light has changed the lifestyle of this population. As a result of this change in lifestyle, people have conceived children at different times than they would have if there had been no heat or light, and their parents went to bed earlier. Thus, the children born after the nuclear accident would not have existed if the government had not switched to nuclear power. They have not been harmed by the switch to nuclear power and the subsequent accident (unless their lives are so bad they are worse than death). If we object to the Nuclear Accident (which most of us would), then we must appeal to some form of harmless wrong-doing. That is, we must claim that a wrong was done, but no one was harmed. We must appeal to something like the Principle of Procreative Beneficence.

AN OBJECTION TO PROCREATIVE BENEFICENCE IN THE SIMPLE CASE

The following objection to Procreative Beneficence is common.

"If you choose Embryo A (without a predisposition to asthma), you could be discarding someone like Mozart or an olympic swimmer. So there is no good reason to select A."

It is true that by choosing A, you could be discarding a person like Mozart. But it is equally true that if you choose B, you could be discarding someone like Mozart without asthma. A and B are equally likely (on the information available) to be someone like Mozart (and B is more likely to have asthma)....

> Savulescu makes a compelling case for screening out disease genes if we are able to. In what follows he argues that if you agree with him about screening out disease genes before implantation, there is no good reason not to move on to non-disease genes. In fact, there are good reasons to select for traits like intelligence because they lead to a better life as defined by three theories of a good life. Ask yourself can you differentiate between these three theories of a good life? Which seems the most compelling?

Moving from Disease Genes to Non-Disease Genes: What Is the "Best Life"?

It is not asthma (or disease) which is important, but its impact on a life in ways that matter which is important. People often trade length of life for non-health related well-being. Non-disease genes may prevent us from leading the best life.

By "best life," I will understand the life with the most well-being. There are various theories of well-being: hedonistic, desire-fulfilment, objective list theories.[4] According to hedonistic theories, what matters is the quality of our experiences, for example, that we experience pleasure. According to desire-fulfilment theories, what matters is the degree to which our desires are satisfied. According to objective list theories, certain activities are good for people, such as achieving worthwhile things with your life, having dignity, having children and raising them, gaining knowledge of the world, developing one's talents, appreciating beautiful things, and so on.

On any of these theories, some non-disease genes will affect the likelihood that we will lead the best life. Imagine there is a gene which contributes significantly to a violent, explosive, uncontrollable temper, and that state causes people significant suffering. Violent outbursts lead a person to come in conflict with the law and fall out of important social relations. The loss of independence, dignity and important social relations are bad on any of the three accounts.

Buchanan et al. argue that what is important in a liberal democracy is providing people with general purpose means, i.e. those useful to any plan of life.[5] In this way we can allow people to form and act on their own conception of the good life. Examples of general purpose means are the ability to hear and see. But similarly the ability to concentrate, to engage with and be empathetic towards other human beings may be all purpose means. To the degree that genes contribute to these, we have reason to select those genes....

On a hedonistic account, the capacity to imagine alternative pleasures and remember the salient features of past experiences is important in choosing the best life. On a desire-fulfilment theory, intelligence is important to choosing means which will best satisfy one's ends. On an objective list account, intelligence would be important to gaining knowledge of the world, and developing rich social relations. Newson has reviewed the empirical literature relating intelligence to quality of life. Her synthesis of the empirical literature is that "intelligence has a high instrumental value for persons in giving them a large amount of complexity with which to approach their everyday lives, and that it equips them with a tool which can lead to the provision of many other personal and social goods."[6]

Socrates, in Plato's Philebus, concludes that the best life is a mixture of wisdom and pleasure. Wisdom includes thought, intelligence, knowledge and memory.[7] Intelligence is clearly a part of Plato's conception of the good life:

> without the power of calculation you could not even calculate that you will get enjoyment in the future; your life would be that not of a man, but of a sea-lung or one of those marine creatures whose bodies are confined by a shell.[8]

CHOICE OF MEANS OF SELECTING

This argument extends in principle to selection of fetuses using prenatal testing and termination of affected pregnancy. However, selection by abortion has greater psychological harms than selection by PGD and these need to be considered. Gametic selection, if it is ever possible, will have the lowest psychological cost.

> Of course, as a philosopher, Savulescu considers objections to his argument. Does Savulescu cover all the objections to selecting for intelligence or some other non-disease trait? Can you think of others?

OBJECTIONS TO THE PRINCIPLE OF PROCREATIVE BENEFICENCE APPLIED TO NON-DISEASE GENES

1. *Harm to the child*: One common objection to genetic selection for non-disease traits is that it results in harm to the child. There are various versions of this objection, which include the harm which arises from excessive and overbearing parental expectations, using the child as a means, and not treating it as an end, and closing off possible future options on the basis of the information provided (failing to respect the child's "right to an open future").

There are a number of responses. Firstly, in some cases, it is possible to deny that the harms will be significant. Parents come to love the child whom they have (even a child with a serious disability). Moreover, some have argued that counselling can reduce excessive expectations.[9]

Secondly, we can accept some risk of a child experiencing some state of reduced well-being in cases of selection. One variant of the harm to child objection is: "If you select embryo A, it might still get asthma, or worse, cancer, or have a much worse life than B, and you would be responsible." Yet selection is immune to this objection (in a way which genetic manipulation is not).

Imagine you select Embryo A and it develops cancer (or severe asthma) in later life. You have not harmed A unless A's life is not worth living (hardly plausible) because A would not have existed if you had acted otherwise. A is not made worse off than A would otherwise have been, since without the selection, A would not have existed. Thus we can accept the possibility of a bad outcome, but not the probability of a very bad outcome. (Clearly, Procreative Beneficence demands that we not choose a child with a low predisposition to asthma but who is likely to have a high predisposition to cancer.)

This is different to genetic manipulation. Imagine you perform gene therapy to correct a predisposition to asthma and you cause a mutation which results in cancer later in life. You have harmed A: A is worse off in virtue of the genetic manipulation than A would have been if the manipulation had not been performed (assuming cancer is worse than asthma).

There is, then, an important distinction between:

> interventions which are genetic manipulations of a single gamete, embryo or fetus selection procedures (e.g., sex selection) which select from among a range of different gametes, embryos and fetuses.

2. *Inequality*: One objection to Procreative Beneficence is that it will maintain or increase inequality. For example, it is often argued that selection for sex, intelligence, favourable physical or psychological traits, etc. all contribute to inequality in society, and this is a reason not to attempt to select the best.

In the case of selection against disease genes, similar claims are made. For example, one version of the *Disability Discrimination Claim* maintains that prenatal testing for disabilities such as Down syndrome results in discrimination against those with those disabilities both by:

> the statement it makes about the worth of such lives and the reduction in the numbers of people with this condition.

Even if the Disability Discrimination Claim were true, it would be a drastic step in favour of equality to inflict a higher risk of having a child with a disability on a couple (who do not want a child with a disability) to promote social equality.

Consider a hypothetical rubella epidemic. A rubella epidemic hits an isolated population. Embryos produced prior to the epidemic are not at an elevated risk of any abnormality but those produced during the epidemic are at an increased risk of deafness and blindness. Doctors should encourage women to use embryos which they have produced prior to the epidemic in preference to ones produced during the epidemic. The reason is that it is bad that blind and deaf children are born when sighted and hearing children could have been born in their place.

This does not necessarily imply that the lives of those who now live with disability are less deserving of respect and are less valuable. To attempt to prevent accidents which cause paraplegia is not to say that paraplegics are less deserving of respect. It is important to distinguish between disability and persons with disability. Selection reduces the former, but is silent on the value of the latter. There are better ways to make statements about the equality of people with disability (e.g., we could direct savings from selection against embryos/ fetuses with genetic abnormalities to improving well-being of existing people with disabilities).

These arguments extend to selection for non-disease genes. It is not disease which is important but its impact on well-being. In so far as a non-disease gene such as a gene for intelligence impacts on a person's well-being, parents have a reason to select for it, even if inequality results.

This claim can have counter-intuitive implications. Imagine in a country women are severely discriminated against. They are abandoned as children, refused paid employment and serve as slaves to men. Procreative Beneficence implies that couples should test for sex, and should choose males as they are expected to have better lives in this society, even if this reinforces the discrimination against women.

There are several responses. Firstly, it is unlikely selection on a scale that contributes to inequality would promote well-being. Imagine that 50% of the population choose to select boys. This would result in three boys to every one girl. The life of a male in such a society would be intolerable.

Secondly, it is social institutional reform, not interference in reproduction, which should be promoted. What is wrong in such a society is the treatment of women, which should be addressed separately to reproductive decision-making. Reproduction should not become an instrument of social change, at least not mediated or motivated at a social level.

This also illustrates why Procreative Beneficence is different to eugenics. Eugenics is selective breeding to produce a better *population*. A *public interest* justification for interfering in reproduction is different from Procreative Beneficence which aims at producing the best child, of the possible children, a couple could have. That is an essentially private enterprise. It was the eugenics movement itself which sought to influence reproduction, through involuntary sterilisation, to promote social goods.

Thirdly, consider the case of blackmail. A company says it will only develop an encouraging drug for cystic fibrosis (CF) if there are more than 100,000 people with CF. This would require stopping carrier testing for CF. Should the government stop carrier testing?

If there are other ways to fund this research (e.g., government funding), this should have priority. In virtually all cases of social inequality, there are other avenues to correct inequality than encouraging or forcing people to have children with disabilities or lives of restricted genetic opportunity....

Conclusions
With respect to non-disease genes, we should provide:

- information (through PGD and prenatal testing)
- free choice of which child to have
- non-coercive advice as to which child will be expected to enter life with the best opportunity of having the best life.

Selection for non-disease genes which significantly impact on well-being is *morally required* (Procreative Beneficence). "Morally required" implies moral persuasion but not coercion is justified.

If, in the end, couples wish to select a child who will have a lower chance of having the best life, they should be free to make such a choice. That should not prevent doctors from attempting to persuade them to have the best child they can. In some cases, persuasion will not be justified. If self-interest or concern to promote equality motivate a choice to select less than the best, then there may be no overall reason to attempt to dissuade a couple. But in cases in which couples do not want to use or obtain available information about genes which will affect well-being, and their desires are based on irrational fears (e.g., about interfering with nature or playing God), then doctors should try to persuade them to access and use such information in their reproductive decision-making.

Notes

1. J. Savulescu. Sex Selection — the case for. *Medical Journal of Australia* 1999; 171: 373–75.
2. E.F. Fugger, S.H. Black, K. Keyvanfar, J.D. Schulman. Births of normal daughters after Microsort sperm separation and intrauterine insemination, in-vitro fertilization, or intracytoplasmic sperm injection. *Hum Reprod* 1998; 13: 2367–70.
3. D. Parfit. 1976. Rights, Interests and Possible People, in *Moral Problems in Medicine*, S. Gorovitz, et al, eds. Englewood Cliffs. Prentice Hall. D. Parfit. 1984. *Reasons and Persons*. Oxford. Clarendon Press: Part IV.
4. Parfit, *op. cit.*, Appendix I, pp. 493–502; Griffin. 1986. *Well-Being*. Oxford. Clarendon Press.
5. A. Buchanan, D.W. Brock, N. Daniels, D. Wikler. 2000. *From Chance to Choice*. Cambridge. CUP: 167. Buchanan and colleagues argue in a parallel way for the permissibility of genetic manipulation

(enhancement) to allow children to live the best life possible (Chapter Five). They do not consider selection in this context.

6. A. Newson. The value of intelligence and its implications for genetic research. *Fifth World Congress of Bioethics*, Imperial College, London, 21–24 September 2000.

7. *Philebus* 21 C 1–12. A.E. Taylor's translation. 1972. Folkstone. Dawsons of Pall Mall: 21 D 11–3, E 1–3.

8. *Philebus* 21 C 1–12.

9. J. Robertson. Preconception Sex Selection. *American Journal of Bioethics* 1:1 (Winter 2001).

Reading 7.2: Sarah E. Stoller, "Why We Are Not Morally Required to Select the Best Children: A Response to Savulescu"

Sarah Stoller responds to Julian Savulescu's argument in favor of procreative beneficence and concludes that Savulescu is wrong. For discussion of PGD, see the introduction to the chapter.

Introduction

The debate about the use of pre-implantation genetic diagnosis (PGD) for non-disease traits has traditionally centered on the moral permissibility of the practice. In an article published in this journal in 2001 entitled "Procreative Beneficence: Why We Should Select the Best Children," Julian Savulescu catapulted the debate to a new level, arguing that testing for non-disease traits of future offspring is not only morally permissible, but morally required.[1] Under a principle he calls "Procreative Beneficence," Savulescu asserts that reproducers have a moral obligation to select the child with the greatest chance of leading the best life. The principle implies that prospective parents are morally required to employ tests such as PGD to select the "best" embryos on the basis of both disease traits and non-disease traits like intelligence. While the Principle of Procreative Beneficence is novel and thought-provoking, it cannot withstand critical analysis.

Several articles have been written in response to Savulescu's paper, each evaluating certain aspects of his argument.[2] None, however, systematically explores the philosophical underpinnings of his theory to demonstrate where it breaks down. In this paper, I argue that the hypothetical examples Savulescu employs to support his theory in fact fail to justify it. He presents these examples as analogous to PGD, when in fact they differ from it in subtle but morally relevant ways. Specifically, Savulescu fails to acknowledge the fact that his examples evoke deontological and virtue ethics concerns that are absent in the context of PGD. These differences turn out to be crucial, so that, in the end, the analogies bear little support for his theory. Given that he bases the crux of his argument on these analogies, Savulescu fails to establish that we are morally obligated to select the best children.

First, Stoller summarizes Savulescu's argument.

Procreative Beneficence: Goods without Benefits and Wrongs without Harms

Although the decision of whether to select the best child may come up in various contexts, Savulescu primarily focuses on PGD. PGD, the technique by which embryos are tested for genetic traits, is performed during in vitro fertilization. Currently, PGD is used to screen embryos for genetic diseases and chromosomal abnormalities, as well as limited non-health related traits such as sex and tissue type. Currently, screening for broad behavioural or psychological non-disease traits like intelligence does not exist, as there is no clear link between such traits and particular genes. As Savulescu points out, however, research programmes are underway to establish these connections. With this research in mind, Savulescu defines the Principle of Procreative Beneficence (henceforth, "the PPB" or "the Principle") as follows: "couples (or single reproducers) should select the child, of the possible children they could have, who is expected to have the best life, or at least as good a life as the others, based on the relevant, available information."[3] The principle demands that, in the absence of some other reason for action, prospective parents use PGD to choose the embryo with the greatest chance of leading the best life (defined as "the life with the most well-being") based on both its disease and non-disease genes.[4] The non-disease trait that Savulescu selects as illustrative of his theory is intelligence, which he believes promotes well-being under any account of what it means to live a good and full life.[5]

The reason that Savulescu believes we ought to select the best children is that such choices will result in more fulfilling lives being led. This belief rests on the idea that we can create a moral good or moral wrong without any particular person benefiting from that good or being harmed by that wrong. That is to say, if we are deciding between Embryos A and B, with A qualifying as the "better" embryo, selecting A does not benefit A—at least, no more so than selecting B benefits B. Conversely, failing to select A does not harm A any more than failing to select B harms B.[6] The point is, rather, that the value of A's life relative to the value of B's life justifies the moral requirement to select A.

Savulescu's Argument for Procreative Beneficence: An Appeal to Intuition

To justify the Principle of Procreative Beneficence [PPB], Savulescu appeals to our intuition about situations involving the creation of better or worse lives. He describes two hypothetical situations, which I will call the "Nuclear Accident" and the "Case of Rubella," that he deems intuitively unethical, despite the fact that no particular person has been harmed. He then suggests that these intuitions can be explained only by a principle like the PPB; if the Nuclear Accident and the Case of Rubella are immoral, he concludes, so too are analogous acts such as foregoing PGD.[7]

In the Nuclear Accident hypothetical, a government opens an old and unsafe nuclear reactor in a poor town to provide its citizens with power during a cold winter. The reactor provides light and heating, a change that leads the townspeople to stay up later than they normally would. Several months later, the reactor melts down and releases large amounts of radiation. The only effect of the accident is that many children are subsequently born with predispositions to childhood malignancy. Because the change in light and heating caused the townspeople to alter their lifestyles, they conceived those children at different times from when they would have had there been no light or heat. As Savulescu explains, the particular children that were born, therefore, would not have been born had the government not switched to nuclear power. Accordingly, we cannot say that the government harmed those children, unless their lives were so bad as to be worse than not living at all.

> Stoller begins to critique Savulescu's analogy between the nuclear accident example and those who would use PPB. She examines the Nuclear Accident story from the views of the three big ethical perspectives mentioned in Chapter 2 (Stoller's argument, whether or not it succeeds, is an excellent example of moral reasoning about a case).

Savulescu goes on to explain how he sees the Nuclear Accident as relating to the PPB. He writes, "If we object to the Nuclear Accident (which most of us would), then we must appeal to some form of harmless wrong-doing. That is, we must claim that a wrong was done, but no one was harmed. We must appeal to something like the Principle of Procreative Beneficence."[8] The analogy is that, like the government's actions, failing to select the best child harms no one but is still unethical because a different, better child could have been born.[9] Savulescu is right to suggest that the government's actions seem intuitively immoral; whether we can extend this intuition to methods of selecting the best children, however, requires a closer analysis. If the Nuclear Accident differs from the failure to select the best children in morally relevant ways, we may condemn the government's actions while still rejecting the PPB.

Pinpointing exactly what is condemnable about the Nuclear Accident requires a brief look at ethical theory. Currently, consequentialism, deontology, and virtue ethics comprise three of the dominant approaches to morality.[10] Consequentialist theories hold that if the good consequences of an act outweigh the bad, the act is morally required, and if the bad outweigh the good, it is morally prohibited.[11] Deontological theories hold that the rightness or wrongness of an action depends not on its consequences, but on whether the actor has adhered to certain moral rules (e.g., "do not lie") that protect the rights of others.[12] Finally, virtue ethics focuses on the agent's character, asking what moral values and motivations are driving his actions.[13] The flaw in Savulescu's analysis of the Nuclear Accident (and the Case of Rubella, described below) is not that he supports one moral theory over the others. Rather, it is that he relies on one theory to explain our intuitions, when the remaining two theories better account for them.

While Savulescu does not explicitly adopt a particular moral theory in his discussion of the Nuclear Accident, he seems to judge it from a consequentialist standpoint. Rather than focusing on the government's intentions or actions, he points to the end result as the objectionable component of the hypothetical; in suggesting what is "wrong" about the Accident, he notes only that children are born with a predisposition to disease. If Savulescu is right to suggest that what we object to about the government's actions is the ultimate product—children born with a predisposition to childhood malignancy rather than different children born without it—then he is right that we must appeal to something like the PPB; if the birth of healthier children is better, in a moral sense, than the birth of less healthy children, we ought to condemn those who opt not to select the best children.

While a consequentialist account of the Nuclear Accident might support the PPB, it is not the only moral theory that can explain our intuition; deontology and virtue ethics can also account for the sense that something unethical has transpired. From a deontological perspective, we would look not at the ultimate consequences, but rather ask whether the government had knowingly broken the moral rule that forbids the harming of others, thereby violating their rights. Although not stated explicitly, Savulescu's hypothetical suggests that the government knew that the reactor was unsafe.[14] If the government did have such knowledge, it knowingly broke the rule against harming others;[15] in causing the emissions that damaged the embryos, it violated the rights of the children those embryos would become.[16] The fact that the children are not ultimately worse off as a result of the government's actions does not alter the fact that, once conceived, their rights were violated. Indeed, deontology is concerned with the rights of people; while no "unconceived" potential person has a right to be conceived, once she *is* conceived, that future person has a right not to be unduly harmed.[17]

If the government did not know the reactor was dangerous, but had been merely negligent in that regard, we may still condemn it from a virtue ethics perspective. Virtue ethicists, appraising the government's character, would reprimand it for not being more scrupulous in its decision to open an unsafe reactor. Like deontologists, virtue ethicists would not credit the fact that the children born as a result of their parents' altered schedules owed their existence to the government. Whether the parents' schedules had been altered or not, whatever children they conceived would have been harmed by the government's negligence; whether the harm accrued to one set of children as opposed to another is irrelevant in assessing the government's character.

> Stoller continues her argument: Savulescu has an unstated bias toward consequentialism, and only from a consequentialist position does the Nuclear Accident example support the PPB.

Approaching the Nuclear Accident either from a deontological or virtue ethics point of view reveals how we could logically and consistently object to the government's actions without supporting the PPB; from these ethical viewpoints, the morally condemnable aspects about the Nuclear Accident are absent in the context of the PPB. Deontology condemns the government for knowingly violating the moral rule against harming others. Parents opting not to employ PGD, however, harm no one. Virtue ethics focuses on the government's character, highlighting its negligence or indifference to harm. With respect to prospective parents refusing PGD, no comparable character flaw exists. Certainly, it is possible to conjure up a condemnable reason for not selecting the best child; parents wishing to have the spotlight on themselves, for example, might not want to be shown up by a more intelligent child. Notwithstanding such farfetched situations, however, parents who refuse PGD probably do so for reasons such as avoiding the burden of deciding which potential child to discard; the virtue ethicist would surely not condemn them for such a motivation. If, then, the reasons we object to the Nuclear Accident are the violation of a moral rule and its reflection on the actor's moral character, our intuition regarding the Nuclear Accident provides no support for the PPB.

Savulescu's Case of Rubella lends itself to similar analysis. He writes, "A woman has rubella. If she conceives now, she will have a blind and deaf child. If she waits three months, she will conceive another different but healthy child."[18] Savulescu concludes that she should choose to wait until the rubella has passed. His suggestion is that this intuition supports the PPB; if we feel that it is wrong to have a blind and deaf child rather than a seeing and hearing one, we are recognizing the moral requirement of having the "best" child.

As with the government's actions in the Nuclear Accident, Savulescu is right to suggest that we might feel troubled by the woman's choice to conceive while still afflicted with rubella (assuming that there is no compelling reason for her not to wait). Again, however, this judgment may not stem from the consequentialist view that it is better to have a child free of handicap. Indeed, our condemnation of the woman may derive primarily from virtue ethics concerns. In making a moral judgment, virtue ethics asks "what kind of person is this?" In the Case of Rubella, this is precisely the question we find troubling. Generally, it is probably fair to assume that a seeing and hearing parent would prefer to have a seeing and hearing child rather than a blind and deaf one; the former would be easier to care for, and the ability to communicate better might allow for a stronger connection between parent and child. Given that it seems counter to one's own interests to choose to have a blind and deaf child over a seeing and hearing one, we automatically ask what kind of person would actively prefer to conceive the former when it would be easy to conceive the latter. Might this woman be a sadist who wants to watch her child suffer? Is she an attention-seeker who desires recognition as a martyr for caring for a handicapped child? It is these kinds of character traits and motivations that a virtue ethicist would denounce.

As with the Nuclear Accident, the condemnable aspects of the Case of Rubella are absent in the context of the PPB. Indeed, opting not to employ PGD does not invite the same questions of dubious motivation as the woman's actions in the Case of Rubella, for several reasons. To begin with, the woman had no apparent reason not to wait until the rubella had passed to conceive, leading us to question her motivation. By contrast, there are various compelling reasons not to undergo PGD—the financial cost, for an example, or an aversion to "playing God"—so that the choice to refuse PGD does not raise the same troubling questions of incentive. Furthermore, in the Case of Rubella, the woman knew that her child would be blind and deaf if she conceived it at that moment, suggesting an active preference for the handicap; leaving a child's genetic make-up to nature, however—especially when there is no particular reason to believe he is at an increased risk of disease or disability—does not suggest an affirmative preference for dealing with pain and suffering. Finally, the analogy between the Case of Rubella and PGD is even weaker in the context of selecting for non-disease traits. Leaving a child's intelligence or athletic ability up to chance suggests none of the quasi-sadistic signs of character that preferring a blind and deaf child does.

Of course, if what is intuitively objectionable about the Nuclear Accident and the Case of Rubella is *not* the violation of moral rules or the actors' motivations, but rather, as Savulescu suggests, the ultimate consequences, then we must appeal to something like the PPB. One way to determine which aspects of Savulescu's hypothetical situations we find intuitively objectionable is to construct another one that is similar to the others in terms of the ultimate consequences (i.e., "worse" children being born rather than "better" children), but without the moral rule violation or the questionable motivations. If we still find the situation intuitively objectionable, it must be the consequences of worse children being born that trouble us; accordingly, we must accept a principle like the PPB. If, however, we find that the new hypothetical situation is *not* objectionable, then what we find troubling about the Nuclear Accident and the Case of Rubella cannot be the fact that children with disease or disability are born instead of healthier children. Accordingly, we would not have to interpret our objection to the Nuclear Accident or Case of Rubella as support for the PPB.

> Having criticized Savulescu's unstated preference for consequentialism, Stoller creates her own analogy.

Imagine that our country is faced with a difficult decision. In recent years, it had been discovered that two planets, millions of miles from earth, have human life on them. The two planets are nearly identical, but one has recently been struck with a temporary bird flu epidemic. The only notable effect of the virus was the possibility of congenital blindness; babies in utero at the time of the epidemic were at an increased risk of being born without vision. Meanwhile, it has come to our country's attention that two meteors are heading towards these two planets, certain to destroy them. Fortunately, our military has the technology to divert a meteor off its path. Unfortunately, it only has the resources to deflect one of the two meteors. Accordingly, our president must decide which of the two planets to save. There is no reason to suspect that we will ever come into contact with either of these planets or that the destruction of one as opposed to the other will affect the earth in any way. The president, however, is still uncomfortable with such a weighty decision in his hands. Feeling that blind children are just as worthy of life as seeing children, he decides to do what he believes to be the fair way of deciding—he flips a coin. As a result of the coin toss, he diverts the meteor heading towards the flu-stricken planet.

In this Meteor Dilemma, the relevant consequences mirror those in the Nuclear Accident and Case of Rubella; in all three situations, a group of less healthy children are born instead of a healthier group of children. Yet it seems to me that the president's course of action is intuitively less reprehensible than both the government's in the Nuclear Accident and the woman's in the Case of Rubella; whether or not we would have made the same decision, we do not condemn the president the way we do the actors in the other hypothetical situations.

The difference in intuition can most plausibly be explained by deontological and virtue ethics concerns. From a deontological point of view, unlike the government in the Nuclear Accident, the president violates no moral rule; in electing to save the flu-stricken planet, the president harms no one. From a virtue ethics point of view, the president's character does not seem worthy of reproach. In the Case of Rubella, the woman's character is questionable because of her seeming preference to give birth to a handicapped child. While a similar (though diluted) argument could be made for the president—not that he prefers the birth of blind children, but that he does not actively prefer the birth of seeing children—the reflection on his character is decidedly different. In the Case of Rubella, we questioned the woman's motivations because self-interest would seem to demand that she wait to conceive. In the Meteor Dilemma, however, given that the president has nothing personal to gain from making either choice, we have no reason to suspect perverse motivations overriding his self-interest. If anything, the motivation for his actions seems commendable, given that he was driven by a sense of fairness to use an objective method to make his decision.

If I am right that the president's decision seems intuitively unobjectionable, it becomes clear how we may oppose the Nuclear Accident and Case of Rubella while still rejecting the PPB. In summary, what troubles us about the Nuclear Accident and Case of Rubella is not the fact that children are born less healthy than other children who might have been born; such was also the case in the Meteor Dilemma, which did not seem unethical. Rather, the two aspects that seem intuitively wrong about the Nuclear Accident and Case of Rubella—the possibility of a moral rule violation and the questionable nature of the actors' characters—are not at issue in the context of the PPB. If the blameworthy aspects of the Nuclear

Accident and Rubella are absent in the context of PGD, Savulescu has failed to establish that our moral views towards them support the PPB.[19]

Ask yourself this: Does Stoller's argument prove that we shouldn't use PGD to produce the best child, or does it actually argue that PGD is not a moral duty in embryo selection? If the latter, then it presents us with a dilemma: accept the duty to pre-implant diagnosis and duty to make the best child follows, or deny both the duty to PGD (for disease traits in embyos) in order to deny procreative beneficence.

Conclusions and Implications

As the foregoing analysis suggests, the Nuclear Accident and Case of Rubella have little bearing on child selection at all. Given that Savulescu relies on these hypothetical cases to justify the PPB, he fails to establish that we have a moral obligation to select the best children. With no persuasive argument to the contrary, we are left with what was perhaps our original intuition—that we have no reason to believe ourselves morally obligated to select the best children....

In the area of procreation, then, when we focus solely on consequences, we ignore key components of our sense of morality. In most contexts, when dealing with a person whose identity is already determined, consequentialist accounts may provide moral answers and possibly encompass deontological and virtue ethics concerns along the way. When, however, we engage in the activity of creating life itself, and the question is not how to treat a particular person but which person if any to create, consequentialist thinking fails to capture all the relevant facets of the issue. Indeed, in the area of procreation, acting beneficently may not require the consequentialist demand of creating the best children; it may instead demand recognition of deontological and virtue ethics as an appropriate moral lens.

Notes

1. J. Savulescu. Procreative Beneficence: Why We Should Select the Best Children. *Bioethics* 2001; 15.
2. See, for example, I. de Melo-Martin. On Our Obligation to Select the Best Children. *Bioethics* 2004; 18; K. Birch. Beneficence, Determinism and Justice: An Engagement with the Argument for the Genetic Selection of Intelligence. *Bioethics* 2005; 19; M. Parker. The Best Possible Child. *J Med Ethics* 2007; 33.
3. Savulescu, *op. cit.* note 1, p. 415.
4. Ibid: 415, 419; While Savulescu believes that employing PGD is morally required, he thinks it should be encouraged rather than coerced. Ibid.

5. The questions of whether intelligence does in fact promote well-being or whether disability detracts from it are open to debate. For the purposes of this paper, however, I will accept those premises.

6. Of course, the *indirect* effects of employing PGD may benefit or harm particular individuals. For example, if fewer disabled persons are born as a result of PGD, the government will spend less money on their care, which will, in turn, benefit taxpayers. In terms of harm, the use of PGD might lead to an increase in social inequality, hurting less fortunate families who cannot afford the cost of PGD. Savulescu acknowledges these effects on third parties and notes that in certain circumstances, the negative effects of PGD might outweigh the benefits; in these cases, PGD might not be morally required (see, for example, his discussion on "Limits of Procreative Beneficence" on pages 424–25). These "third party effects," however, do not relate to the validity of the PPB itself. The PPB states only that the value of the better child's life justifies the moral imperative to use PGD; the speculative indirect effects, be they good (e.g., fewer taxes) or bad (e.g., an increase in inequality) neither support nor weaken the justification for the PPB. Rather, these potential benefits or hardships must be considered *in addition to*, or *as weighed against*, the Principle in determining whether to apply it in a particular situation.

7. Savulescu uses the Nuclear Accident and Case of Rubella to demonstrate why he believes that PGD may be *morally* required; additionally, he presents a hypothetical scenario involving a game of Wheel of Fortune to suggest that PGD may be *rationally* required (Savulescu, *op. cit.* note 1.) This latter claim is certainly subject to critique—prospective parents may have legitimate, rational reasons for not wishing to employ PGD; for example, they may not wish to carry the guilt of having discarded an embryo because of the prediction of a less than stellar IQ. This paper, however, will address only the claim that employing PGD is morally, not rationally, required.

8. Savulescu, *op. cit.* note 1, p. 418.

9. Note that in the Nuclear Accident, despite Savulescu's assertion that 'no one was harmed', there actually *are* victims of the government's actions: the children's parents, who will suffer both emotionally and financially as a result of their children's diseases, and the community as a whole, who may bear part of the cost of the children's healthcare in higher taxes. As explained in footnote 6, however, Savulescu does not rely on effects on third parties to justify the PPB, nor does he rely on effects on the parents or taxpayers to justify why we find the Nuclear Accident morally troublesome. Rather, in both situations, his focus is on the value of the children's lives.

10. B. Gert, C.M. Culver & K.D. Clouser. 1997. *Bioethics: A Return to Fundamentals*. New York: Oxford University Press.

11. Ibid.

12. T. Nagel. 2003. Agent-Relativity and Deontology. In *Deontology*. S. Darwall, ed. Malden, MA: Blackwell Publishing.

13. For a discussion of virtue ethics, see R. Hursthouse. Virtue Theory and Abortion. *Philos Public Aff* 1991.

14. Savulescu writes that "[t]he government decides to open an old and unsafe nuclear reactor," suggesting that the government knew the reactor was unsafe at the time of its decision. Savulescu, *op. cit.* note 1, p. 417.

15. The rule might be more accurately stated as "do not engage in behaviour likely to cause *avoidable* harm to others." Thus, the unavoidable pain that a baby suffers as it is delivered would not be a violation of that baby's rights. In the Nuclear Accident, however, the damage caused by the plant's emissions was not unavoidable; though it was not the case in this particular hypothetical scenario, it is theoretically possible for those children to have been born without the damage caused in utero.

16. Note that whether or not we believe that embryos have rights, the children that are born as a result of the government's actions have been harmed and their rights have been violated; the fact that the harm first accrued to them before birth as opposed to after birth is not morally relevant.

17. Some formulations of deontology, however, hold that to violate a deontological rule, one must violate that rule *intentionally*. See, e.g., Nagel, *op. cit.* note 13. Under this formulation, since the government presumably did not intend to harm the embryos, its actions would be less condemnable.

18. Savulescu, *op. cit.* note 1, p. 417.

19. Of course, if the president's decision *does* seem morally blameworthy, that intuition supports the PPB. In condemning the president, one is necessarily adopting a consequentialist viewpoint; the argument would be that the flu-free planet should have been saved because the existence of seeing children is better than the existence of blind children—an argument that is clearly in line with the PPB.

Reading 7.3: Rebecca Briscoe, "Ethical Considerations, Safety Precautions and Parenthood in Legalising Mitochondrial Donation"

Briscoe argues that there are no good reasons to prevent mitochondrial replacement through donation. She considers several objections based on the worries about three-parent embryos and finds that none of them should prevent legalization.

[...]

Background

The intention of mitochondrial donation is to prevent inheritance through the maternal line of mutations in mitochondrial DNA, while allowing the intended parents to have a child to whom they both genetically contribute. There are currently two techniques proposed for use, which involve manipulation either before or after fertilisation. Both techniques substitute the nucleic DNA of the enucleated donated ovum for the intended mother's nucleic DNA, and combine the intended mother's nucleic DNA with the intended father's nucleic DNA. However, there is presumably no reason why donated sperm cannot also be used in place of the intended father's sperm.

The two potential techniques proposed are:

1. Spindle-chromosome complex transfer (Tachibana *et al.* 2009, 2013), and
2. Pronucleus transfer (Craven *et al.* 2010).

1. *Spindle-chromosome complex transfer*
   a. The donated egg's nucleic DNA is removed;
   b. The intended mother's egg's nucleic chromosomes, along with the associated spindle, are transferred into the enucleated donated egg;
   c. The intended father's sperm is allowed to fertilise the newly created ovum comprising of nucleic DNA from the intended mother and the rest of the cell from the donor of the enucleated egg.

2. *Pronucleus transfer*
   a. Sperm from the intended father or from a donor is used to fertilise the donated egg;
   b. The fertilised donated egg's pronuclei are removed;

c. The intended father's sperm is allowed to fertilise the egg from the intended mother,

d. The pronuclei from the created embryo are transferred into the enucleated donated egg.

Although it may at present be impossible to accurately predict which method will prove easier or safer, and therefore potentially more desirable as a reproductive technology, Craven et al. (2010), having compared their results with those reported by Tachibana et al. (2009), declared a belief that both approaches may be effective in preventing transmission of mitochondrial DNA mutations from mother to child (Craven et al. 2010: 84).

Ethical Considerations of Legalising Mitochondrial Donation

EQUALITY

Arguably, assisted reproductive techniques have offered women more control over their fertility. Evidence suggests that techniques such as intra-cytoplasmic sperm injection have offered men the same increased ability to control their fertility. However, while both sexes may pass on any mutations in their nucleic DNA, only women pass on mitochondrial DNA mutations to their children. Currently this means that if a man has disease-causing mutations in his mitochondrial DNA, he need not worry about conceiving children naturally, but women must use donor eggs if they wish to be certain not to pass on their mitochondrial DNA mutations, thus meaning that they will not be genetically related to their children. Therefore mitochondrial donation arguably offers women the opportunity to rectify this biological inequality between the sexes.

DONORS

Since either proposed method of mitochondrial donation requires modification of a donated ovum *in vitro*, the process of egg donation ought not differ from current practice. One concern may relate to the safety of the donor should greater numbers of ova be required for similar efficacy of fertilisation as compared with current egg donation. This is discussed in more detail in the *Safety Requirements* section, below, but it is important to note that in order to be ethically sound, the safety of the donor must be ensured, and there must be no unreasonable burden placed on the donor beyond that already existing for egg donors. Aside from safety concerns for the donors, it is also important that current guidelines about information provision and counselling (National Institute for Health and Care Excellence 2013, section 1.15.3) are followed for all egg donors, including those specifically for mitochondrial donation. The details about risks of donation should not be different since practice should not change; however the areas discussed during counselling may require modification. These areas relate to "the physical and psychological implications of treatment for themselves and their genetic children" (National Institute for Health and Care Excellence 2013, section 1.15.3.2) and changes would be required in order to incorporate information about unknown health risks to children resulting from mitochondrial donation. Provided that these modifications were made to pre-donation counselling and information provision, and also that the process of egg donation remains in line with current practice, there are no apparent ethical objections to mitochondrial donation specifically from the perspective of the donor, beyond those encountered with current egg donation practices.

DISABILITY

It is not a new proposition to utilise technology to prevent the transmission of inherited diseases, and the arguments for and against this have been well rehearsed. Given the ability to prevent the birth (even if not the conception) of a child with a debilitating condition, there is an argument that it may be immoral to deliberately conceive, and allow to be born, a child who has such a disability (Deech and Smajdor 2007: 50). Parental duties perhaps include preventing the child from inheriting a genetic disorder if this is possible (Glover 2006: 62). Certainly parents who have already had one child with an inherited disorder may feel unable to cope with a second, or simply feel that it would be unfair to wish the same suffering on another child (Glover 2006: 28). However, there is also the risk that a decision not to have a child with a specific condition could cause distress to someone with that condition (Glover 2006: 34), as it may appear that the parents are insulting the quality of that person's life.

While both sides of this debate are very emotive and justifiable, it is legally permissible in the UK to prevent the birth of a child with a serious disability (Abortion Act 1967, section 1(d)). Whatever one's personal views about this, it is likely that most people would prefer to intervene during the conception of the child rather than merely prevent it from being born. Therefore mitochondrial donation is arguably a more ethically justifiable method of creating a child free from a specific inherited disease.

IDENTITY

There is concern that decisions about genetic inheritance should not be made by the parents of the child for the reason that it could appear too much like designing one's children (Glover 2006: 2). Knowledge that they were created in a specific fashion could have a detrimental impact on the self-perceived identity of children (Nuffield Council on Bioethics 2012, section 4.10), as they could feel as though they were created to specific criteria or that they are "puppets of [their] parents" (Glover 2006: 72).

There is also the undeniable fact that a medical condition, whatever its cause, can have an enormous impact on a person's self-image and thus their identity (Nuffield Council on Bioethics 2012, section 4.9). Crucially, this does not mean that a person's self-perceived identity will be positively or negatively affected by the presence or absence of a disorder, and the impact will certainly vary between people. It is also important to note that a disability is not an identity, and a person's self-image, although it may be altered by their disability, is not dependent upon it (Murugami 2009). Therefore, although it is logical to assume that a child born as a result of mitochondrial donation, without an inherited mitochondrial disease, may develop a different self-perceived identity from that which it would otherwise have had, there is no method of determining how much the child's identity would be affected and which identity would be of greater benefit to the child. In the absence of such knowledge, it is illogical to oppose mitochondrial donation on the grounds that it is likely to alter the child's identity.

FUTURE IMPLICATIONS

Although mitochondrial donation has been proposed as a method for allowing a heterosexual couple to create a child to whom they both genetically contribute, while preventing the inheritance of a specific mitochondrial DNA mutation, the technique could have other possible uses in the future. For example, homosexual women who wished to have a child together, to whom they both contributed genetically, could make use of mitochondrial donation alongside sperm donation (Nuffield Council on Bioethics 2012, section 4.141). However, some female homosexual couples may not feel that this would be necessary, as the genetic contributors, whether of nucleic or mitochondrial DNA, are not necessarily regarded in British law as the parents of a child conceived through assisted reproductive technologies. According to the Human Fertilisation and Embryology Act 1990, the woman who carried the child would still be viewed as the child's mother (section 27), and, in line with the 2008 Act amendment, the couple would have to both agree that the other woman was to be the child's other parent (section 43), unless they were in a civil union, in which case this would be assumed (section 42).

The same would apply to people wishing to conceive a child with a genetic link to the three people who intended to act as the child's social parents. With the recent civil union in Brazil between three people (BBC 2012), there is a potential that people in such unions could desire children, and mitochondrial donation offers an opportunity for that child to be genetically connected to all three social parents. However, only one woman may carry the child, and this woman will be considered the child's legal mother under UK law (Human Fertilisation and Embryology Act 1990, section 27).

A child resulting from mitochondrial donation will carry genetic information from three people. This is the first time that such a concept has been a realisable ambition, but potentially it is not the last. Currently, it is neither possible nor legal in the UK (Human Fertilisation and Embryology Act 2008, section 3) to specifically alter the nucleic DNA of a human gamete or embryo and then implant it into a woman for gestation. However, if mitochondrial donation becomes legal as a method of assisted reproduction, it will be the first legal replacement of some of a future child's genetic information, which would also be transmitted to the descendents of any female resultant child. This opens the possibility for legalisation of targeted removal and replacement of nucleic genes, if this were found to be possible. A convention of the Council of Europe currently prohibits interference with the human genome that would cause a change in the genome of the descendents of any resultant children (1997, article 13). Deviation from this convention could seriously impact on how society views humanity's relationship with its genetic history and connection with the rest of the animal kingdom. Historically, the maternal transmission of mitochondrial DNA, along with the wide diversity of this DNA within the human population, has allowed ancestral tracing of humankind back thousands of years, potentially identifying a common mitochondrial ancestor to the current human population (Holt and Jacobs 1994: 31). It is important to note that practices such as adoption and gamete donation have already altered this natural inheritance of mitochondrial DNA, and therefore the risk of replacing one line of mitochondrial DNA with another, through donation, may not appear that significant.

However, given that mitochondrial disorders may arise from mutations in either mitochondrial or nucleic DNA, it would appear unjust to offer assistance for a couple carrying a mutation in mitochondrial DNA but not to one with a nucleic mutation that caused similar symptoms (Nuffield Council on Bioethics 2012, section 3.7). Although present in separate organelles within the human cell, there is no clear distinction between genes on mitochondrial DNA and those on nucleic DNA, meaning that drawing a line at which genetic interference must stop becomes more difficult. It may never become possible to safely modify nucleic genes inside a gamete or an embryo before implantation, but, if mitochondrial donation is legalised as an assisted reproductive technique, there may come a point where this potential will have to be addressed....

Parenthood

IS IT REALLY "THREE PARENT IVF"?

... Genetic and biological parents who have not used any method of assisted reproduction are usually granted the right to retain their child, which is arguably a form of a right to ownership of the child (Barton and Douglas 1995: 20). However, ownership implies possession of goods, which is always in the owner's interests. This is not the case where children are concerned, as the current international emphasis is on children's rights and, specifically, protecting children from harm (United Nations 1989). Therefore, evidence suggests that the reason why natural biological parents are able to retain their children, unless there are concerns about the child's safety, is because it is held to be in the child's best interests not to be separated from its caregivers unnecessarily. Thus the right of natural biological parents to retain their children is only granted in order to provide the best protection to the children concerned (Barton and Douglas 1995: 23)....

The traditional view that parenthood is dependent upon a genetic contribution made to the child has been challenged repeatedly by adoption, artificial insemination, gamete donation, and embryo donation. As a result of this, genetic contribution has been downplayed in importance in the legal recognition of parenthood. Concurrently, more assisted reproductive techniques have been developed to allow people to create a child with whom there is some genetic link between the child and the intended social parents. The resulting paradox is that genetic contribution is held to be as important as the adults contributing the genetic information believe it to be (Nuffield Council on Bioethics 2012, section 4.143). Although it can be argued that this has led to a move towards supporting social parenthood over genetic parenthood (Barton and Douglas 1995: 89), the application of assisted reproductive law to surrogacy shows that it is gestational parenthood that has been emphasized....

Although it has previously been possible to create a child with three biological parents, using gametes from two people and implanting the resultant embryo into another woman, mitochondrial donation presents the first opportunity for a child to be born with three genetic parents....

A NEW PARENTHOOD?

... Thus there is a potential for more than two people to be viewed in law as the parents of a child. While it is unlikely that full parenthood roles will be applied to more than two people in the near future, it is possible that the social parents will be called the child's parents and other contributors (genetic or gestational) will have a different role. The proposal about "limited" parents (Shanley 2001: 143) raises the issue of rights and duties of parenthood; should every person with the title of parent, or limited parent, have the same rights over, and duties towards, "their" child? (Barton and Douglas 1995: 18). With the proposal of other contributors being recognised in law, it seems unrealistic to endow all contributors to a child with the same rights and responsibilities. The title given to these "extra" parents, how they could be identified and categorised, and the rights and responsibilities that accompany the title are yet to be determined and are unlikely to be agreed immediately. However, since mitochondrial donation can be understood in the context of full egg donation, perhaps full gamete donors and mitochondrial donors alike could be accorded a new "semi-parental" status. The proposal to introduce mitochondrial donation could therefore be seen as a welcome opportunity to discuss the potential for children to have more than two parents.

Conclusion

This discussion of some of the ethical considerations arising from the proposal to legalise mitochondrial donation has revealed no clear objections to its introduction as an assisted reproductive technique. Therefore, although there also remain the well-traversed arguments surrounding the existing techniques of IVF and gamete donation, which would also apply to mitochondrial donation, this article finds no new ethical objection specifically contesting legalisation of this technique. However, it cannot claim to be a full discussion about all of the potential problems that may arise, and care must be taken to ensure that there is an ongoing ethical reflection if this technology is used....

Furthermore, since parenthood can only be understood in relation to contribution to a child, be it a genetic, gestational or social contribution, existing and emerging assisted reproductive technologies, alongside increasing acceptance of changing societal family structures, may necessitate a degree of recognition of more than two contributors to a child. The proposal for legalising mitochondrial donation provides an opportunity for consideration of how parenthood is viewed and defined in British law and culture, and whether there is a potential for change. Whether or not this opportunity is seized, logic dictates that it is in the interests of children to begin these discussions sooner rather than later.

Bibliography [for this extract]

Barton, C., and G. Douglas., 1995. *Law and Parenthood*. London: Butterworths.

BBC, 2012. Three-Person Civil Union Sparks Controversy in Brazil. *BBC News*. Available at: http:// www.bbc. co.uk/news/world-latin-america-19402508 (accessed 28 August 2012).

Council of Europe, 1997. *Convention for the Protection of Human Rights and Dignity of the Human Being with regard to the Application of Biology and Medicine: Convention on Human Rights and Biomedicine*.

Craven, L., H.A. Tuppen, G.D. Greggains, S.J. Harbottle, *et al.*, 2010. Pronuclear Transfer in Human Embryos to Prevent Transmission of Mitochondrial DNA Disease. *Nature*, 465, pp. 82–85.

Deech, R., and A. Smajdor, 2007. *From IVF to Immortality: Controversy in the Era of Reproductive Technology*. Oxford: Oxford University Press.

Glover, J., 2006. *Choosing Children: Genes, Disability, and Design*. Oxford: Oxford University Press.

Holt, I.J., and H.T. Jacobs, 1994. The Structure and Expression of Normal and Mutant Mitochondrial Genomes. In V. Darley-Usmar, and A. H. V. Schapira, eds. *Mitochondria: DNA, Proteins and Disease*. London: Portland Press, pp. 27–54.

Murugami, M.W., 2009. Disability and Identity. *Disability Studies Quarterly*, 29.4. Available at: http://dsq-sds.org/article/view/979/1173 (accessed 1 September 2012).

National Institute for Health and Care Excellence, 2013. *Fertility (CG156)*.

Nuffield Council on Bioethics, 2012. *Novel Techniques for the Prevention of Mitochondrial DNA Disorders: An Ethical Review*.

Shanley, M.L., 2001. *Making Babies, Making Families: What Matters Most in an Age of Reproductive Technologies, Surrogacy, Adoption, and Same-Sex and Unwed Parents*. Boston: Beacon Press.

Tachibana, M., M. Sparman, H. Sritanaudomchai, H. Ma, *et al.*, 2009. Mitochondrial Gene Replacement in Primate Offspring and Embryonic Stem Cells. *Nature*, 461, pp. 367–72.

Tachibana, M., P. Amato, M. Sparman, J. Woodward, *et al.*, 2013. Towards Germline Gene Therapy of Inherited Mitochondrial Diseases. *Nature*, 493, pp. 627–31.

United Nations, 1989. *Convention on the Rights of the Child*.

Reading 7.4: Katarina Lee, "Ethical Implications of Permitting Mitochondrial Replacement"

Katarina Lee disagrees with Briscoe and argues that mitochondrial replacement should not be legalized.

Mitochondrial replacement techniques made headlines in February 2015 when the United Kingdom became the first country "to approve laws to allow the creation of babies from three people."[1] MRTs are meant to create what is colloquially known as three-parent embryos. The purpose of this technology is to assist women with severe mitochondrial disease to have children without the disease.[2] Essentially, the mtDNA (mitochondrial DNA) of an ovum or embryo is removed and replaced with the mtDNA of a donor.[3] The first report of a baby born by this technique was made public in September 2016.[4] While the United Kingdom has a tendency to pass legislation regarding assisted reproductive technologies before other nations, in February 2016, American ethicists also argued that in limited circumstances MRTs would be ethically permissible.[5] ...

Brief History of Mitochondrial Manipulation

... In 2013, the FDA also asserted jurisdiction over OvaScience's Augment procedure, in which mitochondria from a woman are inserted into her own ova to "revitalize" them. The FDA deemed this a form of genetic therapy that required an investigational new drug application. As a result, OvaScience halted development of Augment in the United States and began using the technique abroad. At least one birth has been reported following its use.

The FDA took a more proactive approach to three-parent embryos. In February 2016, the Institute of Medicine published a report titled *Mitochondrial Replacement Techniques: Ethical, Social and Policy Considerations*.[6] The report, sponsored by the FDA, resulted from a study conducted by prominent bioethicists, physicians, lawyers, and scientists regarding the ethical feasibility of MRTs. The committee concluded that investigative studies of these therapies are permissible as long as specific conditions are met. The report highlights many of the ethical issues and federal concerns with MRTs, but fails to comprehensively address the effect of MRTs on parentage laws.[7]

While an extended discussion is outside the scope of this paper, several legal parentage questions would have to be adequately addressed prior to permitting MRTs. Legal parentage in the United States is granted through genetic or gestational ties to children as well as through intention.[8] Historically, children had two legal parents: a legal mother and a legal father. Legal parentage was granted either through state law or through the Uniform Parentage Act. With the advent of nontraditional family structures and the legalization of same-sex marriage, individual states have had to amend their traditional notions of a legal father and legal mother to allow for two legal mothers or two legal fathers.[9] Generally, states are still reluctant to recognize three legal parents, although a small but growing number of courts and legislative bodies have done so.[10]

Lastly, while the bioethics committee suggested that MRTs may be ethically permissible, Congress's 2016 budget bill prohibits the government from funding "research in which a human embryo is intentionally created or modified to include a heritable genetic modification"—that is, any experiment that genetically alters a human embryo.[11] Additionally, the Dickey–Wicker amendment "prohibits *federal funds* being used for any research in which a human embryo is either created for research purposes or destroyed as part of the research."[12]

Mitochondrial Disease and the MRT Process

Before describing MRTs, it is important to understand what mitochondrial diseases are. Essentially they "occur when mitochondria fail to produce enough energy for the body to function properly."[13] This results from a mutation of either nuclear DNA or mitochondrial DNA.[14] Mitochondrial diseases vary in severity and can affect a variety of cells, including those of the eyes, ears, brain, nerves, muscles, heart, and other organs. Additionally, if mitochondria do not behave normally, they may cause secondary mitochondrial dysfunction leading to other diseases, including Parkinson's, Alzheimer's, Lou Gehrig's, autism, cancer, and diabetes....

Ethical Arguments in Opposition to MRTs

> Below is Lee's thesis paragraph. Which of our ethical principles does Lee appeal to in her four reasons that mitochondrial replacement should not be legalized?

While MRTs may give women the opportunity to have genetically related children who will not inherit their mitochondrial diseases, there are several ethical arguments against these practices. In this portion of the paper, I will discuss (1) medical risks associated with the procedures, (2) informed consent concerns, (3) resource allocation issues, and (4) the effect MRTs will have on the assisted reproductive technology market. I have excluded a discussion of the ethical and moral permissibility of destroying embryos, as this debate, while important, is applicable to many reproductive technologies that do not use MRTs. It is important to note, however, that the potential destruction of embryos raises significant ethical questions about duties to future persons as well as the rights of embryos.[15] Additionally, I will not argue that one form of MRT is more ethically permissible than another, but will note that the manipulation of ova rather than embryos poses fewer ethical quandaries.

MEDICAL RISKS ARE TOO DANGEROUS

Potentially the most persuasive argument against MRTs is based on the medical risks associated with the procedure. Medical risks exist for the intended mother, the ova donor, a gestational surrogate (if used), the embryo, and the children he or she may have after reaching adulthood. The medical concerns are mostly speculative at this time, because the limited available data, which come mostly from nonhuman studies, are inconclusive about the safety of these procedures.[16] Importantly, studies conducted with mice have shown an increase in exhaustion as well as a change in learning capabilities and behavior in mice with mismatched nuclear and mitochondrial DNA.[17] Moreover, the data on human zygotes and embryos are unclear because the subjects were abnormally fertilized, as they were unipronuclear and tripronuclear.[18]

While these embryos may be gestated by the intended mothers, it is also possible that surrogates will be employed. As a result, it is important to acknowledge potential health risks to both groups of gestating women as well as both groups of ova donors. As with other IVF procedures, the intended mother and the ova donor will have to undergo ova retrieval so that the intended mother's nDNA can be removed from her ovum and placed into the ovum with healthy mtDNA. Ova retrieval involves two main steps: In the first, the woman ingests a number of drugs to stimulate her ovaries and mature the ova; then clinicians retrieve the ova. Retrieval is typically done by transvaginal ultrasound aspiration, in which a needle inserted through the vagina punctures the ovary to retrieve matured ova.[19] "Potential side effects of this process include bruising, nausea, allergic reactions, injury to adjacent organs, infection, and ovarian hyperstimulation syndrome, which in rare cases can lead to blood clots and kidney failure."[20] If the intended mother also wishes to gestate the embryo, she must undergo an additional drug regimen to prepare her uterus for embryo transfer.[21] Notably, this process increases the risk of ectopic pregnancy.[22] If a surrogate gestates the embryo instead, she will face this risk as well....

While there are potential medical consequences for the women who participate in MRTs, arguably the greatest health risks will be faced by the embryos and by future generations. As will be addressed, the most persuasive arguments in support of MRTs are that individuals have the right to choose autonomously to procreate in this way and that the assumption of potential risks is an extension of their autonomous decision-making capacity. There are some procedures, however, to which individuals should not be able to consent, because they are simply too risky.

INFORMED CONSENT CONCERNS

... Compared to the sperm provider and the ova donor, the intended mother bears significantly greater risk and responsibility. First, while both she and the ova donor must consent to undergoing the ova retrieval process, the intended mother is in most cases the one accepting the risks associated with gestation and consenting to the creation of the three-parent embryo. Given the limited data, it may be difficult for her to accurately consent to these procedures. Another concern, especially with the intended mother, is that her emotional desire to have a disease-free child may unduly motivate her to consent to the creation of the embryos. This is not to suggest that women cannot consent to procedures in which they are emotionally invested, but the desire to have a disease-free child to whom she is genetically tied arguably makes obtaining truly informed consent difficult, if not impossible. Intended mothers cannot consent objectively. Moreover, the intended mother bears the burden of consenting to a procedure that may, in fact, have negative health consequences for her future child. While several of these concerns are relevant in other assisted reproductive technologies, the limited data as well as disease prevention make obtaining informed consent from intended mothers more difficult....

If the intended mother enters into a three-parent arrangement with the intended father, he should be a part of the consent process. Notably, he may be the sperm generator or the legal father of the future child. In every case, he should be required to consent to the procedure. Like the intended mother, the intended father may have difficulty understanding the medical risks and may oppose a procedure that could harm the child created by MRT....

[It] should be acknowledged that while embryos cannot consent to their creation, questions about whether intended parents should be able to consent to the creation of embryos using risky procedures are open to ethical debate. Most of this debate centers on duties to future persons, often referenced as the non-identity problem.[23] While it is extremely difficult to argue that an embryo is better off not existing than existing, some would argue that intended parents have a duty to not subject their future children to the undue risks posed by MRTs. Opponents of this concern would argue that individual autonomy permits intended parents to create children by the use of MRTs: given that the animal data are highly inconclusive and that individuals can create families by a variety of means, intended parents who use MRTs are not exposing their children to extraordinary risk. In light of the sheer number of parties involved in the creation of three-parent embryos as well as the medical risks and emotional ties associated with consenting to this practice, gaining truly informed consent is extremely difficult if not impossible.

RESOURCE ALLOCATION

Some general concerns with experimental procedures are (1) whether resources should be spent on a given protocol and (2) who should fund it. Since Congress has prohibited governmental funding, MRT procedures, if permitted by the FDA, would have to be privately funded. One of the largest concerns is that from a utilitarian perspective, investing in MRTs benefits a very small portion of the population. As Jeffrey Kahn highlights, only a few hundred individuals in the United States would even be eligible to use these technologies, as the condition and the odds of severe mitochondrial defects are rare.[24] Conceivably, the procedure's resource cost is greater than its benefit to a few hundred individuals. Additionally, MRTs circumvent and, in theory, could eventually eradicate mitochondrial disease. They are not in fact treating mitochondrial disease. Arguably, resources should be spent on curing, not bypassing, disease. If MRT research is privately funded, additional concerns arise about insurance coverage as well as adverse-event protections. The United States offers very weak protections for individuals who experience an adverse event after engaging in experimental research.[25] If the research is government funded, there is likely to be significant discord, since many taxpayers believe that experiments on embryos are morally impermissible. Given the common practice of assisted reproduction in the United States, which is generally paid for out of pocket or through an employee compensation package, it is reasonable to expect that individuals who wish to undergo MRT treatments would pay for it in the same ways.[26]

Relevant Slippery Slope Concerns

> Recall the discussion of slippery slopes at the beginning of this chapter. Notice that Lee employs a similar argument. Do you think this line of argument is compelling? Why or why not?

While slippery slope arguments are fallible, because the permissibility of any given procedure will not necessitate a "jump" to another procedure, it is important to address the effect MRTs could have on assisted reproductive technologies. MRTs raise the question about the permissibility of other forms of genetic manipulation, especially in the context of eradicating disease. However, defining the difference between disease and enhancement further complicates the ethical debate surrounding genetic engineering. Moreover, if only the gestation of male embryos is supported, as recommended by the authors of the National Academies report, additional concerns about sex selection arise. Lastly, like all assisted reproductive technologies, MRTs could create an additional divide between the wealthy and the poor, since only the wealthy are likely to have access to such techniques and the ability to pay for them. While some of these concerns are secondary to the ethical permissibility of MRTs, they should be fully analyzed before the techniques are permitted in the United States.

Relevant Counterarguments

> Notice how Lee considers objections to her thesis. Pay close attention to how she answers these objections. Ask yourself: Has the author done a

> good job of answering potential criticisms? Did she leave out some objection that is more important? (Whether you ultimately agree with Lee or not, her technique here of the defense phase of the 5 Ds is a good one to emulate.)

While unknown and known medical risks, obstacles to informed consent, concerns about resource allocation, and slippery slope concerns preclude the use of MRTs, three counterarguments should also be considered, namely, (1) autonomy, (2) beneficence, and (3) the advancement of science.

AUTONOMY

The strongest argument in favor of MRTs maintains that individual autonomy should be protected. The four traditional bioethical principles promulgated by Tom Beauchamp and James Childress are autonomy, beneficence, non-maleficence, and justice. If a given medical or research practice accords with these principles, it generally is considered ethically permissible. Autonomy, or "the obligation to respect the decision making capacities of autonomous persons," has become the most highly regarded of these principles.[27] Thus, the argument goes, if consenting adults decide to create embryos using MRTs, then scientists, medical researchers, and ethicists should support their decision. Proponents argue that this is especially true in this situation, since for a woman with mitochondrial disease, MRTs provide the only opportunity for her to have a healthy child who is genetically related to her.

However, autonomy has limits. Generally, autonomous choices are permissible if the individual can consent and the decision does not harm the individual or others.[28] As argued above, gaining truly informed consent from all parties involved in MRT procedures is difficult if not impossible, and considering the medical risks to both the gestating mother and the child, the autonomy argument is not persuasive. Moreover, as mentioned above, the creation of embryos in a laboratory setting is rejected on moral grounds by many ethicists, including those in the Roman Catholic tradition.

BENEFICENCE

Beneficence, or the "obligations to provide benefits and to balance benefits against risks," is the second most compelling argument for permitting MRTs.[29] Mitochondrial diseases are terrible life-altering diseases that may result in death. Using MRTs will conceivably eradicate these diseases from the population, and eradicating disease provides a benefit to future children as well as to society. Moreover, proponents argue that society has an obligation to assist individuals in having children, as procreation is a natural human function.

While eradicating disease is clearly a benefit, the beneficence argument is not compelling because (1) the benefit of eradicating disease does not clearly outweigh the potential risks of MRTs; (2) practically, for inheritable mitochondrial defects to be eradicated, everyone with the condition would have to undergo MRTs or refrain from having children; (3) the MRT process is arguably eugenic, because it does not treat a disease but simply breeds it out; and (4) individuals have other opportunities to become parents.

ADVANCEMENT OF SCIENCE

A less compelling argument in favor of MRTs is that the development of this technology is a positive scientific advancement. Not only will the technology help eradicate disease, but it also may aid further scientific advancement. Its development could provide insight into how genetic manipulation can be used to eradicate other diseases. Additionally, it will provide valuable information about the interactions between nDNA and mtDNA. Lastly, MRTs, if deemed safe and efficacious, may enable individuals to create children with genetic ties to three parents without a medical need. For example, female homosexual couples may wish to create a child that has genetic material from both partners. While scientific advancement is generally a positive goal, it is not a sufficient condition for permitting a practice that has significant medical risk.

…

Notes

1. James Gallagher, "UK Approves Three-Person Babies," *BBC News*, February 24, 2015, http://www.bbc.com/.
2. Ian Sample, "'Three-Parent' Babies Explained: What Are the Concerns and Are They Justified?," *Guardian*, February 2, 2015, https://www.theguardian.com/.
3. Margaret Marsh, "'Three Parent Embryos' Back in the News," February 18, 2016, http://mmarsh.camden.rutgers.edu/.
4. American Society for Reproductive Medicine (ASRM), "Report of First Baby Born Using Spindle Nuclear Transfer to Prevent Mitochondrial Disease," news release, September 27, 2016, https://www.asrm.org/.
5. Anne B. Claiborne, Rebecca A. English, and Jeffrey P. Kahn, "Finding an Ethical Path Forward for Mitochondrial Replacement," *Science* 351.6274 (February 12, 2016), doi: 10.1126/science.aaf3091.
6. National Academies of Science, Engineering and Medicine, *Mitochondrial Replacement Techniques: Ethical, Social, and Policy Considerations* (Washington, DC: National Academies Press, 2016).
7. Ibid., 79–112; see also the briefing slides (February 2, 2016) at http://www.national academies.org/.
8. Katarina Lee, "Shifting Surrogacy Laws and Legal Parenthood," *Voices in Bioethics*, August 26, 2015, https://voicesinbioethics.net/.
9. See Douglas NeJaime, "With Ruling on Marriage Equality, Fight for Gay Families Is Next," *Los Angeles Times*, June 26, 2015, http://www.latimes.com/.
10. Ian Lovett, "Measure Opens Door to Three Parents, or Four," *New York Times*, July 13, 2012, http://www.nytimes.com/; Gabrielle Emanuel, "Three (Parents) Can Be a Crowd, but for Some It's a Family,"

NPR, March 30, 2014, http://www.npr.org/; and Patrick McGreevy and Melanie Mason, "Brown Signs Bill to Allow Children More Than Two Legal Parents," *Los Angeles Times*, October 4, 2013, http://articles.latimes.com/.

11. Consolidated Appropriations Act of 2016, Pub. L. 114-113, sec. 749. See also Joel Achenbach, "Ethicists Approve '3 Parent' Embryos to Stop Diseases, but Congressional Ban Remains," *Washington Post*, February 3, 2016, https://www.washingtonpost.com/; and Ike Swetlitz, "FDA Urged to Approve 'Three-Parent Embryos,' a New Frontier in Reproduction," *STAT*, February 3, 2016, https://www.statnews.com/.

12. Marsh, "'Three Parent Embryos' Back in the News," original emphasis; and Megan Kearl, "Dickey-Wicker Amendment, 1996," *Embryo Project Encyclopedia*, August 27, 2010, https://embryo.asu.edu/.

13. "What Are Mitochondrial Diseases?," Cleveland Clinic, reviewed October 9, 2014, http://my.clevelandclinic.org/.

14. Patrick F. Chinnery, "Mitochondrial Disorders Overview," National Center for Biotechnology Information, August 14, 2014, https://www.ncbi.nlm.nih.gov/.

15. Notably in the Roman Catholic tradition, the instruction *Dignitas personae*, by the Congregation for the Doctrine of the Faith (September 8, 2008), provides clear ethical and moral arguments supporting respect for the embryo from the beginning of its existence.

16. Rebecca Taylor, "UK Scientists Close to Creating Three-Parent Babies: Creating Children with Three Genetic Parents," *LifeNews*, November 2, 2015, http://www.lifenews.com/.

17. Swetlitz, "FDA Urged to Approve 'Three-Parent Embryos.'"

18. Lyndsey Craven et al., "Pronuclear Transfer in Human Embryos to Prevent Transmission of Mitochondrial DNA Disease," *Nature* 465.7294 (May 6, 2010): 82, doi: 10.1038/nature08958; and Neva Haites and Robin Lovell-Badge, "Scientific Review of the Safety and Efficacy of Methods to Avoid Mitochondrial Disease through Assisted Conception," Human Fertilisation and Embryology Authority, April 2011, 17, http://www.hfea.gov.uk/.

19. "In Vitro Fertilization (IVF): What You Can Expect," Mayo Clinic, June 16, 2016, http://www.mayoclinic.org/.

20. "Risks of In Vitro Fertilization," ASRM fact sheet, revised 2014, https://www.asrm.org/.

21. "In Vitro Fertilization," Mayo Clinic; and "Drugs Commonly Used for Women in Gestational Surrogacy Pregnancies," Center for Bioethics and Culture Network, accessed February 8, 2017, http://www.breeders.cbc-network.org/.

22. "Risks of In Vitro Fertilization," ASRM.

23. David Boonin, "How to Solve the Non-identity Problem," *Public Affairs Quarterly* 22.2 (April 2008): 129–59.

24. William Brangham, "Three-Parent DNA Treatment for Rare Defect Raises Debate," *PBS NewsHour*, February 3, 2016, http://www.pbs.org/.

25. See "Protection of Human Subjects" in the *Code of Federal Regulations*, specifically, 22 CFR §225.101.

26. Katarina Lee, "A Comparison of Canadian and American ART Law," *Voices in Bioethics*, October 14, 2015, http://voicesinbioethics.net/.

27. T.L. Beauchamp, "Methods and Principles in Biomedical Ethics," *Journal of Medical Ethics* 29.5 (October 2003): 269, doi: 10.1136/jme.29.5.269.

28. See Andrew G. Shuman and Andrew R. Barnosky, "Exploring the Limits of Autonomy," *Journal of Emergency Medicine* 40.2 (February 2011): 229–232, doi: 10.1016/j.jemermed.2009.02.029; and Rebecca L. Volpe et al., "Exploring the Limits of Autonomy," *Hastings Center Report* 42.3 (May–June 2012): 16–18, doi: 10.1002/hast.46.

29. Beauchamp, "Methods and Principles in Biomedical Ethics," 269.

ETHICS COMMITTEE

Linda Huff Wants a Dwarf Child

Linda and her husband have a form of pituitary dwarfism (PD). Pituitary dwarfism is less debilitating than achondroplastic dwarfism. It does carry increased risks for heart disease, hip dysplasia, depression, hypoglycemia (low blood sugar), and other conditions. In some cases, those with this kind of dwarfism cannot have children, though they can have normal sex lives. These risks are comparable to other life long, treatable diseases such as arthritis, auto-immune disorders, and diabetes in "normal" sized people. The Huffs come to the Hillview Wellness Center for IVF treatment. They request the following screenings:

1. They would like to screen out embryos that show Tay-Sachs disease, as it runs in Linda's family. Tay-Sachs disease is a rare disorder passed from parents to child. In the most common form, a baby about 6 months old will begin to show symptoms. As the disease progresses, the child's body loses function, leading to blindness, deafness, paralysis, and death.
2. They would like to screen out embryos that show markers for obesity. Obesity is a problem for pituitary dwarves slightly more than for "normal" sized people.
3. Linda and her husband specifically want to select fertilized eggs that have a greater chance of PD. They understand that the clinic cannot guarantee such a thing, but "while you are doing the screening, if it shows up, please implant those embryos."

Linda explains that she and her husband have been very active in the Little People of America organization. Linda has even been the national spokesperson and testified before Congress to dispel the stigma of dwarfism as a disease. She has publically protested the selective abortion of pituitary dwarf children. The Huffs have worked tirelessly to show that PD is not a disease but a viable way of life.

> As a committee, decide which (if any) of the three requests the clinic should agree to.

CHAPTER 8

Dilemmas for Patients and Families

Duty to Vaccinate?*

At the height of the pandemic surge, not a single ICU bed could be found in Alabama. Bad news for Ray DeMonia, who was having a heart attack. From his home in Cullman, Ray's family called 43 hospitals in three states. Finally they found one over two hundred miles away in Mississippi. Ray was airlifted but died shortly after arriving—three days shy of his 73rd birthday. Ray's obituary asks that everyone get vaccinated so that more resources are available for those who need it. His daughter said, "If people would just realize the strain on hospital resources that's happening right now, then that would be really amazing. But I don't know if that'll ever happen."

Who's to blame for Ray DeMonia not having an ICU bed? Is it the people who didn't get vaccinated because they just didn't want to?

WHAT'S AT STAKE?

Bioethics is not just about what medical providers do. Patients and family members often have to face tough ethical dilemmas as well. In this chapter, we will

---

* Adapted from Timothy Bella, "Alabama man dies after being turned away from 43 hospitals as covid packs ICUs, family says," *The Washington Post*, Sept. 12, 2021, https://www.washingtonpost.com/health/2021/09/12/alabama-ray-demonia-hospitals-icu/.

consider the difficult bioethical dilemmas faced by family members and patients. If you are reading this textbook and you have no intention of going into any sort of health-care field, the information can still be of use to you, for there are two things you can be almost assured of: you will be a patient at some time and you will probably have to make medical decisions for a loved one. Even the decision to get a vaccine can be an ethical decision that affects others. We will consider a patient's rights and responsibilities (or duties) as well as patient virtues.

Patient Rights

Bioethics as a discipline can trace its roots to a sea-change in medical care in the late 1970s and the early 1980s. Part of that change was the result of investigations into unethical research methods (e.g., the Tuskegee Syphilis study in Chapter 4). Another part of that change was several high-profile court cases and media coverage of paternalism by health-care providers (e.g., Jerry Canterbury in Chapter 3). When you combine these high-profile events with a general distrust of elites and reinvigorated social ethics due to a greater social focus on rights during the 1970s and 1980s (civil rights, women's rights, LGBTQ rights, for example), you have a recipe for patients' rights becoming a major focus of health care.

It may be difficult for those born after this sea-change to appreciate how health-care providers could deny the rights of patients in favor of doing what is in the patient's best interest. To understand just how significant the patients' rights movement was, we have to go back in time to understand the role of the patient prior to this paradigm shift.

Before the patient's rights movement, patients and family members did not face bioethical dilemmas very much because patients were expected to acquiesce to the wishes of the provider, especially the physician. The word "patient" is connected to "passive," after all. Sociologist Talcott Parsons (1902–79) translated this idea into the "sick role," a set of expectations surrounding patients while under the care of a doctor. For Parsons, sickness was a deviancy—that is, outside the bounds of societal norms. As a result, patients had certain privileges due to their vulnerable state, but they also had expectations. Those privileges and expectations are summarized in Parsons's four elements of the sick role:

1. The person is not responsible for assuming the sick role.
2. The sick person is exempted from carrying out some or all of the normal social duties (e.g., work, family).
3. The sick person must try to get well; the sick role is only a temporary phase.

4. In order to get well, the sick person needs to seek and submit to appropriate medical care.

Element 1 says the sick person is not at fault for this deviancy; it is something that happens to them. They are passive in assuming the sick role, so they are patients. Parsons makes clear that someone is declared a part of the sick role by some authority, usually a medical doctor. They are subsequently declared well by an authority. Element 2 says that patients are exempted from certain societal functions (note that Parsons sees work and family as the hallmarks of a functioning member of society). Element 3 says that the main obligation of the patient is to get well. Finally, element 4 says that the patient's primary role is one of complying with medical care; their primary duty is to seek out and follow medical care.

Parsons's sick role has not fared well in the history of medicine. You can see several reasons for this just by asking some probing questions. Is it always the case that the sick person is not responsible for their illness? Are all sick people excused from societal norms because they are sick? Parsons's third element implies that the only options are sick and well. Is that true? What about terminal illnesses and chronic illnesses? Do people have an obligation to seek out medical care to get well? Consider cancer patients who do not want to go through the second round of chemotherapy. Most people would say they are not obligated to do so. Parsons would seem to disagree.

Parsons's sick role made patients passive. Their only obligations were compliance and telling the truth to their doctor, their only goal being to get well and their only duty to seek out medical treatment. Of course, medicine and medical care have changed quite a bit since Parsons. Not all that comes under the heading of medical care or treatment is even about sick people getting well. What about fertility clinics? What about cosmetic surgery? Occupational therapy? Not only is the "sick role" problematic; it is also limited.

Parsons's sick role in medical sociology has largely been abandoned, for the reasons mentioned above. However, to see how it might work, consider someone who is declared mentally incompetent. People are declared mentally incompetent by a professional. Thereafter they assume a certain role, for example "mental patient." They are excused from societal functions and given leeway with regard to punishment, neglect, and so on. The patient is expected to comply with all medical treatment in order to get well. This includes medication and therapy, for example. Finally, the patient is declared mentally well by a professional.

> ### Questions Good Patients Ask Their Provider
> 1. What is the test for?
> 2. How many times have you done this procedure?
> 3. When will I get the results?
> 4. Why do I need this treatment?
> 5. Are there any alternatives?
> 6. What are the possible complications?
> 7. Which hospital is best for my needs?
> 8. How do you spell the name of that drug?
> 9. Are there any side effects?
> 10. Will this medicine interact with medicines that I'm already taking?
>
> Source: *The 10 Questions You Should Know* (Rockville, MD: Agency for Healthcare Research and Quality), https://www.ahrq.gov.

Some important cases of patients' rights are discussed in other chapters, but it will be helpful to review the sorts of rights patients have as a result of these cases. The evolution of patient rights began with perhaps the strongest right: the right to refuse treatment. This was followed by the right to be informed of all medical interventions including the risks, benefits, and alternatives. Finally came the right and authority to consent to treatment or withdraw that consent. These are the three categories of rights that patients or designated decision makers have.

You might not be surprised, then, to note that these rights are accompanied by a set of corresponding responsibilities or duties. These duties are far more controversial. Perhaps because of the passive status of the patient that stems from Parsons's sick role, medical providers are reticent about applying too many or too stringent duties on patients. If you buy into Parsons's passive role of the patient, you might think that the primary duties of patients are only two: truthfulness about their illness and compliance with the medical treatment provided.

There is a certain appeal to this idea. If the end of medicine is getting patients well, then truthfulness and compliance are just about all that patients need to do to help the physician reach that end. On this view, the patient is what the late bioethicist Edmund Pellegrino (1920–2013) called "wounded humanity." The patient's duty, therefore, is to contribute to the end result of getting well. Truthfulness and compliance do that.

There are worries about this sort of picture, however. One worry is paternalism: overriding a patient's autonomy for their own good becomes much less problematic if the patient's duties are merely to tell the truth and comply with what the doctor or nurse requires of them. Dax Cowart tells of doctors who wanted to amputate his hands to prevent the spread of infection. When he told them they would have to get a court order to do this, the doctors tried other treatments and Dax had the partial use of his hands until his death, something he would not have had if he had simply complied with the treatment asked of him.*

A second worry is that Parsons's picture of the truthful and compliant patient does not fit with the modern world of managed health care, where patients may have six or seven different specialists, each with different ideas about what "getting well" might mean. Consider the patient with a chronic disease like lupus who has a primary physician, a rheumatologist, an orthopedic surgeon, and so on. While all of them may pursue the health of the patient as the end, they may have very different ideas of what "health" looks like. Furthermore, consider what "health" or "recovery" might mean when the patient has a terminal illness rather than a chronic illness. The expectations are different, and thus so are the duties toward both medical providers, family members, and oneself.

Patient Obligations or Duties

The AHA Patient Bill of Rights also mentions a separate set of patient duties to health-care providers. Notice that most of these can be grouped into compliance and truth-telling. As the Bill of Rights states,

> Patients are responsible for providing information about past illnesses, hospitalizations, medications, and other health-related matters.

There was a television show in the early 2000s called *House M.D.* House was a Sherlock Holmes (House/Holmes—get it?) of medicine, diagnosing mysterious medical illnesses with an acerbic wit and a complete disregard for the standards of bioethics or the law. House refused to participate in taking a medical history, leaving it to his much-abused interns. His reason was that "everyone lies." House expected patients to lie about their medical history, so he never accepted it. The show often featured patients who lied to House and his team, and House, in turn, had no qualms about lying to patients. In the real world, patients have a moral obligation to be truthful in their medical history, because otherwise the providers may harm the patient by accident. It might be said that this moral duty

---

* Dax Cowart, "Patient Autonomy: One Man's Story," *Journal of the Arkansas Medical Society* 85, no. 4 (1988): 165–69. See also *Dax Cowart—40 Years Later* [video] (Cosmic Light Productions, 2012), https://vimeo.com/64585949.

comes from entering into a contract with the medical team. The patient has an obligation to not waste the medical providers' time.

Ethicists are divided about whether the patient-provider relationship is essentially a contract, but one thing is for sure: it is at least a contract, if not something more. As such, the patient has obligations to uphold their side of the relationship or get out of the relationship. Most would think it is wrong to keep things from their doctor that might affect how treatment goes, just as we would think it is wrong for a research participant to fail to disclose side effects when their experience might disqualify them from being in the research study. For instance, if a requirement for being in a clinical trial is that you stop taking a particular medicine but you start taking that medicine again, it seems you have a moral duty to tell the research investigators, because there is an implied two-way trust.

Doubled Agency

Larry Churchill and his co-authors call this two-way relationship "doubled agency." To be someone's agent is to have authority. I have "agency" when I act on my own behalf rather than remain passive; likewise, I can appoint an agent to act on my behalf. Churchill and colleagues argue that when we enter into the provider-patient relationship, there is a change of agency: "The practitioner [i.e., 'medical provider'] becomes our agent, acting on our behalf and in our place in certain prescribed areas related to health and illness."* Churchill et al.'s idea is that patients lose some of their agency when they get sick. They respond to that loss by authorizing an agent (the medical provider) to augment their agency—augment, not replace. The patient and the provider work together to respond to the illness with their doubled agency.

The AHA Patient Bill of Rights continues:

> Patients must take responsibility for requesting additional information or clarification about their health status or treatment when they do not fully understand the current information or instructions.

This one is difficult because patients and family members may not know what to ask, and many are intimidated by doctors, merely complying with whatever the doctor wants because just being in the presence of a medical professional raises blood pressure for some people (often called the "white coat effect").

---

* Larry R. Churchill, Joseph B. Fanning, and David Schenck, *What Patients Teach: The Everyday Ethics of Health Care* (Oxford: Oxford University Press, 2013).

Just as medical providers have a duty to speak to patients in a way they can understand, do patients have a duty to learn to converse with their providers in a competent way?

The AHA Bill of Rights goes on:

> Patients are responsible for making sure that the health care institution has a copy of their written advance directive if they have one.

> Patients also should be aware that the hospital has to be reasonably efficient and equitable in providing care to other patients and the community.

Here the patient's bill of rights and responsibilities charges patients and family members with upholding the principle of justice. Almost all resources in health care are scarce resources, and patients (and family members) have a moral obligation not to take up more resources than their fair share. This means that patients have obligations not to monopolize the time of nurses or doctors.

Prepare for the Visit

I once asked some doctors what they wished patients would do to improve the regular office visit. Several pointed out that they wished patients would prepare for their visit. They should come with a list of questions (since the white coat effect causes people to forget what they were going to say), and realize that it may take more than one visit to deal with every complaint they have. What do you think about this?

The Bill of Rights concludes,

> Patients and their families are responsible for being considerate of and making reasonable accommodations to the needs of the hospital, other patients, medical staff, and hospital employees.

> Patients are responsible for providing necessary information for insurance claims and for working with the hospital as needed to make payment arrangements.

> A patient's health depends on much more than health-care services. Patients are responsible for recognizing the impact of their lifestyles on their personal health.

This last one is quite a claim. It seems to imply that patients have an obligation to pursue a healthy lifestyle beyond any specific medical intervention. Do patients have a moral obligation to seek to be healthy? Is it a moral failure if patients do not devote some of their efforts to being healthy? Some of our readings will explore this claim.

WHAT'S THE DEBATE?

Reading 8.1: Leonard C. Groopman et al., "The Patient's Work"

In this article, the authors consider what it means for patients in their care to have responsibilities. If medical care is a "two-way street," then what is the patient's part? What is the work that patients must do in their relationship with medical providers?

In *The Healer's Power*, Howard Brody placed the concept of power at the heart of medicine's moral discourse. Struck by the absence of "power" in the prevailing vocabulary of medical ethics, yet aware of peripheral allusions to power in the writings of some medical ethicists, he intuited the importance of power from the silence surrounding it. He formulated the problem of the healer's power and its responsible use as "the central ethical problem in medicine."[1] Through the prism of power he refracted a wide range of ethical problems, from informed consent to truth-telling, from confidentiality to futility, from the physician's fantasies to the physician's virtues. At times this prism shed new light on old problems, enabling us to see from an unexpected angle the elements of which the problem was composed. At other times it exposed issues of ethical significance that had been neglected in the bioethics literature.

Brody argued that without power physicians cannot heal. The healer, therefore, cannot relinquish his power—it "irreducibly remains with the physician"[2]—so he must be aware of and acknowledge the uses he makes of it. He then is obliged to share that power with his patient by means of "transparency"—"thinking out loud"[3]—in the service of the patient's life plans. Writing from the perspective of a primary care physician, Brody adopted the metaphor of the doctor-patient relationship as an ongoing conversation between two people who come to know and trust each other, and who construct a meaningful narrative of the patient's life through the course of their common experience and their extended conversation. Doctor and patient collaborate in the ongoing process of healing.

Yet if the healer, in order to heal, is called on to make proper use of his power, we may ask what the sufferer, the sick person, the patient—in order to be healed, cured, or treated—is called on to do. If the healing process should be collaborative, then both parties are working.

Does the concept of the patient's work make sense? The very notion of the patient's work may seem surprising if not self-contradictory. The patient, by virtue of his medical condition, generally enjoys a reduced work load, not an increased one. And it is the doctor, not the patient, who is at work when they meet. The hospital, the clinic, and the office are the workplaces of the doctor, not the patient. Medical ethics has been concerned with defining and prescribing the proper conditions of the *doctor's* work, not the patient's. Or has it? The patient's work—not unlike the healer's power—has been a subject whispered about and alluded to, but not openly and fully explored within medical ethics.[4] Like power, work is a category that social scientists are more comfortable with than ethicists. As with power, so with work; the silence surrounding it draws our attention to it.

> In an effort to find some concept of the patient's part in recovery, the authors draw an analogy between what we think of as ordinary patients (those temporarily sick with some ailment that is treated) and patients who are in psychotherapy and physical rehab. Ask yourself whether this analogy holds. Are there significant differences between mental therapy or rehab and the typical patient with the flu?

Work in Psychotherapy and Rehabilitation

Although in general the concept of the patient's work has been absent from the discourse of medical ethics, there are two fields within medicine in which the notion that the patient is working is not alien. In psychiatry—at least in psychotherapy—and in rehabilitation medicine, we commonly speak of the patient working. In the former the work is emotional and cognitive; in the latter it is primarily physical. In both fields the process of treatment depends fundamentally on the patient's active participation and on a collaborative interaction between therapist and patient. The patient's motivation is considered crucial to the treatment process, and resistance to the process is commonly encountered—even expected—in both fields. Engagement of the patient in the treatment process is an essential condition for both psychotherapy and rehabilitation—in a way that it may not be in other medical fields—although recognition of and respect for the need for disengagement may in some cases also be essential to maintaining a therapeutic alliance.

Psychotherapy and rehabilitation medicine also share as primary goals—alongside the alleviation of symptoms—the enhancement of the patient's functional capacity (emotional or physical functioning) and, more broadly, the enhancement of the patient's sense of autonomy—that is, his ability to direct himself either physically or psychologically. All of these goals require an active, participating—working—patient. Psychotherapy and rehabilitation medicine occupy peripheral regions of the medical map as we currently conceive it. They can be and often are practiced by non-physician therapists. Rehabilitation takes place after the properly medical work of surgery is done or after the acute treatment of stroke or trauma or other medical illness is complete. And although psychiatry has in recent decades become increasingly "medicalized" through psychopharmacology, psychotherapy remains ancillary to the prevailing conceptions of organicist medicine. Yet just as Brody argued that primary care is more an attitude than a specialty, and that that attitude can and should be imported into the relationship between doctor and patient, so we argue that the patient's work is a useful concept not only in psychotherapy and rehabilitation medicine, but within the doctor-patient relationship more generally.

Work in Doctor-Patient Models

> The authors now consider two models of doctor-patient interaction. For discussion of Talcott Parsons's sick roles see this chapter. Jay Katz's autonomy model has not been discussed but should be clear from the summary provided here.

Has the concept of the patient's work truly been foreign to the ethics of the doctor-patient relationship? Insofar as the patient's work has been discussed in the ethics of the doctor-patient relationship, it has been buried under other names than "work" or it has been found outside medical ethics itself. In the paternalistic paradigm of the doctor-patient relationship, the patient has had a role, most thoroughly described by the sociologist Talcott Parsons. In the autonomy paradigm the patient has had a responsibility, most strongly articulated by Jay Katz. Role and responsibility have been the disguised forms taken by the patient's work in these models.

Parsons described the sick role and the social and psychological expectations that accompanied it. He taught us that "being sick" is not simply a natural fact, but a social role, with an "institutionalized expectation system" that is "not only a right of the sick person but an obligation upon him." The exemption from normal responsibility, for example, is accompanied by the obligation to stay in bed. The sick role further relieves the sick person from responsibility for being sick—he is not to blame for his condition—but requires him to want to get well, to seek technically competent help, and to cooperate with the helper. Failure to do so would raise questions of malingering and of the "secondary gain" from illness, and would abrogate the person's exemptions from his usual responsibilities. Of the obligation to cooperate in the treatment, Parsons writes, "it is here, of course, that the role of the sick person as patient becomes articulated with that of the physician in a complementary role structure."[5] For the doctor to do his work, the patient must do his—which is to perform his socially assigned sick role.

The theorists of patient autonomy rejected this definition of the sick role, which they criticized for its dependency features. The patient in this role was deferential, compliant, and regressed. Katz writes:

> It is not surprising that this model has been instinctively embraced by physicians and patients alike. Doctors embraced it because it called for unquestioning compliance, unilateral trust, and verbal silence. It appealed to patients, engulfed by pain and suffering, because surrender to powerful, wise, and soothing caretakers was strongly fostered by memories of earlier days when a parent satisfied all discomforting bodily needs. Thus, the regression to more childlike functioning that can result from illness becomes augmented by a patient's wish for caretaking by a parent-physician who, as memory informs, will immediately alleviate all suffering. The regression is also reinforced by doctors' proclivities to view patients as helpless and incompetent children.[6]

In reaction to this image of the infantilized patient, Katz painted a picture of the independent adult patient, allowed to exercise his "right to self-determination"[7] by making well-informed decisions about his medical treatment. But this right became, in Katz's influential work, a right that the bearer had a duty to exercise:

> Indeed, I take a further step and postulate a duty to reflection that cannot be easily waived. Asserting such a duty sounds strange. We are accustomed to recognizing a right to choice as an aspect of the

right to self-determination, but a duty to reflection as a component of autonomy is quite another matter. Yet, if my views on psychological autonomy have merit, then respect for the right of self-determination requires respect for human beings' proclivities to exercise this right in both rational and irrational ways. Doctors are obliged to facilitate patients' opportunities for reflection to prevent ill-considered rational and irrational influences on choice.

Patients, in turn, are obligated to participate in the process of thinking about choices. In arguing that both parties make every effort to facilitate reflection in order to sort out the rational and irrational expectations that eventually can converge on choice, I express a value preference for the enhancement of individual psychological autonomy.[8]

The patient might have to be encouraged to be autonomous and free. The exercise of choice, the making of one's own decisions, has become a duty.[9] Informed choice is the patient's work. Moreover, it is part of the physician's moral function to lead the patient toward greater autonomy through the process of informed consent.

Behind the movement for patient autonomy lay not only reactions against dependency, distrust of authority, and an ideology of self-determination, but also an understanding of the psychology of illness. The control over bodily functions—from the regulation of excretory functions to speech and the purposive use of the limbs—is an early and significant developmental achievement, which is a source of childhood self-esteem as well as a precondition for socialization. The loss of bodily control is a frequent, if not a universal, feature of physical illness, which, depending on the nature and severity of the illness as well as the life situation and personality of the patient, is often accompanied by feelings of shame and helplessness, and at times depression. Loss of bodily control involves a degree of loss of self-control because our sense of self is woven into our relationship to our bodies. A burgeoning psychological literature from the 1960s and 1970s based on a "learned helplessness" model of depression argued for the importance of active control over one's environment as a key to maintaining self-esteem in the face of adversity or failure.[10]

In the face of physical illness, the patient's "taking control" became a therapeutic act. For some proponents of patient autonomy, control involved not only becoming informed—understanding one's illness and knowing what to expect—but making decisions as well. Controlling one's own treatment decisions was part and parcel of overcoming one's illness. The duty to control was simultaneously a moral duty to make one's own decisions, a therapeutic requirement for psychological health, and part of the social obligation to get well.

> The authors critique the autonomy model and offer some middle ground between the completely passive patient of Parsons and Katz's fully engaged patient from other ethicists. Is it unrealistic to expect patients in pain or suffering to exercise autonomous decision making? Is the alternative called "mutuality" presented by the authors of this article an improvement on Katz's model, or just another version of it?

In retrospect, the psychological assumptions underpinning the autonomy model can seem naive. How can Katz's patient, who he describes as "engulfed by pain and suffering," be expected to exercise his right—his duty—to self-determination by making complex medical decisions? Should we condemn the dependency needs—or wishes—of sick people or assume that those needs are a form of false consciousness created by an authoritarian social structure of which the traditional doctor-patient relationship forms a part? Moreover, even if assuming active control helps many people cope with the psychological threats of illness, what of those patients to whom such control is psychologically unwelcome or emotionally detrimental? Should they be manipulated, cajoled, coerced, forced to decide? Carl Schneider, who in *The Practice of Autonomy* critically examines the vaunted benefit as well as the assumed desire of the sick to be in control of medical decision making, concludes:

> Real people are stubbornly more complicated than this model supposes. Some people may behave as autonomists imagine, but an imposing number of them act quite differently. Their desire for information is more equivocal than the model assumes; their taste for rational analysis is less pronounced; their personal beliefs are not as well developed, relevant, or strong; and their desire for control is more partial, ambivalent, and complex.[11]

Dissatisfaction with the simplifications and excesses of an individualist, autonomy-centered ethical model, and with the contractual and consumerist conception of medical treatment that usually accompanies it, has led to alternative methodological approaches to medical ethics and alternative models of the doctor-patient relationship.

Some of these newer models expand upon the concept of autonomy to encompass more than the mere exercise of control through decision making. Ezekiel and Linda Emanuel, for example, recognized that the paternalistic model of the doctor-patient relationship in which autonomy had meant patient assent had been replaced in practice by an informative model in which "the conception of patient autonomy is patient control over decision making."[12] They favored interpretive and deliberative forms of autonomy, in which patient self-understanding and moral development, rather than patient control, were the central moral ends that emerged from the doctor-patient relationship. And Brody, as we have seen, situated himself within an emerging medical ethics of collaboration and mutuality in the doctor-patient relationship, in contrast to both the medical ethics of paternalism and the medical ethics of rights-centered autonomy. This mutualist medical ethics, emphasizing the collaboration between doctor and patient, included a "renewed sense of the values of the profession of medicine as well as a more communitarian ethic generally."[13]

If the patient's work in the paternalistic ethic is the performance of a sick role and in the autonomy ethic the making of decisions and taking of control, then what is the patient's work in the mutualist ethic? Brody, as we have seen, wishes the doctor-patient relationship to resemble an ongoing dialogue through which patient and physician place the patient's medical choices within the context of the patient's life plans. And Arthur Frank, a sociologist of illness and advocate for the ethical importance of illness narratives, writes of one type of illness narrative—the "quest stories"—that they "meet suffering head on; they accept illness and seek to *use* it. Illness is the occasion of a journey that becomes a quest."[14] The mutualist patient's work appears to be engagement in a conversation, construction of a meaningful life narrative, and the use of illness as a means of self-understanding and change. The hard-working mutualist patient uses his illness and suffering to create something—a narrative that bears witness to his experience or a tool in his struggle with suffering. The successful mutualist patient transforms his illness, and himself, into a "good story," as the writer Anatole Broyard wished himself—and his case of prostate cancer—to become.[15] Although these literary products may represent exceptional results of the patient's work, it is useful to see them as examples of what the mutualist ethic calls for from the patient.

The patient's work recognizes the psychological importance for the patient of having an activity, of participating in the process of treatment, of exercising control in a situation of loss of control. The autonomy model recognizes that one way that people achieve a sense of control is by being informed and making decisions. Unfortunately, it fails to appreciate that other ways that people achieve a sense of control may include obedience or distraction or denial or telling stories. These ways are recognized by the other models.

Comparing the Models

To view these models through the prism of the concept of the patient's work, we compare them (Table 1) in terms of the characteristic activities of the doctor and the characteristic activities of the patient.

TABLE 1			
Comparison of Three Models of the Doctor-Patient Relationship			
	Paternalism	**Autonomy**	**Mutuality**
M.D.	Diagnoses	Presents choices	Contextualizes
	Prescribes	Informs	Converses
	Protects	Leaves alone (doesn't interfere)	Empowers
		Executes/complies	Interprets
			Constructs
Patient	Defers	Questions	Collaborates
	Complies	Chooses	Converses
		Decides	Constructs
		Controls	Changes

In many obvious ways the three models conflict: The deferential, compliant patient of the paternalistic model is incompatible with the questioning, choosing, deciding, controlling patient of the autonomy model. From another perspective, they are related dialectically—as thesis, antithesis, and synthesis, with the mutualist synthesis combining elements of the first two to produce something different from either. Yet in another respect, they are disjunctive—and therefore not in conflict—in that they apply under different medical circumstances and in different social contexts. We generally accept that in emergency situations doctors can behave paternalistically, attending first and foremost to diagnosing and treating the medical condition—serving the patient's immediate health interests—and taking the patient's autonomy rights and life plan into consideration only secondarily, unless they are clearly known ahead of time. Similarly, a consultation with a specialist unknown to the patient who recommends an invasive treatment might best fall under an autonomy model, in which the patient questions, gathers information, solicits different opinions, and decides for himself.

The treatment of insulin-dependent diabetes in a primary care setting, on the other hand, might best be understood as an ongoing dialogue between doctor and patient in which an understanding of the meaning to and impact upon the patient of the illness and its treatment form the context within which choices are made and the treatment is conducted.

Yet another way of understanding these three models is that they correspond to different psychological types of patients, which we might call the dependent patient, the "take charge" patient, and the conversational or meaning-seeking patient. Different personality styles and psychological needs will fit best with each of the models. And if patient empowerment and avoidance of patient coercion by the physician are ethical aspects of all doctor-patient relationships, then adaptation of the relationship to fit patient styles and needs would place each model on an equal ethical plane. When it comes to doctor-patient relationships, one size does not fit all, and insisting that they do disrespects the individuality of the patient.

Each of these three relational models may come into play in one and the same treatment. Consider, for example, the treatment by a psychiatrist of a patient with bipolar disorder—a chronic, remitting, and recurring illness—that involves both psychopharmacology and psychotherapy. During asymptomatic periods the focus of the treatment will most resemble a conversation in which perceptions, meanings, and life plans will be explored, contextualized, interpreted, and constructed. When medications are changed, the psychiatrist is likely to present the patient with information, choices, and a recommendation, leaving the patient to decide, although a discussion of the meaning of the medication change to the patient may be a part of the process. At times of crisis, such as an acute manic episode in which the patient has lost any insight into his illness, the psychiatrist will behave paternalistically, prescribing a treatment—hospitalization, for example—with limited if any choice or discussion.

Do you agree with the authors that these models represent different sorts of patients? Could you describe the differences between the paternalist patient, the autonomous patient, and the mutual patient? If so, which kind of patient are you when you are sick? What does that say about your duties as a patient? How would medical providers help patients identify what kind of patient they are?

What does this example tell us? First, it implies again that the different models apply in different clinical situations and that treatment situations are constantly evolving.[16] Moreover, it helps us see that all three models (and perhaps others as well) are in play simultaneously in the complex reality of many treatment situations. Because these models are ideal types that are heuristically useful rather than empirical descriptions of actual relationships, it is not surprising that they are found to coexist in the "real world" of doctors and patients. The patient's "own good"—his health interests—coexists with his right to self-determination, which lives alongside his overarching life plans. At times, the patient is obeying, at times, choosing and deciding, at times, formulating, narrating, and making meaning. Or, rather, he may be doing all these things simultaneously.

The notion of the patient's work implies that the patient can fail to perform his work or work badly.[17] Noncompliance is the best known form of the patient's failure to do his work in the paternalistic model.[18] Passivity, dependence, and indecisiveness would represent poor work for the autonomist's patient. Resistance to conversation, narrative incoherence, or an absence of life plans would constitute poor work in the mutualist paradigm. All three paradigms therefore seem to *prescribe* the nature of the patient's work, as either compliance with doctor's orders or active control over medical decision making or engagement in ongoing exploration of the meaning and place of illness in the patient's life.

In addition to prescribing forms of work to the patient, each of the three models assigns the physician a moral function alongside his technical function. The paternalistic model assigns the doctor the moral function of trustee of the patient's health interests. In the autonomy model, the physician is the facilitator of the patient's autonomy, as epitomized in the process of informed consent, through which, when properly enacted, the patient is engaged as a moral agent in his own treatment.[19] In the mutualist model, the doctor's moral function is as interlocutor in a conversation on the meaning and living of the patient's life.

All three models, then, give both doctor and patient moral work to do with the aim of restoring the patient's health or relieving suffering. They allow the doctor to be engaged with the patient but at the same time detached from him, as in Renee Fox's classic formulation of "detached concern" and, more recently, Brody's notion of the physician's "empathic curiosity."[20] Similarly, our concept of the patient's work allows the patient to be engaged with his illness yet not under its sway. If the patient has work to do, then the patient is not defined entirely by his illness. His illness becomes the object of his work, and he the subject. At the very least, the patient's work—whether enacting the sick role, participating in decision making, or narrating his experience—provides the patient with an organizing set of responses to the condition of illness and, therefore, a framework within which to live in relation to it.

Ethical Implications

The notion that the patient has work to do is commonly accepted in end-of-life medical situations. Indeed, one of the justifications for truth-telling of terminal diagnoses is the importance for the patient of completing whatever "unfinished business" is left. We expect dying patients to complete their work. Such unfinished business generally involves getting one's house in order, both materially and emotionally. It might involve "finding meaning" at the end of life. "If a patient does not know he is dying, he will not be able to find meaning in the dying process," writes Fins.[21] The patient is responsible for a part of the dying process, just as the physician is responsible for a part. The patient has his work to do in the process.

Our pluralistic view of the three models of the doctor-patient relationship, which places them all on an equal ethical plane, reopens the debate on the morality, as well as the wisdom, of this accepted American practice of informing patients when they are dying. If one doctor-patient relationship does not fit all patient types and clinical situations, then one rule cannot necessarily be universally correct. One could argue that, just as in the emergency situation, the paternalistic model should be in place barring some compelling reason to the contrary, so in the dying situation, the autonomy model should be in place barring some compelling reason to the contrary. But this is a subject for ongoing debate.

Maintaining personal dignity in the face of illness is an important ethical issue in contemporary medicine. The critically ill patient hooked up to pumps, catheters, and respirators has become an image not only of the loss of control but also of the loss of dignity. Medical disability, with the concomitant incapacity to participate fully in social and family functions, has long incurred damage to a person's social status and has become the occasion for a movement to reclaim the dignity of the handicapped. And stigma, which adheres to certain diseases—from AIDS to cancer to epilepsy to schizophrenia—spoils the social identity of the sick person and does further injury to his dignity.

In our society, work is an important source of personal and social dignity. Conceiving of the patient as having work to do is a means of dignifying the patient's activities, of thinking about the patient as an active agent, engaged in directed, purposive activity toward an end. Seeking empathically to understand what the patient is engaged in during the process of his illness can enable those involved in treating him to see the person beneath and beyond the patient. This can help the patient maintain a sense of himself as a person during a life-altering experience such as serious illness and, therefore, maintain a sense of his dignity despite the indignities inflicted by disease.

But this requires that those treating him understand that individual psychologies can differ significantly, and that one person's way of working at maintaining his personal dignity (by making his own decisions, for example) may be quite different from another's (by obediently following doctor's orders, for example). We should not make metaphysical assumptions about the universally valid goods of life, which both the autonomy model and the mutualist model seem to make, implying that the work of making one's own decisions or of finding meaning is the proper work of humans.

Indeed, the invisibility of the patient's work—its hitherto absence from the conceptual lexicon of medical ethics—may derive in part from the fact that the healthy take health for granted and have difficulty seeing the work involved in coping with illness. Especially for people with serious or chronic illnesses, which may have a profound impact on global functioning—such as the bipolar patient we described earlier—to accept and stick with a treatment regimen despite distressing side effects and to be willing to experiment to find acceptable, if not optimal, therapy all involve work on the part of the patient.

The concept of the patient's work can serve as an organizing metaphor for physician and patient as they forge a therapeutic relationship. It reminds the physician that the patient is an active participant in the process of treatment, even if that activity may take various forms, from compliance to decision making to conversing. It encourages the doctor to understand the patient's particular manner of working and to work with it himself. It can also serve as a heuristic device in educating medical students and house staff. We hope that the concept and the attendant clinical skills will help physicians integrate as part of *their* work the facilitation of the patient's work. This can enhance the doctor's ability to see beyond the patient to the person and improve the quality of medical care by rendering it both psychologically richer and morally more dignity preserving and, therefore, more humane.

Notes

1. Brody H. *The Healer's Power.* New Haven, CT: Yale University Press; 1992:36.
2. See note 1, Brody 1992:132.
3. See note 1, Brody 1992:116.
4. In one of the rare essays directly addressing the question of the obligations of the patient, Martin Benjamin, in "Lay Obligations in Professional Relations," simply "requires lay people to honor commitments and disclose relevant information." Benjamin M. Lay obligations in professional relations. *Journal of Medicine and Philosophy* 10;1985:85–103. See also Brody H. Patients' responsibilities. In: *Encyclopedia of Bioethics.* New York: Macmillan; 1995.
5. Parsons T. *The Social System.* New York: Free Press; 1951:436–37.

6. Katz J. *The Silent World of Doctor and Patient.* New York: Free Press; 1984:100–01.

7. See note 6, Katz 1984:122–23.

8. See note 6, Katz 1984:104.

9. Schneider CE. *The Practice of Autonomy: Patients, Doctors, and Medical Decisions.* New York: Oxford University Press; 1998:9–32.

10. For an overview see Seligman MEP. *Helplessness: On Depression, Development, and Death.* San Francisco: Freeman; 1975.

11. See note 9, Schneider 1998:229.

12. Emanuel EJ, Emanuel LL. Four models of the physician-patient relationship. *JAMA* 1992;267:2221.

13. See note 1, Brody 1992:162. See also Dochin A. Understanding autonomy relationally: Toward a reconfiguration of bioethical principles. *Journal of Medicine and Philosophy* 2001;26:365–68.

14. Frank A. *The Wounded Storyteller.* Chicago: University of Chicago Press; 1995:115.

15. Broyard A. *Intoxicated by My Illness.* New York: Clarkson Potter; 1992:45.

16. In this case, as in many psychiatric cases, the evolving treatment situation includes changes in the patient's mental state or state of self.

17. Brody H. *Stories of Sickness.* New Haven, CT: Yale University Press; 1987:128–42.

18. Although, of course, noncompliance may be a sign of the doctor's failure to do his work of engaging the patient in the treatment process. In the paternalistic model, however, engaging the patient in the treatment does not form part of the doctor's work.

19. Despite the oft-noted resistance by many doctors to informed consent, there is evidence that what Robert Zusman has called "the culture of rights" has permeated into the medical world. See Zusman R. *Intensive Care: Medical Ethics and the Medical Profession.* Chicago: University of Chicago Press; 1992:219–29.

20. Fox RC. Training for uncertainty. In: Schwartz H, Kart C. *Dominant Issues in Medical Sociology.* Reading, MA; 1978; see note 1, Brody 1992:260–67.

21. Fins JJ. Truth-telling and reciprocity in the doctor-patient relationship: A North American perspective. In: Portenoy RK, Bruera E, eds. *Topics in Palliative Care*, vol. 5. New York: Oxford University Press; 2001:92.

Reading 8.2: Susan M. Wolf et al., "Sources of Concern about the Patient Self-Determination Act"

A host of bioethicists and doctors express concern about the Patient Self-Determination Act of 1991.

On December 1, 1991, the Patient Self-Determination Act of 1990 (PSDA)[1] went into effect. This is the first federal statute to focus on advance directives and the right of adults to refuse life-sustaining treatment. The law applies to all health care institutions receiving Medicare or Medicaid funds, including hospitals, skilled-nursing facilities, hospices, home health and personal care agencies, and health maintenance organizations (HMOs).

The statute requires that the institution provide written information to each adult patient on admission (in the case of hospitals or skilled-nursing facilities), enrollment (HMOs), first receipt of care (hospices), or before the patient comes under an agency's care (home health or personal care agencies). The information provided must describe the person's legal rights in that state to make decisions concerning medical care, to refuse treatment, and to formulate advance directives, plus the relevant written policies of the institution. In addition, the institution must document advance directives in the person's medical record, ensure compliance with state law regarding advance directives, and avoid making care conditional on whether or not patients have directives or otherwise discriminating against them on that basis. Finally, institutions must maintain pertinent written policies and procedures and must provide staff and community education on advance directives. The states must help by preparing descriptions of the relevant law, and the Secretary of Health and Human Services must assist with the development of materials and conduct a public-education campaign. The Health Care Financing Administration has authority to issue regulations.

> In this section, the authors lay out the goals of the Patient Self-Determination Act (PSDA). How do you think these goals (now over 20 years old) have fared?

A goal of the statute is to encourage but not require adults to fill out advance directives—treatment directives (documents such as a living will stating the person's treatment preferences in the event of future incompetence), proxy appointments (documents such as a durable power of attorney appointing a proxy decision maker), or both. There is widespread agreement that directives can have many benefits.[2,3,4,5] These include improved communication between doctor and patient, increased clarity about the patient's wishes, and ultimately greater assurance that treatment accords with the patient's values and preferences. Yet few Americans have executed advance directives. Estimates range from 4 to 24 percent [6,7,8] (and Knox RA: personal communication).

A second goal of the PSDA is to prompt health professionals and institutions to honor advance directives. The U.S. Supreme Court's Cruzan decision suggests that advance directives are protected by the federal constitution.[9] The great majority of states and the District of Columbia also have specific statutes or judicial decisions recognizing treatment directives.[10] In addition, all states have general durable-power-of-attorney statutes, and most states further specify how this or another format can be used to appoint a proxy for health care decisions.[10] Patients thus have a right to use directives that is based in constitutional, statutory, and common law, and others must honor the recorded choices.[11] There is evidence, however, that advance directives are ignored or overridden one fourth of the time.[12]

Why do you suppose that advance directives are ignored or not implemented? Doctors have a saying, "Dead people don't sue," and this affects decisions to honor advance directives. When there is a conflict between an advance directive and a living family member, who will doctors defer to most often?

Efforts to educate patients about directives and to educate health care professionals about their obligation to honor them thus seem warranted. But the PSDA has caused concern.[6,13,14] Implementation may result in drowning patients in written materials on admission, insensitive and ill-timed inquiry into patients' preferences, and untrained bureaucrats attempting a job that should be performed by physicians. Indeed, one can favor directives yet oppose the PSDA because of these dangers. The question is how to accomplish the statute's positive underlying goals while minimizing the potential adverse effects.

The key to avoiding an insensitive and bureaucratic process is to ensure that physicians integrate discussion of directives into their ongoing dialogue with patients about current health status and future care. Many have urged that doctors do this.[4,6,15] Yet the literature shows that physicians still have reservations about advance directives,[6,12,13,16,17,18,19] and some remain reluctant to initiate discussion.[7,15,20,21] Only by forthrightly addressing these reservations can we successfully make directives part of practice, realize the potential benefits for all involved, and avoid implementing the PSDA in a destructive way.

Our multidisciplinary group—including physicians, a nurse, philosophers, and lawyers—convened to address those reservations in order to dispel doubts when appropriate and delineate continuing controversy where it exists.

Reservations about Treatment Directives

Patients do not really want to discuss future incompetence and death, and so would rather not discuss advance directives. Future incompetence, serious illness, and death are not easy topics to discuss for either patients or physicians. Yet studies indicate that most patients want to discuss their preferences for future treatment [4,7,18,22] and that such discussion usually evokes positive reactions and an enhanced sense of control.[18,23]

Misconceptions nonetheless remain and may produce anxiety in some patients. Some people wrongly assume that treatment directives are used only to refuse treatments and thus shorten life.[24] But people use directives to request treatments as well.[4,25] Such a demand for treatment can raise important ethical problems later if the physician becomes concerned that the treatment may be medically inappropriate or futile for that patient. These problems are currently being debated.[26,27,28,29] Yet they are not peculiar to advance directives; they can arise whenever a patient or surrogate demands arguably inappropriate treatment. The point is that treatment directives are a way to express the patient's preferences for treatment, whatever they may be.

> Given the value of advance directives for making decisions when patients cannot, do you think there is any moral duty for patients to make their end-of-life wishes known through some kind of advance directive? Which principles might justify this moral duty?

There are substantial advantages to both patients and doctors in discussing and formulating treatment directives. A discussion of future medical scenarios can reduce the uncertainty of patients and physicians, strengthen rapport, and facilitate decision making in the future.[16,23,30] Beyond their clinical advantages, directives are one way to fulfill the legal requirement in some states that there be "clear and convincing evidence" of the patient's wishes before life-sustaining treatment is withdrawn.[31,32] The state statutes on treatment directives also generally give physicians a guarantee of civil and criminal immunity when they withhold or withdraw life-sustaining treatment relying in good faith on a patient's directive.

Some debate remains, however, about when directives should first be discussed and with which patients.[4,21,33] The PSDA requires giving information to all adults when they first enter a relevant institution or receive care. This will involve some healthy patients and patients who are expected to return to good health after treatment for a reversible problem. Yet even healthy persons and young people wish to engage in advance planning with their physicians.[4]

Concern nonetheless persists about whether the time of admission or initial receipt of treatment is an appropriate moment to broach the topic of directives. Ideally, initial discussion should take place in the outpatient setting, before the patient experiences the dislocation that often attends inpatient admission. Many patients, however, will reach admission without the benefit of such discussion. If the discussion on admission is handled sensitively and as the first of many opportunities to discuss these matters with the physician and other care givers, admission is an acceptable time to begin the process. For patients who already have directives, admission is a logical time to check the directives in the light of their changed medical circumstances.

Discussion of advance directives takes too much time and requires special training and competence. The discussion of advance directives is an important part of the dialogue between doctor and patient about the patient's condition, prognosis, and future options. But the physician need not discharge this function alone. Others in the health care institution may play an important part in answering questions, providing information, or assisting with documents. The PSDA helpfully makes health care institutions and organizations responsible for the necessary staff education. However, because patients considering treatment directives need to understand their health status and treatment options, physicians have a central role.

Physicians may nonetheless harbor understandable concern about the amount of time that will be required to counsel each patient. An initial discussion of directives structured by a document describing alternative medical scenarios can be accomplished in 15 minutes,[4] but some will undoubtedly find that the initial discussion takes longer, and further discussion is also necessary in any case. Institutions may want to acquire brochures, videotapes, and other materials to help educate patients, and may enlist other personnel in coordinated efforts to assist patients. In addition, the PSDA requires institutions and organizations to engage in community education, which may reach patients before they are admitted. All these efforts promise to facilitate the discussion between doctor and patient.

Treatment directives are not useful, because patients cannot really anticipate what their preferences will be in a future medical situation and because patients know too little about life-support systems and other treatment options. The first part of this objection challenges the very idea of making decisions about medical situations that have not yet developed. Patients who make such decisions will indeed often be making decisions that are less fully informed than those of patients facing a current health problem.[6] Yet the decisions recorded in directives, even if imperfect, give at least an indication of what the patient would want. If the goal is to guide later treatment decisions by the patient's preferences, some indication is better than none.

The question, then, is not whether the decisions embodied in directives are just as informed as those made contemporaneously by a competent patient. It is instead whether the recorded decisions accurately indicate the patient's preferences as best he or she could know them when competent. The answer to that question depends largely on how skillful physicians are in explaining possible medical scenarios and the attendant treatment options. There are many spheres in which we ask people to anticipate the future and state their wishes—wills governing property and most contracts are examples. But in each case the quality of their decisions depends a good deal on the quality of the counseling they receive. It is incumbent on physicians to develop their skills in this regard. Several instruments have been described in the literature to help them communicate successfully with patients.[19,34,35] In addition, the patient's designation of a proxy can provide a person to work with the physician as the medical situation unfolds.

Good counseling by physicians is the best remedy for patients' ignorance about life-support systems, too. Patients need to understand these treatments in order to judge whether the expected burdens will outweigh the benefits in future medical circumstances. Yet a patient choosing in advance will usually have a less detailed understanding than a patient facing an immediate and specific decision, who may even try the treatment for a time to gain more information.[3] This too supports the wisdom of designating a proxy to work with the medical team.

Treatment-directive forms are too vague and open to divergent interpretations to be useful guides to treatment decisions later. Some forms do contain outmoded language. Terms such as "extraordinary" treatment and "heroic" care have been widely discredited as being overly vague [3,36] (even though "extraordinary" is used in some state laws [37]), and patients should be discouraged from using such generalities. Instead, patients who wish to use treatment directives should be encouraged to specify which treatments they wish to request or refuse, and the medical circumstances under which they want those wishes to go into effect. Although such specification has been challenged,[17] it is a more effective way for patients to communicate their wishes than a general refusal of life-sustaining treatment. The desire for a particular treatment may well vary according to diagnosis and prognosis [4,38]—for instance, artificial nutrition may be desired if the patient is conscious and has a reversible condition, but unwanted if the patient is in a persistent vegetative state. Another way to communicate wishes is for patients to state their preferred goals of treatment, depending on diagnosis [39]—for example, in case of terminal illness, provide comfort care only.

It is nonetheless almost impossible to write a directive that leaves no room for interpretation. Whatever language the patient uses, the goal is to try to determine the patient's intent. Often family members or other intimates can help. Even a vague directive will usually provide some guidance. Some patients will choose to avoid problems of interpretation and application by appointing a proxy and writing no treatment directive. The proxy can then work with the physician as circumstances unfold. Yet the proxy must still strive to choose as the patient would. If the patient has left a treatment directive or other statement of preferences, it will fall to the proxy to determine what the patient intended. The incompetent patient's best interests should take precedence over even the most thoughtful choices of a patient while competent. Some people argue that the choices stated in a directive are sometimes less relevant than the current experience of the now incompetent patient.[40,41] In the vast majority of cases, this problem does not arise, because the patient's earlier decisions do not conflict with his or her best interests when incompetent. Yet some demented patients, in particular, may seem to derive continued enjoyment from life, although they have a directive refusing life-sustaining treatment. The argument for discounting the directive is that these patients are now such different people that they should not be bound by the choices of their earlier selves, they may no longer hold the values embodied in the directive, and they may appear to accept a quality of life they formerly deemed unacceptable.

> The authors now come to a disagreement among them. Should the wishes expressed in an advance directive while the patient had decisional capacity override the best interests of the patient who now lacks decisional capacity? This is particularly important with regard to dementia.

Our group did not reach agreement on this argument for overriding some directives. Members who rejected it argued that it is essential that competent patients who record their wishes know those wishes will be followed later, a person's values and choices should govern even after loss of competence because he or she remains essentially the same person, and to recognize the proposed exception would invite widespread disregard of treatment directives. Although we did not resolve this controversy, we did agree on certain procedural safeguards. A treatment directive should not be overridden lightly. In cases in which this controversy arises, only the patient's appointed proxy, a court, or a court-appointed decision maker should be able to consider overriding the directive. Finally, physicians should specifically discuss with patients what the patients' preferences are in the event of dementia.

Even if a directive is valid in all other respects, it is not a reliable guide to treatment because patients may change their minds. Patients may indeed change their minds as their circumstances change. Physicians should therefore reexamine directives periodically with their patients. Data suggest, however, that there is considerable stability in patients' preferences concerning life-sustaining treatment.[16,42,43,44] In one study of hospitalized patients, 65 to 85 percent of choices did not change during a one-month period, the percentage depending on the illness scenario presented (kappa = 0.35 to 0.70, where 0 represents random and 1 perfect agreement).[42] In another study there was 58 and 81 percent stability in patients' decisions over a six-month period when they were presented with two scenarios (kappa = 0.23 and 0.31).[43] Further research is necessary, but in any case, patients are always free to change or revoke earlier directives. Once a patient has lost competence and the physician can no longer check with the patient about treatment preferences, a directive becomes the most reliable guide to what the patient would want. Physicians cannot justifiably disregard directives because the patient might hypothetically have changed his or her mind.

> The authors now turn to concerns about family members or other proxies following advance directives or living wills. What sorts of conflicts can arise even if a patient has expressed their wishes in an advance directive? For the family member or proxy, which principles should guide their decisions: the patient's wishes or the best interests of the patient?

Reservations about Proxy Appointments

Patients may appoint a proxy to make treatment decisions in the event of incompetence, using a durable power of attorney or other document. Some patients both appoint a proxy and execute a treatment directive. Proxy appointments raise some different sources of concern than treatment directives.

The appointed proxy may later seem to be the wrong surrogate decision maker. This concern may arise for one of several reasons. The proxy may have had no involvement in the patient's health planning and may not even realize that the patient has chosen him or her as proxy. To avoid this problem the physician should encourage the patient both to secure the proxy's acceptance of the appointment and to consider involving the proxy in the process of making decisions about future care. The proxy will then be prepared to discharge the function and will have some knowledge of the patient's wishes. The physician should also encourage the patient to tell family members and other intimates who the chosen proxy is, especially since some patients will prefer to designate a proxy from outside their families. This will reduce the chance of surprise and disagreement later.

Physicians may nonetheless encounter appointed proxies with little previous involvement in the patient's planning process and daily life. Yet a patient's designation of a proxy is an exercise in self-determination. The physician is bound to contact that person if the patient loses competence and the appointment goes into effect, rather than ignore the appointment and simply turn to someone else. There may be no further problems, because everyone may agree anyway on what course of treatment the patient would wish. But uncertainty or disagreement about the right choice of treatment may force the resolution of questions about who the most appropriate proxy is. If the medical team or the patient's relatives or other intimates have serious doubts about whether the designated proxy can fulfill the required functions, it is their responsibility to address these doubts through discussion. If the problem cannot be resolved in this way, they may need to seek judicial resolution and the appointment of an alternate.

Sometimes the designated proxy seems inappropriate not because the person is too remote but because the person is so involved that his or her own wishes and interests seem to govern, rather than the patient's. Family members and other intimates almost always have to deal with their own emotional and financial issues in serving as a proxy decision maker, and the mere existence of such issues does not disqualify them. Physicians and other members of the medical team have a responsibility to work with proxies, helping them to identify their own matters of concern, to separate those from the patient's, and to focus on the patient's wishes and interests in making decisions about treatment. Occasionally, the medical team will encounter a proxy who simply cannot do this. If efforts among the involved parties to remedy the problem fail, then care givers may have to seek judicial scrutiny and the appointment of another proxy.

Even a diligent proxy cannot tell what the patient wanted without an explicit treatment directive, so a proxy's choice should carry no particular weight. Family members, other intimates, and physicians often fail to select the same treatment the patient chooses when asked.[45,46,47,48,49] In one study there was 59 to 88 percent agreement, depending on the illness scenario the researchers posed (kappa = ≤0.3 in all cases)[45]; in another study, agreement was 52 to 90 percent (kappa = ≤0.4 in all cases).[49] Advising the proxy to choose as the patient would, rather than simply asking for a recommendation, seems to act as a partial corrective.[46]

These data should come as no surprise. Even a person's relatives and other intimates are not clairvoyant and may not share identical values. Moreover, proxies are not always adequately informed that their choices for the patient must be based on the patient's wishes and interests, even when those do not accord with the proxy's. Yet there is often no one better informed about the patient's past values and preferences than the proxy, and the patient in any case has manifested trust by appointing that person. Physicians should encourage patients not only to appoint a proxy, but also to provide instructions to guide the proxy. Physicians should also explicitly clarify for the proxy the primacy of the patient's wishes and interests.

The proxy may make a treatment choice contrary to the patient's treatment directive, claiming that the proxy appointment takes precedence over the directive. Some patients will appoint a proxy and leave no treatment directive or other instructions to limit the proxy's authority. Others will guide their proxy by writing a treatment directive or other record of preferences.[5] Problems may then arise if the proxy tries to override the preferences. The law in individual states often directly addresses the relation between proxy appointments and treatment directives.[50,51,52,53] In general, the proxy is ethically and legally bound to effectuate the patient's treatment choices. When the patient has failed to make explicit treatment choices, either in a treatment directive or orally, the proxy is bound to extrapolate from what is known of the patient's values and preferences to determine as best he or she can what the patient would want; this is typically labeled an exercise in "substituted judgment." If not enough is known of the patient's values and preferences to ground such a judgment, the proxy is bound to decide in the patient's best interests. A proxy's authority is thus governed by certain decision-making standards, and the proxy is obligated to honor the patient's wishes, whether stated in a treatment directive or elsewhere. One caveat has been noted: there is some disagreement over whether a proxy can override a treatment directive that seriously threatens an incompetent but conscious-patient's best interests.

The proxy may make a decision with which the physician or institution disagrees. This is not a problem peculiar to appointed proxies or advance directives. Disagreement surfaces with some frequency between physicians and patients, families, other intimates, and proxies. As always, it is crucial for the physician to discuss the disagreement with the relevant decision maker, attempting to understand the source and resolve the matter. If resolution is elusive, others within the institution can sometimes assist. Judicial resolution is available if all else fails.

One source of disagreement deserves special mention. The proxy (or for that matter, the treatment directive itself) may state a treatment choice that the individual physician believes he or she cannot carry out as a matter of conscience or that violates the commitments and mission of the institution. There has been scholarly discussion [54,55] and some adjudication [56] of the circumstances under which institutions and physicians or other care givers can exempt themselves from carrying out treatment choices. Care givers and institutions are not free to impose unwanted treatment. The PSDA recognizes, however, that a number of states (such as New York) allow providers to assert objections of conscience.[57] Before a patient is admitted, institutions should give notice of any limitation on their willingness to implement treatment choices. Similarly, an individual physician should give as much notice as possible and should assist in the orderly transfer of the patient to a physician who can carry out those choices.

Conclusion

Advance directives have provoked a number of reservations. As the PSDA goes into effect, requiring discussion and implementation of directives, it will be essential to address physicians' further reservations as they arise.

Yet that necessary step will not be sufficient to ensure that the PSDA produces more benefit than harm. There is a risk that written advance directives may wrongly come to be viewed as the only way to make treatment decisions for the future. Physicians and other care givers may improperly begin to require an advance directive before treatment may be forgone for incompetent patients. To avoid this, staff education must include discussion of the various ways to decide about life-sustaining treatment and plan future care. Even under the PSDA, not all patients will use advance directives.

There is a further risk of confusion about the procedures and materials to use in implementing the PSDA. All personnel in the relevant institutions will need clarification of the step-by-step process to be followed with patients, the written materials to use, and how to resolve specific questions. The information conveyed to patients must be understandable, accurate in summarizing the patients' rights, and sensitively communicated. All staff members who are involved must be trained. Institutions must design appropriate protocols.

Finally, there is a risk that the PSDA will reduce the discussion of treatment options and directives to a bureaucratic process dominated by brochures and forms. To avoid this, the discussion of advance directives must be part of an ongoing dialogue between physician and patient about the patient's health status and future. Doctors must accept responsibility for initiating these discussions and conducting them skillfully. Such discussions should begin early in the patient's relationship with the doctor, and the content of directives should be reviewed periodically. Institutions and organizations should set up complementary systems to support this effort. The PSDA's requirements must become not a ceiling but a floor—a catalyst for broader innovation to integrate directives into good patient care.

References

1. Omnibus Budget Reconciliation Act of 1990. Pub. L. No. 101-508 §§ 4206, 4751 (codified in scattered sections of 42 U.S.C., especially §§ 1395cc, 1396a (West Supp. 1991))

2. President's Commission for the Study of Ethical Problems in Medicine and Biomedical and Behavioral Research. Making health care decisions: the ethical and legal implications of informed consent in the patient-practitioner relationship. Vol. 1. Report. Washington, D.C.: Government Printing Office, 1982.

3. Guidelines on the termination of life-sustaining treatment and the care of the dying. Bloomington, Ind.: Indiana University Press and the Hastings Center, 1987

4. Emanuel LL, Barry MJ, Stoeckle JD, Ettelson LM, Emanuel EJ. Advance directives for medical care—a case for greater use. N Engl J Med 1991; 324:889-95

5. Annas GJ. The health care proxy and the living will. N Engl J Med 1991; 324:1210-13

6. La Puma J, Orentlicher D, Moss RJ. Advance directives on admission: clinical implications and analysis of the Patient Self-Determination Act of 1990. JAMA 1991;266:402-05

7. Gamble ER, McDonald PJ, Lichstein PR. Knowledge, attitudes, and behavior of elderly persons regarding living wills. Arch Intern Med 1991;151:277-80

8. Knox RA. Poll: Americans favor mercy killing. Boston Globe. November 3, 1991:1, 22

9. Cruzan v. Director, Mo. Dep't of Health, 110 S. Ct. 2841 (1990)

10. Society for the Right to Die. Refusal of treatment legislation: a state by state compilation of enacted and model statutes. New York: Society for the Right to Die, 1991

11. Meisel A. The right to die. New York: John Wiley, 1989

12. Danis M, Southerland LI, Garrett JM, et al. A prospective study of advance directives for life-sustaining care. N Engl J Med 1991;324:882-88

13. White ML, Fletcher JC. The Patient Self-Determination Act: on balance, more help than hindrance. JAMA 1991;266:410-12

14. Greco PJ, Schulman KA, Lavizzo-Mourey R, Hansen-Flaschen J. The Patient Self-Determination Act and the future of advance directives. Ann Intern Med 1991;115:639-43

15. Teno J, Fleishman J, Brock DW, Mor V. The use of formal prior directives among patients with HIV-related diseases. J Gen Intern Med 1990;5:490-94

16. Davidson KW, Hackler C, Caradine DR, McCord RS. Physicians' attitudes on advance directives. JAMA 1989;262:2415-19

17. Brett AS. Limitations of listing specific medical interventions in advance directives. JAMA 1991;266:825-28

18. Lo B, McLeod GA, Saika G. Patient attitudes to discussing life-sustaining treatment. Arch Intern Med 1986;146:1613-15

19. Emanuel LL, Emanuel EJ. The medical directive: a new comprehensive advance care document. JAMA 1989;261:3288-93

20. Kohn M, Menon G. Life prolongation: views of elderly outpatients and health care professionals. J Am Geriatr Soc 1988;36:840-44

21. McCrary SV, Botkin JR. Hospital policy on advance directives: do institutions ask patients about living wills? JAMA 1989;262:2411-14

22. Shmerling RH, Bedell SE, Lilienfeld A, Delbanco TL. Discussing cardiopulmonary resuscitation: a study of elderly outpatients. J Gen Intern Med 1988;3:317-21

23. Finucane TE, Shumway JM, Powers RL, D'Alessandri RM. Planning with elderly outpatients for contingencies of severe illness: a survey and clinical trial. J Gen Intern Med 1988;3:322-25

24. Ackerman F. Not everybody wants to sign a living will. New York Times. October 13, 1989:A32

25. Molloy DW, Guyatt GH. A comprehensive health care directive in a home for the aged. Can Med Assoc J 1991;145:307-11

26. Callahan D. Medical futility, medical necessity: the-problem-without-a-name. Hastings Cent Rep 1991;21(4):30-35

27. Youngner SJ. Futility in context. JAMA 1990;264:1295-96

28. Youngner. Who defines futility? JAMA 1988;260:2094-95

29. Lantos JD, Singer PA, Walker RM, et al. The illusion of futility in clinical practice. Am J Med 1989;87:81-84

30. Emanuel LL. Does the DNR order need life-sustaining intervention? Time for comprehensive advance directives. Am J Med 1989;86:87-90

31. Orentlicher D. The right to die after Cruzan. JAMA 1990;264:2444-46

32. Weir RF, Gostin L. Decisions to abate life-sustaining treatment for nonautonomous patients: ethical standards and legal liability for physicians after Cruzan. *JAMA* 1990;264:1846–53

33. Hardin SB, Welch HG, Fisher ES. Should advance directives be obtained in the hospital? A review of patient competence during hospitalizations prior to death. *Clin Res* 1991;39:626A. abstract

34. Doukas DJ, McCullough LB. The values history: the evaluation of the patient's values and advance directives. *J Fam Pract* 1991;32:145–53

35. Gibson JM. National values history project. *Generations* 1990;14:Suppl:51–64

36. Eisendrath SJ, Jonsen AR. The living will: help or hindrance? *JAMA* 1983;249:2054–58

37. North Carolina Gen. Stat. § 90–321(a)(2) (1991)

38. Forrow L, Gogel E, Thomas E. Advance directives for medical care. *N Engl J Med* 1991;325:1255

39. Emanuel L. The health care directive: learning how to draft advance care documents. *J Am Geriatr Soc* 1991;39:1221–28

40. Dresser RS. Advance directives, self-determination, and personal identity. In: Hackler C, Moseley R, Vawter DE, eds. *Advance directives in medicine.* New York: Praeger Publishers, 1989:155–70

41. Buchanan AE, Brock DW. *Deciding for others: the ethics of surrogate decision making.* New York: Cambridge University Press, 1989:152–89

42. Everhart MA, Pearlman RA. Stability of patient preferences regarding life-sustaining treatments. *Chest* 1990;97:159–64

43. Silverstein MD, Stocking CB, Antel JP, Beckwith J, Roos RP, Siegler M. Amyotrophic lateral sclerosis and life-sustaining therapy: patients' desires for information, participation in decision making, and life-sustaining therapy. *Mayo Clin Proc* 1991;66:906–13

44. Emanuel LL, Barry MJ, Stoeckle JD, Emanuel EJ. A detailed advance care directive: practicality and durability. *Clin Res* 1990;38:738A. abstract

45. Seckler AB, Meier DE, Mulvihill M, Paris BEC. Substituted judgement: how accurate are proxy predictions? *Ann Intern Med* 1991;115:92–98

46. Tomlinson T, Howe K, Notman M, Rossmiller D. An empirical study of proxy consent for elderly persons. *Gerontologist* 1990;30:54–64

47. Zweibel NR, Cassel CK. Treatment choices at the end of life: a comparison of decisions by older patients and their physician-selected proxies. *Gerontologist* 1989;29:615–21

48. Ouslander JG, Tymchuk AJ, Rahbar B. Health care decisions among elderly long-term care residents and their potential proxies. *Arch Intern Med* 1989; 149:1367–72

49. Uhlmann RF, Pearlman RA, Cain KC. Physicians' and spouses' predictions of elderly patients' resuscitation preferences. *J Gerontol* 1988;43:M115–M121

50. Kansas Stat. Ann. § 58–629 (Supp. 1990)

51. Vermont Stat. Ann. tit. 14, §§ 3453, 3463 (Supp. 1991)

52. West Virginia Code § 16–30A–4 (Supp. 1991)

53. Wisconsin Stat. Ann. § 155.20 (1989–90)

54. Annas GJ. Transferring the ethical hot potato. *Hastings Cent Rep* 1987;17(1):20–21

55. Miles SH, Singer PA, Siegler M. Conflicts between patients' wishes to forgo treatment and the policies of health care facilities. *N Engl J Med* 1989;321:48–50

56. In re Jobes, 529 A.2nd 434 (N.J. 1987)

57. New York Pub. Health Law § 2984 (McKinney Supp. 1991)

Reading 8.3: J.K. Miles, "Taking Patient Virtue Seriously"

Chapter 2 introduced virtue ethics as a theory for practical bioethics. In this article I consider virtue ethics applied to patients. What are the virtues of a good patient? How do we figure out what makes some patients better at being patients than others? How do we cultivate those virtues?

What is it that makes some people better patients than others? Even correcting for socioeconomic factors, why do some people flourish despite their chronic illness while others languish? Healthcare providers are asking these important questions. Literature on patient self-management has ballooned as healthcare professionals have come to recognize that patients who can take responsibility for their care are less expensive and contribute to increased morale among healthcare providers [1]. It is also an important question for public health policy. Recognizing what makes certain people better at recovering from illness and keeping themselves healthy could help with education initiatives and overall healthcare costs.

Here I am after a theory of how one can develop the virtues necessary to be a good patient. So far attempts to teach and mentor patients about how to be a good patient, such as Britain's Expert Patient Programme, have seen mixed results [2–4]. The most successful programs rely on more than instruction and mentoring. They create a culture where patients develop self-efficacy, which I argue stands in for a bundle of virtues associated with being a good patient.

> In the next section, I consider why the virtues of patients are under-explored, including objections to the idea of applying virtues to patients at all.

My title implies that the medical community has yet to take patient virtue theory seriously. If it did, the virtues of a good patient would occupy the same status as the virtues of a good physician or a good nurse. Extended discussion of the virtues of a good physician [5] and a good nurse [6] have informed discussions of healthcare ethics.

One reason for the asymmetry between ethical theory on provider (physician and nurse) virtue and ethical theory on patient virtue may not be a matter of negligence as much as a matter of priority. Medical professionals and bioethicists, not patients, are the predominant readers of bioethics literature, so one would expect the bulk of theory to be about the provider in the provider–patient relationship [7]. The recent trend toward patient self-management and the public health emphasis on self-care and patient responsibility, however, mean that bioethics must broaden its concerns to encompass the patient as well as the clinician [8].

Second, there is the worry that delving into patient virtue could be detrimental to actual patient care. Given patients' dependence on medical professionals and their vulnerable state due to illness, clinicians may think it is wrong-headed to apply virtue theory to patients because they are not fully autonomous agents. An emphasis on patient virtue could, the objection goes, cause healthcare providers to think less of patients who do not exhibit the expected virtues and result in a diminished provider–patient relationship.

It seems presumptuous, if not paternalistic, to assume that the burdens of illness render moral reflection and cultivation impossible. Larry Churchill et al. suggest a "reciprocal set of patient values, principles, and virtues" to complement both patients' rights and the traditional values of the physician [8, p. 151]. Bioethicists can correct this asymmetry in a way that provides a practical theory for patient-centered medicine—something clinicians and administrators can take seriously. Failure to provide such a theory risks widening the gap between clinical and moral reasoning....

> The first reason seems understandable. Bioethics literature is written mostly for the medical establishment, so philosophizing about patient virtues is not a priority. The second reason, however, is more controversial. Do you agree with my claim that it is paternalistic to avoid any discussion of patient virtue for fear that it might harm vulnerable patients? What do you think of Larry Churchill's call for a reciprocal set of values, principles, and virtues for patients and providers?

Strategies for Finding Patient Virtues

There is a definite trend in contemporary medical theory toward patient empowerment, self-management, and shared decision-making. Studies of patients with chronic conditions show that character and outlook are key to coping with illness [9, 10]. Efforts to construct a patient virtue theory seem to use two basic strategies. The first is a role-based strategy, whereby patient virtue derives from an extended examination of the role of the patient in the provider–patient relationship. Virtuous patients are those who exemplify the right attitudes and actions within that role. The alternative is a duty-based strategy.

Just as doctors and other healthcare professionals have duties toward their patients, so do patients have duties toward themselves and their healthcare team. The virtuous patient is one who discharges those duties with excellence. Both strategies show promise, but I will make the case that the role-based strategy has the advantage.

> I do a lot of philosophical name dropping or referencing in this section. Note the discussion of Parsons's "sick role" from earlier readings in this chapter. I present two different strategies for figuring out the virtues of a good patient, role-based and duty-based, but I think there are problems with each. A couple of questions to ask yourself: Why do I think both strategies have problems? Why do I favor the "bottom-up" role-based approach? Have I left out any objections?

THE ROLE-BASED STRATEGY

In 1985, Karen Lebacqz broached the subject of patient virtue by arguing that one cannot talk about patient virtue without first understanding the role of the patient and the circumstances by which a patient can be excellent in her role: "We cannot speak of a virtuous 'patient' until we speak of the 'sick role'. 'Patient' is a role, and the virtues of a patient have to do with excellence in the role as well as responses to pain and personal change" [11, p. 77]. Edmund Pellegrino and David Thomasma consider patient virtue in *For the Patient's Good*, writing "in so far as patients are patients, four virtues are particularly required: truthfulness, probity (compliance), tolerance of others, and trust" [12, p. 107]. However, Pellegrino admits that only truthfulness and compliance are necessary to the end of healing. Tolerance and trust enhance the provider–patient relationship.

The trouble with this description of the sick role is that it assumes that healing is within the purview of the physician. The patient's part in healing is to give the doctor the information needed to diagnose and treat (truthfulness) and then to adhere to the treatment provided (compliance). This may work well if a patient has an acute case of strep throat or appendicitis where the definition of healing is clear. However, it may not suffice for a patient facing a healthcare environment in which she must interact with as many as twelve different healthcare providers.

Pellegrino and Thomasma's account of the patient's role risks obscuring their point about virtue as applied to medicine [12]. Healing as an end can look very different depending on the overall ends of individuals outside their role as patient. Consider the difference between what healing means for a chronic patient versus what it means for a terminal patient. Both patients are concerned with self-maintenance and both have obligations to their physician regarding the virtues of veracity and compliance, but they attend to these obligations in different contexts.

Instead of defining the "sick role" from the top down, a more promising method for picking out patient virtues is to observe those patients who seem to be flourishing and find their common character traits. Alastair Campbell and Teresa Swift derive "the personal qualities that a chronically ill person must draw on or develop in order to live a happy or fulfilling life despite physical disability" [13]. The subjects were patients with chronic but treatable diseases—specifically, rheumatoid arthritis and endometriosis—alongside patients with terminal end-stage renal disease and patients with mental illness (mood disorder). Patients were interviewed about "living well" with their conditions. What emerged were several key virtues including self-regarding virtues (maintaining self-respect, being realistic) and other-regarding virtues (maintaining good relationships, taking part in the community, being courageous). Swift et al. did a more extensive study of the virtues found in interviews with chronic osteoarthritis patients, with narratives coalescing around the thematic foci of courage, prudence, gratitude, and self-worth [10].

Wim Dekkers and colleagues used similar methods to identify virtues for end-stage renal disease patients [9]. The authors identify twelve thematic clusters that constitute virtuous coping with illness. Not surprisingly, these attitudes overlap with previous data. Dekkers et al. mention both self-regarding virtues such as perseverance, acceptance, and vitality and other-regarding virtues such as a sense of community and gratitude. This bottom-up approach seems to present a more promising track for bioethics to insert itself into the clinical conversation. It is patient-centric in a way that the top-down approach is not. It also fits more comfortably within evidence-based medicine because the approach lends itself to empirical study. As Stanford's successful chronic disease self-management program (CDSMP) has shown, clinicians steeped in evidence-based medicine are more receptive to patient studies than to philosophical reasoning alone [14].

While this bottom-up role-based strategy gives useful insight into what virtues manifest in narrative, it does not by itself offer direction as to how virtues might be encouraged, depicting only what they look like when they are present. The mixed results of the United Kingdom's expert patient program suggest that education is not sufficient for patient self-efficacy [2]. In successful programs like Stanford's long-running CDSMP, patients are seen to develop self-efficacy not only by taking courses but also by adopting a culture in which self-effective habits are encouraged, practiced, and mentored [14]. In the next section, I suggest that casting self-efficacy in terms of virtue would improve the general thinking about patient self-management.

THE DUTY-BASED STRATEGY

Another way to identify patient virtues is to begin with something that is slightly easier to nail down—such as patient duties. The duty-based approach might be called quasi-Kantian, since, for Kant, virtue is the strength of will a person possesses to fulfill her duties [15].

Patients have duties to be truthful with their physicians or nurses and to comply with agreed upon treatment plans. It might be said that the virtuous patient is the one who discharges those duties with excellence. Such patients are, for instance, truthful without being overweening and compliant without being obsequious.

The most articulate attempt to derive patient virtue from duty is Candace Cummins Gauthier's patient virtue of moral responsibility [16]. Within the healthcare system, patients have obligations to individual caregivers, family members, providers, and the medical community as a whole. The American Medical Association Code of Ethics derives patient responsibility from the principle of autonomy [17]. Gauthier, however, thinks autonomy is insufficient to ground a patient's other-regarding duties: "What we are looking for is a way to justify the move from respect for patient autonomy, with its focus on individual self-determination, to patient responsibilities that have either an indirect or a direct impact on others, such as family members and the community as a whole" [16, p. 155]. While Gauthier recognizes the problem of laying strong moral requirements on a sick individual, as Pellegrino does when he speaks of wounded humanity and Dan English does when he speaks of patient feasibility [12, 18], she is not willing to absolve sick people of their moral duties to others. In her words: "My own conclusion is that while the exercise of autonomy, without consideration of the impact of one's choices on others is certainly possible and even understandable, it is also morally wrong in the sense of being morally irresponsible" [16, p. 158]. By developing a virtue of moral responsibility for patients, Gauthier attempts to bridge the gap between patient autonomy and the social good of healthcare: "To be morally responsible, as a virtue of character, one must be properly responsive to the outcomes of one's choices and actions, and their impact in the world" [16, p. 160]. Patients who possess the virtue of moral responsibility act autonomously in light of their care for others and their recognition of their place in a social order.

This approach seems right. Patients who do not adequately consider their relationship to others in terms of justice lack virtue. Gauthier's emphasis on other-regarding moral responsibility undermines what might be called the "squeaky wheel objection." What if, the objection goes, being an ornery difficult patient steeped in denial actually gets patients more attention from medical staff and this leads to better health outcomes? In other words, what if the squeaky wheel gets the best care? Would this change our concept of patient virtue?

There are two problems with this line of thinking. First, the squeaky wheel objection assumes that more attention leads to better care. In the clinical setting, there is evidence that quantity does not entail quality. Difficult patients do not just exhaust healthcare providers; they cause them to make more errors in diagnosis [19]. Second, Gauthier's morally responsible patient theory contradicts this conclusion. Virtuous patients consider the impact of their individual healthcare decisions on the other stakeholders, such as their family, medical team, and community. They do not take up more resources than necessary because such resources may be needed for others. A morally responsible patient will make end-of-life treatment known ahead of time with clear advance directives [16, p. 277]. Family members of patients that lack decisional capacity should take into consideration the interests of others when they believe others' interests would be important to the patient.

Gauthier does not mention duties to one's own health in her sketch of moral responsibility. This omission may represent an attempt at maintaining distance from the American Medical Association's autonomy-based conception of responsibility. However, what happens when such duties to one's own health conflict with one's moral responsibility to others in a clinical setting? Samuel Gorovitz argues that patients do not have a duty to seek their own health [20]. Roger Sider and Colleen Clements argue that they do have such a duty [21]. Surely, though, if moral responsibility is a virtue, then it encompasses both self-regarding and other-regarding dimensions. This is demonstrated by the role-based strategy. There is a balance to be struck—one that practical wisdom or prudence would go a long way to illuminate if moral responsibility were interpreted as a virtue.

Toward a Patient Virtue Theory

Of course, as a moral philosopher, I am not going to pick a theory of patient virtue from those above. I am going to combine the best elements and sketch my own theory.

With these strategies in mind, I am able to make several claims about how a patient virtue theory might proceed. To implement a theory of patient virtue that can inform the provider–patient relationship, one should begin by addressing the virtue theory on the other side—that is, the virtues of clinicians.

The virtues of good doctors or nurses are inextricable from their role in the clinical setting. Ethicists began by identifying the professional role played by physicians. This was accomplished from the top down by Pellegrino and Thomasma [12], but also from the bottom up by observing exemplars of physician virtue put forth by early medical humanities contributors like William Osler [4]. The bioethics literature has distilled the character traits that allow clinicians to perform their role with excellence. Clinical education has, in turn, sought to train physicians and evaluate them according to how they exhibited those virtues. This educational process uses exemplars of physician virtue without demanding a formalized list of virtues or dictating how they were to be applied in medicine. Such training is more than just instruction in the virtues; it is a forum in which the virtues were modeled, rehearsed, and practiced.

Likewise, it seems that virtues are inextricable from the role of the patient. Reliance on the "sick role" reduces patient virtue to compliance and truth-telling. Those skills/virtues do not pick out what it means to say that some patients are better at being patients than others. They do not get at the heart of what is meant by self-management or shared decision-making.

The narrative studies by Campbell and Swift suggest that the best approach may be from the bottom up [13]. More studies need to be conducted to elucidate the common experiences among patients who manage their disorders well. An illness or disorder is an obstacle or impediment to a person's good. It does not just impede one's good of health; it impedes one's entire flourishing.

... If illness is an impediment to flourishing, patient virtues are those character traits that enable the patient to recover as well as possible from this impediment.... Some impediments can be removed completely, as a broken bone that heals or a sinus infection that is cured with antibiotics. Other impediments cannot be removed; they can only be tolerated, as when someone has a knee injury that heals but forces him to live with a persistent limp. Still other impediments dramatically alter what flourishing means for a given person. A traumatic brain injury for the professor or a terminal illness for the stay-at-home parent combines elements of chronic malady with a fundamental change in what flourishing can be.

Coping is not merely a social skill; it is a habitual bringing to bear of character traits to negotiate an impediment to flourishing.... Recovery entails far more than the virtues of compliance and honesty.

What stands out in the empirical studies is practical wisdom or prudence. This virtue allows successful patients to adjust their sense of good in light of their illness. Virtuous patients adjust their expectations and find ways to continue flourishing even when their prior state cannot be recovered. For instance, a patient diagnosed with rheumatoid arthritis can display practical wisdom by recognizing that recovery may not mean that she is able to do all the things she used to do (e.g., weightlifting), given her propensity for joint damage and the fact that rheumatoid arthritis is incurable.

Not all patient virtues are self-regarding, however, as recognized by the duty-based strategy. The virtue of justice is applicable to the patient's relationship with her physician. The successful patient recognizes that resources in healthcare are limited. Patients should not expect more or less than they deserve from healthcare providers. Furthermore, virtuous patients recognize that they are in a sharing relationship that generates obligations if they are to be just in their dealings. As Gauthier and the duty-based strategy highlight, fairness dictates truthful disclosure because without truthful disclosure clinicians make mistakes, misdiagnose, or waste scarce resources [16]....

More research needs to be done, but it seems plausible that patients would develop virtues in the same way that doctors and nurses do. They simulate, emulate, and evaluate encounters. To this end, patient education programs that take patient virtue seriously would do well to simulate encounters where good patients excel, such as the initial provider–patient encounter or the follow-up visit. Good patients know how to talk to doctors about their illnesses. They are not completely passive, but neither are they belligerent and demanding. Patient education that takes virtue seriously is also apt to find mentoring extremely important, as it fulfills the role-model method of cultivating virtues. If those patients who handle terminal or chronic illness well can be identified, then they can serve as models for others to emulate. So-called expert patients can help other patients and medical staff in their representation of an ideal.

People developing virtues benefit from friendships and reflection. Reaping these benefits will require a new level of commitment within healthcare. There are classes to prepare people to drive defensively, administer cardiopulmonary resuscitation, and render first aid, since these are skills that they might need. And yet people are not taught how to be good patients—a skill that they will almost certainly need....

References

1.   Redman, Barbara K. 2004. *Patient self-management of chronic disease: The health care provider's challenge*. Boston: Jones and Bartlett.

2. Griffiths, Chris, Gill Foster, Jean Ramsey, Sandra Eldridge, and Stephanie Taylor. 2007. How effective are expert patient (lay led) education programmes for chronic disease? *BMJ* 334: 1254–56.

3. Hardy, Pip. 2004. *The Expert Patient Programme: A critical review*. Pilgrim Projects. www.pilgrimprojects.co.uk/papers/epp_msc.pdf. Accessed March 8, 2019.

4. Shaw, Joanne, and Mary Baker. 2004. "Expert patient"—dream or nightmare? *BMJ* 328: 723–24.

5. Marcum, James A. 2012. *The virtuous physician: The role of virtue in medicine*. Dordrecht: Springer.

6. Sellman, Derek. 2011. *What makes a good nurse: Why the virtues are important for nurses*. London: Jessica Kingsley.

7. Draper, Heather, and Tom Sorell. 2002. Patients' responsibilities in medical ethics. *Bioethics* 16: 335–52.

8. Churchill, Larry R., Joseph B. Fanning, and David Schenck. 2013. *What patients teach: The everyday ethics of healthcare*. Oxford: Oxford University Press.

9. Dekkers, Wim, Inez Uerz, Jean-Pierre Wils. 2005. Living well with end stage renal disease: Patients' narratives interpreted from a virtue perspective. *Ethical Theory and Moral Practice* 8: 485–506.

10. Swift, Teresa L., Richard E. Ashcroft, Win Tadd, Alastair V. Campbell, and Paul A. Dieppe. 2002. Living well through chronic illness: The relevance of virtue theory to patients with chronic osteoarthritis. *Arthritis and Rheumatism* 47: 474–78.

11. Lebacqz, Karen. 1985. The virtuous patient. In *Virtue and medicine: Explorations in the character of medicine*, ed. Earl E. Shelp, 275–88. Dordrecht: Reidel.

12. Pellegrino, Edmund D., and David C. Thomasma. 1988. *For the patient's good: The restoration of beneficence in health care*. New York: Oxford University Press.

13. Campbell, Alastair V., and Teresa Swift. 2002. What does it mean to be a virtuous patient? Virtue from the patient's perspective. *Scottish Journal of Healthcare Chaplaincy* 5: 29–35.

14. Lorig, Kate. 2014. Chronic disease self-management program: Insights from the eye of the storm. *Frontiers in Public Health* 2: 253. https://doi.org/10.3389/fpubh.2014.00253.

15. Hill, Thomas E., Jr., and Adam Cureton. 2018. Kant on virtue: Seeking the ideal in human conditions. In *The Oxford handbook of virtue*, ed. Nancy E. Snow, 263–280. Oxford: Oxford University Press.

16. Gauthier, Candace Cummins. 2005. The virtue of moral responsibility and the obligations of patients. *Journal of Medicine and Philosophy* 30: 153–66.

17. American Medical Association. 2016. AMA Code of Medical Ethics. https://www.ama-assn.org/sites/ama-assn.org/files/corp/media-browser/principles-of-medical-ethics.pdf. Accessed March 8, 2019.

18. English, Dan C. 2005. Moral obligations of patients: A clinical view. *Journal of Medicine and Philosophy* 30: 139–52.

19. Schmidt, H.G., Tamara van Gog, Stephanie C.E. Schuit, Kees Van den Berge, Paul L.A. Van Daele, Herman Bueving, Tim Van der Zee, Walter W. Van den Broek, Jan L.C.M. Van Saase, and Sílvia Mamede. 2017. Do patients' disruptive behaviours influence the accuracy of a doctor's diagnosis? A randomised experiment. *BMJ Quality and Safety* 26: 19–23.

20. Gorovitz, Samuel. 1984. Why you don't owe it to yourself to seek health. *Journal of Medical Ethics* 10: 143–46.

21. Sider, Roger C., and Colleen D. Clements. 1984. Patients' ethical obligation for their health. *Journal of Medical Ethics* 10: 138–42.

...

ETHICS COMMITTEE

The Ashley Treatment*

Ashley is a nine-year-old girl who has static encephalopathy—a severe brain impairment. She cannot walk or talk. She has the mental capacity of a 1-year-old. She cannot keep her head up, roll over, or sit up by herself. She is fed with a tube. Her parents call her "Pillow Angel" because she stays right where they place her, usually on a pillow.

In an unusual case stirring ethical debate, doctors at Seattle Children's Hospital and Ashley's parents are describing how she received treatment over the past few years designed to stunt her growth radically. Her treatment has involved several major medical interventions:

1. hysterectomy (to prevent menstruation and pregnancy),
2. surgery to remove her breast buds (to provide comfort and to desexualize her to care givers),
3. subsequent high doses of estrogen and growth-stopping hormones.

The treatment, known as growth attenuation, is expected to keep Ashley's height at about 1.3 meters and her weight at about 34 kilograms for life. Had she not been treated, doctors estimate, she would have attained a woman's average weight and height.

The treatment has outraged some doctors and caregivers, who say it is a violation of a person's dignity to impose such impairment on their growth. Some say it is also a violation of non-maleficence. Others object that while some elements of what is being called the "Ashley Treatment" are justified for Ashley's health, others are simply convenient for the parents and should not be provided.

But Ashley's parents, who do not want to be publicly identified, say it allows her to have more interaction with her parents and younger siblings and provides the best options for Ashley's health.

---

* This is a summary of the real-world case of "Ashley X," which was widely covered in the media. For a visual summary, see pillowangel.org/AT-Summary.pdf.

Do a full case-study analysis per our usual procedure, and in that analysis be sure to answer the following questions:

Suppose your hospital is approached (or as a parent the option of having the "Ashley Treatment" is presented to you for your child): Would you allow the procedure? Would you modify it (only do some of the procedure but not all of it), or would you flatly refuse?

CHAPTER 9

Dilemmas with Abortion

Choosing for Two?*

It was one of the toughest decisions Danielle had ever had to make. Just a few weeks ago she came in to see her OB for a check-up and pap smear at the end of her first trimester. She was so happy that she was finally pregnant after hoping and praying for so long. She'd been a little anxious every day since her doctor found some abnormalities and sent them off to be checked—in fact, she was very anxious. Then came the bad news like a hammer. The abnormalities were stage II cervical cancer. Her husband would have her on chemo and radiation *yesterday* if he could. But the baby. She wanted this baby. Wanted it like nothing else. She had names picked out: Randall or Rene. Would the cancer treatments hurt the baby? "We just don't know," the doctor said. There were studies of treating *stage I* cervical cancer without any ill effects on the fetus, but nothing with stage II. Her doctor would have her get an abortion and a hysterectomy: "That's the standard course of treatment in this scenario." But it wasn't a scenario. It was her body and her baby, and therefore her choice. Danielle had always been pro-choice—no one should tell a woman what to do with her body. Her husband agreed with the doctor: "I want this baby but if it's a choice between you and it, I choose you." But the 21-week-old on the ultrasound mattered too, right?

---

* This case is adapted from information and concepts in "Cervical Cancer in Pregnant Women: Treat, Wait or Interrupt? Assessment of Current Clinical Guidelines, Innovations and Controversies," *Therapeutic Advances in Medical Oncology* 5.4 (July 2013): 211–19.

Her best friend, Sheila, was adamant: "It's not like it's a baby. Not yet." Was she right? The fetus didn't say. Just jostled inside her. She would have to choose for both.

WHAT'S AT STAKE?

The decision Danielle has to make in the opening gambit is one that many women face: have an abortion to save her own life. Furthermore, Danielle's decision affects more than herself; it affects her doctor, her husband, and the fetus. Many people think that banning abortion completely would affect only those who want to end an unwanted pregnancy; however, abortion is not always elective, as Danielle's decision shows.

The decision to undertake an abortion is inescapably a moral decision. Abortion ends a life, but so does every factory farm where cows are slaughtered for meat. Why is one a common, albeit controversial, practice and the other is the most contentious issue in politics today? When people argue over abortion, they aren't arguing over taking a "life" but rather about the moral status of some kinds of life. Animal rights activists do the same when they argue that eating meat is wrong because animals have rights. Only creatures with moral status can have rights. More people believe unborn fetuses have moral status than people believe animals do. But what is the mysterious "moral status"?

The easiest way to think of moral status is to ask what the difference is between how we can treat rabbits, robots, rocks, and Danielle's future child Randall or Rene.

Rocks have zero moral status. You can kick them, crack them, build with them without any concern that you are doing wrong. Any wrong I do with rocks would have to be using rocks to harm or hurt something else *with* moral status. Can I throw rocks at a robot? "As long as it's yours," you might say. Robots don't seem to have much more moral status than rocks. What if the robot could think pretty sophisticatedly, like IBM's Watson, who beat two *Jeopardy!* champions hands down? If you think it would be wrong to throw rocks at a computer that exhibited that sort of sophisticated thinking, then you are giving Watson more moral status than a rock.

Moral status indicates what is ethically permitted. Rocks have no moral status. A robot you buy from Walmart does not either. But human beings named Randall or Rene *do* have moral status. I should not be able to own people named Randall. But the sixty-four-million-dollar philosophical question is why? It's the job of ethics to seek a justification. What is it about guys named Randall that means I can't own them or throw them off a cliff like a rock or a robot I own? Whatever that is, it is a clue to moral status.

There are several candidates for what makes for the ground of moral status. You might think that the first major difference between rocks, robots, rabbits, and Randalls is the capacity for pain and suffering. Even super-smart Watson the Artificial Intelligence does not feel pain when it is unplugged. This capacity for experiencing pain (and/or pleasure) is what Peter Singer calls "sentience."* If this is what gives Randall more moral status than robots or rocks, then what about the fetus that will be Randall? The fetus can feel pain early in its development, so according to Singer it would have moral status. So does a rabbit. On Singer's account, rabbits and the fetus have the *same* moral status because they feel the same pain.

Singer uses this moral status claim to argue that animals have the same moral status as human beings, that we should not eat them, and that if we are going to experiment on them, we should spread the wealth and experiment on humans in the same way as we do rats, cats, and especially the intelligent primates like chimpanzees. (Fish are a tough case because it is not clear that fish feel pain as mammals do.)

Is there any reason to give fetus Randall or fully grown Randall more moral status than a rabbit, robot, or rock? Don Marquis has argued for the idea that fetus Randall has a future experience of life with desires, goals, projects, and sophisticated thinking that the rabbit will never have.† This gives fetus Randall a future-like-ours that the rabbit, robot, or rock doesn't have. This "future-like-ours" is a catch-all for the sort of moral life that humans have with desires (I want an ice-cream tomorrow), goals (I want to lose weight so I won't eat the ice cream I want), and long-term projects (If I lose that 10 pounds I can go to my class reunion and meet that special someone who got away).

Are there problems with this "future-like-ours" argument? Sure. The first is a sort of objection that says, "Why is this sophisticated mental activity you call 'future-like-ours' so valuable in itself?" In other words, the "future-like-ours" folks have identified this rich cognitive experience and said, "This is what gives moral status," but they have not said what justifies this set of capacities over any other features.

It seems arbitrary. If I wanted to argue that human beings have full moral status (rights and so forth), then I could find some trait that all humans have but no rabbit, robot, or rock has. Humans have 46 chromosomes. Then I can decree that having 46 chromosomes and no fewer gives moral status. I could just as

---

* Peter Singer, "All Animals Are Equal," *Philosophic Exchange* 5, no. 1, Article 6, 1974.
† Don Marquis, "Why Abortion Is Immoral," *The Journal of Philosophy* 86, no. 4 (1989): 183–202.

easily decide that only those with XX chromosomes have full moral status and it would be just as justified.

Second, there are human beings who do not fit the future-like-ours criteria that we might not want to exclude from having full moral status. Some of these people, to make matters more complicated, *did* have a future like ours, but due to some sort of injury or illness they can no longer expect to have a future like ours. Think of people in persistent vegetative states. Do they lose their moral status as soon as they permanently lose those future capacities? Can we treat them like rocks or robots or rabbits? Can we harvest their organs? Test drugs on them?

The future-like-ours argument would seem to give full moral status to embryos, fetuses, and human beings (don't forget any intelligent alien species from sci-fi as well). But it would exclude people in persistent vegetative states or with cognitive impairment. Furthermore, if this sort of complex inner life is the *sine qua non* ("that without which," i.e., the main requirement) of moral status, doesn't that mean if someone has less of it, they have less moral status? Does the "future-like-ours" argument open up the possibility of degrees of moral status?

Where you stand on the question of moral status affects a lot of your views on today's hot-button public policy issues. It affects how you look at embryonic stem-cell research. Are embryos more like rocks and robots or rabbits and Randalls? It affects your views on cloning. Is cloning wrong because it violates something about moral status? The same is true about the status of persons in persistent vegetative states.

How you think about moral status certainly affects your views on abortion, but it does not settle the question. Even if you argue compellingly that fetuses have full moral status, this does not automatically imply that fetuses have rights to not be aborted. Or so says bioethicist Judith Jarvis Thomson (1929–2020), in the first reading below. If the fetus has moral status, is abortion automatically murder or homicide? There may be good reasons to think that whatever abortion is, it's not murder *even if* the fetus has full moral status as a person. Unlike many who argue for the legality of abortion, Thomson, assumes, for the sake of argument, that *the fetus has the same moral status* as a fully grown adult. She compares pregnancy to waking up to find a world-famous violinist attached to you because he needs your kidneys. The violinist has full moral status but needs your kidneys to survive, much like a fetus needs a womb to gestate. Does the violinist's dependence on you mean they have the right to your kidneys for the next nine months? Moral status does not automatically imply a right to gestation, says Thomson.

You might think "waking up attached to a violinist" is a strange way to describe the normal process of consensual sex leading to accidental pregnancy.

Some have noted that Thomson's analogy fits better with pregnancy due to rape. Thomson, however, wants the argument to apply to all cases of pregnancy, and she adds other analogies that are not as convincing as the violinist analogy. Francis Beckwith (b. 1960) analyzes Thomson's argument in the second reading.

WHAT'S THE DEBATE?

Reading 9.1: Judith Jarvis Thomson, "A Defense of Abortion"

Thomson gives perhaps the most famous argument in favor of keeping abortion legal. Often anti-abortion arguments rely on the rights of the fetus to life. Thomson concedes that fetuses have full moral status but argues that this does not imply the right to be brought to term.

Most opposition to abortion relies on the premise that the fetus is a human being, a person, from the moment of conception. The premise is argued for, but, as I think, not well. Take, for example, the most common argument. We are asked to notice that the development of a human being from conception through birth into childhood is continuous; then it is said that to draw a line, to choose a point in this development and say "before this point the thing is not a person, after this point it is a person" is to make an arbitrary choice, a choice for which in the nature of things no good reason can be given. It is concluded that the fetus is, or anyway that we had better say it is, a person from the moment of conception. But this conclusion does not follow. Similar things might be said about the development of an acorn into an oak tree, and it does not follow that acorns are oak trees, or that we had better say they are. Arguments of this form are sometimes called "slippery slope arguments"—the phrase is perhaps self-explanatory—and it is dismaying that opponents of abortion rely on them so heavily and uncritically.

I am inclined to agree, however, that the prospects for "drawing a line" in the development of the fetus look dim. I am inclined to think also that we shall probably have to agree that the fetus has already become a human person well before birth. Indeed, it comes as a surprise when one first learns how early in its life it begins to acquire human characteristics. By the tenth week, for example, it already has a face, arms and legs, fingers and toes; it has internal organs, and brain activity is detectable. On the other hand, I think that the premise is false, that the fetus is not a person from the moment of conception. A newly fertilized ovum, a newly implanted clump of cells, is no more a person than an acorn is an oak tree. But I shall not discuss any of this. For it seems to me to be of great interest to ask what happens if, for the sake of argument, we allow the premise. How, precisely, are we supposed to get from there to the conclusion that abortion is morally impermissible? Opponents of abortion commonly spend most of their time establishing that the fetus is a person, and hardly anytime explaining the step from there to the impermissibility of abortion. Perhaps they think the step too simple and obvious to require much comment. Or perhaps instead they are simply being economical in argument. Many of those who defend abortion rely on the premise that the fetus is not a person, but only a bit of tissue that will become a person at birth; and why pay out more arguments than you have to? Whatever the explanation, I suggest that the step they take is neither easy nor obvious, that it calls for closer examination than it is commonly given, and that when we do give it this closer examination we shall feel inclined to reject it.

I propose, then, that we grant that the fetus is a person from the moment of conception. How does the argument go from here? Something like this, I take it. Every person has a right to life. So the fetus has a right to life. No doubt the mother has a right to decide what shall happen in and to her body; everyone would grant that. But surely a person's right to life is stronger and more stringent than the mother's right to decide what happens in and to her body, and so outweighs it. So the fetus may not be killed; an abortion may not be performed.

> Did you notice the argument made in the last paragraph? That is the argument Thomson is trying to argue against.

It sounds plausible. But now let me ask you to imagine this. You wake up in the morning and find yourself back to back in bed with an unconscious violinist. A famous unconscious violinist. He has been found to have a fatal kidney ailment, and the Society of Music Lovers has canvassed all the available medical records and found that you alone have the right blood type to help.

> Is it far-fetched that you would have the only right blood type? Sure, but remember this is a thought experiment. Thomson is making an analogy between waking up attached to the violinist and finding oneself pregnant.

They have therefore kidnapped you, and last night the violinist's circulatory system was plugged into yours, so that your kidneys can be used to extract poisons from his blood as well as your own. The director of the hospital now tells you, "Look, we're sorry the Society of Music Lovers did this to you—we would never have permitted it if we had known. But still, they did it, and the violinist is now plugged into you. To unplug you would be to kill him. But never mind, it's only for nine months. By then he will have recovered from his ailment, and can safely be unplugged from you." Is it morally incumbent on you to accede to this situation? No doubt it would be very nice of you if you did, a great kindness. But do you have to accede to it? What if it were not nine months, but nine years? Or longer still? What if the director of the hospital says. "Tough luck, I agree, but now you've got to stay in bed, with the violinist plugged into you, for the rest of your life. Because remember this. All persons have a right to life, and violinists are persons. Granted you have a right to decide what happens in and to your body, but a person's right to life outweighs your right to decide what happens in and to your body. So you cannot ever be unplugged from him." I imagine you would regard this as outrageous, which suggests that something really is wrong with that plausible-sounding argument I mentioned a moment ago.

In this case, of course, you were kidnapped, you didn't volunteer for the operation that plugged the violinist into your kidneys. Can those who oppose abortion on the ground I mentioned make an exception for a pregnancy due to rape? Certainly. They can say that persons have a right to life only if they didn't come into existence because of rape; or they can say that all persons have a right to life, but that some have less of a right to life than others, in particular, that those who came into existence because of rape have less. But these statements have a rather unpleasant sound. Surely the question of whether you have a right to life at all, or how much of it you have, shouldn't turn on the question of whether or not you are a product of a rape. And in fact the people who oppose abortion on the ground I mentioned do not make this distinction, and hence do not make an exception in case of rape.

> Do you agree with Thomson's last statement that her argument should have its bite regardless of whether the unwanted fetus is the result of rape?

Nor do they make an exception for a case in which the mother has to spend the nine months of her pregnancy in bed. They would agree that would be a great pity, and hard on the mother; but all the same, all persons have a right to life, the fetus is a person, and so on. I suspect, in fact, that they would not make an exception for a case in which, miraculously enough, the pregnancy went on for nine years, or even the rest of the mother's life.

Some won't even make an exception for a case in which continuation of the pregnancy is likely to shorten the mother's life, they regard abortion as impermissible even to save the mother's life. Such cases are nowadays very rare, and many opponents of abortion do not accept this extreme view. All the same, it is a good place to begin: a number of points of interest come out in respect to it.

> In the following section (1.), Thomson considers what she calls the extreme view. What reasons does she give for the extreme view being the least effective view regarding abortion?

1.

Let us call the view that abortion is impermissible even to save the mother's life "the extreme view." I want to suggest first that it does not issue from the argument I mentioned earlier without the addition of some fairly powerful premises. Suppose a woman has become pregnant, and now learns that she has a cardiac condition such that she will die if she carries the baby to term. What may be done for her? The fetus, being a person, has a right to life, but as the mother is a person too, so has she a right to life. Presumably they have an equal right to life. How is it supposed to come out that an abortion may not be performed? If mother and child have an equal right to life, shouldn't we perhaps flip a coin? Or should we add to the mother's right to life her right to decide what happens in and to her body, which everybody seems to be ready to grant—the sum of her rights now outweighing the fetus's right to life?

The most familiar argument here is the following. We are told that performing the abortion would be directly killing the child, whereas doing nothing would not be killing the mother, but only letting her die. Moreover, in killing the child, one would be killing an innocent person, for the child has committed no crime, and is not aiming at his mother's death. And then there are a variety of ways in which this might be continued. (1) But as directly killing an innocent person is always and absolutely impermissible, an abortion may not be performed. Or, (2) as directly killing an innocent person is murder, and murder is always and absolutely impermissible, an abortion may not be performed. Or,

(3) as one's duty to refrain from directly killing an innocent person is more stringent than one's duty to keep a person from dying, an abortion may not be performed. Or, (4) if one's only options are directly killing an innocent person or letting a person die, one must prefer letting the person die, and thus an abortion may not be performed.

Some people seem to have thought that these are not further premises which must be added if the conclusion is to be reached, but that they follow from the very fact that an innocent person has a right to life. But this seems to me to be a mistake, and perhaps the simplest way to show this is to bring out that while we must certainly grant that innocent persons have a right to life, the theses in (1) through (4) are all false. Take (2), for example. If directly killing an innocent person is murder, and thus is impermissible, then the mother's directly killing the innocent person inside her is murder, and thus is impermissible. But it cannot seriously be thought to be murder if the mother performs an abortion on herself to save her life. It cannot seriously be said that she must refrain, that she must sit passively by and wait for her death.

Let us look again at the case of you and the violinist. There you are, in bed with the violinist, and the director of the hospital says to you, "It's all most distressing, and I deeply sympathize, but you see this is putting an additional strain on your kidneys, and you'll be dead within the month. But you have to stay where you are all the same. because unplugging you would be directly killing an innocent violinist, and that's murder, and that's impermissible." If anything in the world is true, it is that you do not commit murder, you do not do what is impermissible, if you reach around to your back and unplug yourself from that violinist to save your life.

The main focus of attention in writings on abortion has been on what a third party may or may not do in answer to a request from a woman for an abortion. This is in a way understandable. Things being as they are, there isn't much a woman can safely do to abort herself. So the question asked is what a third party may do, and what the mother may do, if it is mentioned at all, if deduced, almost as an afterthought, from what it is concluded that third parties may do. But it seems to me that to treat the matter in this way is to refuse to grant to the mother that very status of person which is so firmly insisted on for the fetus. For we cannot simply read off what a person may do from what a third party may do. Suppose you find yourself trapped in a tiny house with a growing child. I mean a very tiny house, and a rapidly growing child—you are already up against the wall of the house and in a few minutes you'll be crushed to death. The child on the other hand won't be crushed to death; if nothing is done to stop him from growing he'll be hurt, but in the end he'll simply burst open the house and walk out a free man. Now I could well understand it if a bystander were to say. "There's nothing we can do for you. We cannot choose between your life and his, we cannot be the ones to decide who is to live, we cannot intervene." But it cannot be concluded that you too can do nothing, that you cannot attack it to save your life. However innocent the child may be, you do not have to wait passively while it crushes you to death. Perhaps a pregnant woman is vaguely felt to have the status of house, to which we don't allow the right of self-defense. But if the woman houses the child, it should be remembered that she is a person who houses it.

I should perhaps stop to say explicitly that I am not claiming that people have a right to do anything whatever to save their lives. I think, rather, that there are drastic limits to the right of self-defense. If someone threatens you with death unless you torture someone else to death, I think you have not the right, even to save your life, to do so. But the case under consideration here is very different. In our case there are only two people involved, one whose life is threatened, and one who threatens it. Both are innocent: the one who is threatened is not threatened because of any fault, the one who threatens does not threaten because of any fault. For this reason we may feel that we bystanders cannot interfere. But the person threatened can.

In sum, a woman surely can defend her life against the threat to it posed by the unborn child, even if doing so involves its death. And this shows not merely that the theses in (1) through (4) are false; it shows also that the extreme view of abortion is false, and so we need not canvass any other possible ways of arriving at it from the argument I mentioned at the outset....

3.

Where the mother's life is not at stake, the argument I mentioned at the outset seems to have a much stronger pull. "Everyone has a right to life, so the unborn person has a right to life." And isn't the child's right to life weightier than anything other than the mother's own right to life, which she might put forward as ground for an abortion?

This argument treats the right to life as if it were unproblematic. It is not, and this seems to me to be precisely the source of the mistake.

For we should now, at long last, ask what it comes to, to have a right to life. In some views having a right to life includes having a right to be given at least the bare minimum one needs for continued life. But suppose that what in fact IS the bare minimum a man needs for continued life is something he has no right at all to be given? If I am sick unto death, and the only thing that will save my life is the touch of Henry Fonda's cool hand on my fevered brow, then all the same, I have no right to be given the touch of Henry Fonda's cool hand on my fevered brow. It would be frightfully nice of him to fly in from the West Coast to provide it. It would be less nice, though no doubt well meant, if my friends flew out to the West coast and brought Henry Fonda back with them. But I have no right at all against anybody that he should do this for me. Or again, to return to the story I told earlier, the fact that for continued life the violinist needs the continued use of your kidneys does not establish that he has a right to be given the continued use of your kidneys. He certainly has no right against you that you should give him continued use of your kidneys. For nobody has any right to use your kidneys unless you give him this right—if you do allow him to go on using your kidneys, this is a kindness on your part, and not something he can claim from you as his due. Nor has he any right against anybody else that they should give him continued use of your kidneys. Certainly he had no right against the Society of Music Lovers that they should plug him into you in the first place. And if you now start to unplug yourself, having learned that you will otherwise have to spend nine years in bed with him, there is nobody in the world who must try to prevent you, in order to see to it that he is given some thing he has a right to be given.

Some people are rather stricter about the right to life. In their view, it does not include the right to be given anything, but amounts to, and only to, the right not to be killed by anybody. But here a related difficulty arises. If everybody is to refrain from killing that violinist, then everybody must refrain from doing a great many different sorts of things. Everybody must refrain from slitting his throat, everybody must refrain from shooting him—and everybody must refrain from unplugging you from him. But does he have a right against everybody that they shall refrain from unplugging you from him? To refrain from doing this is to allow him to continue to use your kidneys. It could be argued that he has a right against us that we should allow him to continue to use your kidneys. That is, while he had no right against us that we should give him the use of your kidneys, it might be argued that he anyway has a right against us that we shall not now intervene and deprive him of the use of your kidneys. I shall come back to third-party interventions later. But certainly the violinist has no right against you that you shall allow him to continue to use your kidneys. As I said, if you do allow him to use them, it is a kindness on your part, and not something you owe him.

The difficulty I point to here is not peculiar to the right of life. It reappears in connection with all the other natural rights, and it is something which an adequate account of rights must deal with. For present purposes it is enough just to draw attention to it. But I would stress that I am not arguing that people do not have a right to life—quite to the contrary, it seems to me that the primary control we must place on the acceptability of an account of rights is that it should turn out in that account to be a truth that all persons have a right to life. I am arguing only that having a right to life does not guarantee having either a right to be given the use of or a right to be allowed continued use of another person's body—even if one needs it for life itself. So the right to life will not serve the opponents of abortion in the very simple and clear way in which they seem to have thought it would.

4.

There is another way to bring out the difficulty. In the most ordinary sort of case, to deprive someone of what he has a right to is to treat him unjustly. Suppose a boy and his small brother are jointly given a box of chocolates for Christmas. If the older boy takes the box and refuses to give his brother any of the chocolates, he is unjust to him, for the brother has been given a right to half of them. But suppose that, having learned that otherwise it means nine years in bed with that violinist, you unplug yourself from him. You surely are not being unjust to him, for you gave him no right to use your kidneys, and no one else can have given him any such right. But we have to notice that in unplugging yourself, you are killing him; and violinists, like everybody else, have a right to life, and thus in the view we were considering just now, the right not to be killed. So here you do what he supposedly has a right you shall not do, but you do not act unjustly to him in doing it.

The emendation which may be made at this point is this: the right to life consists not in the right not to be killed, but rather in the right not to be killed unjustly. This runs a risk of circularity, but never mind: it would enable us to square the fact that the violinist has a right to life with the fact that you do not act unjustly toward him in unplugging yourself, thereby killing him. For if you do not kill him unjustly, you do not violate his right to life, and so it is no wonder you do him no injustice.

But if this emendation is accepted, the gap in the argument against abortion stares us plainly in the face: it is by no means enough to show that the fetus is a person, and to remind us that all persons have a right to life—we need to be shown also that killing the fetus violates its right to life, i.e., that abortion is unjust killing. And is it?

I suppose we may take it as a datum that in a case of pregnancy due to rape the mother has not given the unborn person a right to the use of her body for food and shelter. Indeed, in what pregnancy could it be supposed that the mother has given the unborn person such a right? It is not as if there are unborn persons drifting about the world, to whom a woman who wants a child says "I invite you in."

> Thomson's violinist argument, it seems, works best when the violinist is an intruder analogous to the case of rape or incest. In this next set of paragraphs, she considers the objection that a woman who engages in consensual sex also does not owe the fetus the use of her body. Do you think this part of the argument is weaker than, as strong as, or stronger than her argument about pregnancy from rape or incest?

But it might be argued that there are other ways one can have acquired a right to the use of another person's body than by having been invited to use it by that person. Suppose a woman voluntarily indulges in intercourse, knowing of the chance it will issue in pregnancy, and then she does become pregnant; is she not in part responsible for the presence, in fact the very existence, of the unborn person inside? No doubt she did not invite it in. But doesn't her partial responsibility for its being there itself give it a right to the use of her body? If so, then her aborting it would be more like the boy's taking away the chocolates, and less like your unplugging yourself from the violinist—doing so would be depriving it of what it does have a right to, and thus would be doing it an injustice.

And then, too, it might be asked whether or not she can kill it even to save her own life: If she voluntarily called it into existence, how can she now kill it, even in self-defense?

The first thing to be said about this is that it is something new. Opponents of abortion have been so concerned to make out the independence of the fetus, in order to establish that it has a right to life, just as its mother does, that they have tended to overlook the possible support they might gain from making out that the fetus is dependent on the mother, in order to establish that she has a special kind of responsibility for it, a responsibility that gives it rights against her which are not possessed by any independent person—such as an ailing violinist who is a stranger to her. On the other hand, this argument would give the unborn person a right to its mother's body only if her pregnancy resulted from a voluntary act, undertaken in full knowledge of the chance a pregnancy might result from it. It would leave out entirely the unborn person whose existence is due to rape. Pending the availability of some further argument, then, we would be left with the conclusion that unborn persons whose existence is due to rape have no right to the use of their mothers' bodies, and thus that aborting them is not depriving them of anything they have a right to and hence is not unjust killing.

And we should also notice that it is not at all plain that this argument really does go even as far as it purports to. For there are cases and cases, and the details make a difference. If the room is stuffy, and I therefore open a window to air it, and a burglar climbs in, it would be absurd to say, "Ah, now he can stay, she's given him a right to the use of her house—for she is partially responsible for his presence there, having voluntarily done what enabled him to get in, in full knowledge that there are such things as burglars, and that burglars burgle." It would be still more absurd to say this if I had had bars installed outside my windows, precisely to prevent burglars from getting in, and a burglar got in only because of a defect in the bars. It remains equally absurd if we imagine it is not a burglar who climbs in, but an innocent person who blunders or falls in. Again, suppose it were like this: people-seeds drift about in the air like pollen, and if you open your windows, one may drift in and take root in your carpets or upholstery. You don't want children, so you fix up your windows with fine mesh screens, the very best you can buy. As can happen, however, and on very, very rare occasions does happen, one of the screens is defective, and a seed drifts in and takes root. Does the person-plant who now develops have a right to the use of your house? Surely not—despite the fact that you voluntarily opened your windows, you knowingly kept carpets and upholstered furniture, and you knew that screens were sometimes defective. Someone may argue that you are responsible for its rooting, that it does have a right to your house, because after all you could have lived out your life with bare floors and furniture, or with sealed windows and doors. But this won't do—for by the same token anyone can avoid a pregnancy due to rape by having a hysterectomy, or anyway by never leaving home without a (reliable!) army.

It seems to me that the argument we are looking at can establish at most that there are some cases in which the unborn person has a right to the use of its mother's body, and therefore some cases in which abortion is unjust killing. There is room for much discussion and argument as to precisely which, if any. But I think we should sidestep this issue and leave it open, for at any rate the argument certainly does not establish that all abortion is unjust killing.

> In Section 5 Thomson draws on a distinction, considered in Chapter 2, to make a case for why the fetus does not have a right to be brought to term even if the mother perhaps has a duty to provide a womb for the child. Does this strengthen the argument? Why or why not?

5.

There is room for yet another argument here, however. We surely must all grant that there may be cases in which it would be morally indecent to detach a person from your body at the cost of his life. Suppose you learn that what the violinist needs is not nine years of your life, but only one hour: all you need do to save his life is to spend one hour in that bed with him. Suppose also that letting him use your kidneys for that one hour would not affect your health in the slightest. Admittedly you were kidnapped. Admittedly you did not give anyone permission to plug him into you. Nevertheless it seems to me plain you ought to allow him to use your kidneys for that hour—it would be indecent to refuse.

Again, suppose pregnancy lasted only an hour, and constituted no threat to life or health. And suppose that a woman becomes pregnant as a result of rape. Admittedly she did not voluntarily do anything to bring about the existence of a child. Admittedly she did nothing at all which would give the unborn person a right to the use of her body. All the same it might well be said, as in the newly amended violinist story, that she ought to allow it to remain for that hour—that it would be indecent of her to refuse.

Now some people are inclined to use the term "right" in such a way that it follows from the fact that you ought to allow a person to use your body for the hour he needs, that he has a right to use your body for the hour he needs, even though he has not been given that right by any person or act. They may say that it follows also that if you refuse, you act unjustly toward him. This use of the term is perhaps so common that it cannot be called wrong; nevertheless it seems to me to be an unfortunate loosening of what we would do better to keep a tight rein on. Suppose that box of chocolates I mentioned earlier had not been given to both boys jointly, but was given only to the older boy. There he sits stolidly eating his way through the box, his small brother watching enviously. Here we are likely to say, "You ought not to be so mean. You ought to give your brother some of those chocolates." My own view is that it just does not follow from the truth of this that the brother has any right to any of the chocolates. If the boy refuses to give his brother any he is greedy, stingy, callous—but not unjust. I suppose that the people I have in mind will say it does follow that the brother has a right to some of the chocolates, and thus that the boy does act unjustly if he refuses to give his brother any. But the effect of saying this is to obscure what we should keep distinct, namely the difference between the boy's refusal in this case and the boy's refusal in the earlier case, in which the box was given to both boys jointly, and in which the small brother thus had what was from any point of view clear title to half.

A further objection to so using the term "right" that from the fact that A ought to do a thing for B it follows that B has a right against A that A do it for him, is that it is going to make the question of whether or not a man has a right to a thing turn on how easy it is to provide him with it; and this seems not merely unfortunate, but morally unacceptable. Take the case of Henry Fonda again. I said earlier that I had no right to the touch of his cool hand on my fevered brow even though I needed it to save my life. I said it would be frightfully nice of him to fly in from the West Coast to provide me with it, but that I had no right against him that he should do so. But suppose he isn't on the West Coast. Suppose he has only to walk across the room, place a hand briefly on my brow— and lo, my life is saved. Then surely he ought to do it—it would be indecent to refuse. Is it to be said, "Ah, well, it follows that in this case she has a right to the touch of his hand on her brow, and so it would be an injustice in him to refuse"? So that I have a right to it when it is easy for him to provide it, though no right when it's hard? It's rather a shocking idea that anyone's rights should fade away and disappear as it gets harder and harder to accord them to him.

So my own view is that even though you ought to let the violinist use your kidneys for the one hour he needs, we should not conclude that he has a right to do so—we should say that if you refuse, you are, like the boy who owns all the chocolates and will give none away, self-centered and callous, indecent in fact, but not unjust. And similarly, that even supposing a case in which a woman pregnant due to rape ought to allow the unborn person to use her body for the hour he needs, we should not conclude that he has a right to do so; we should say that she is self-centered, callous, indecent, but not unjust, if she refuses. The complaints are no less grave; they are just different. However, there is no need to insist on this point. If anyone does wish to deduce "he has a right" from "you ought," then all the same he must surely grant that there are cases in which it is not morally required of you that you allow that violinist to use your kidneys, and in which he does not have a right to use them, and in which you do not do him an injustice if you refuse. And so also for mother and unborn child. Except in such cases as the unborn person has a right to demand it—and we were leaving open the possibility that there may be such cases—nobody is morally required to make large sacrifices, of health, of all other interests and concerns, of all other duties and commitments, for nine years, or even for nine months, in order to keep another person alive.

6.

We have in fact to distinguish between two kinds of Samaritan: the Good Samaritan and what we might call the Minimally Decent Samaritan. The story of the Good Samaritan, you will remember, goes like this:

> A certain man went down from Jerusalem to Jericho, and fell among thieves, which stripped him of his raiment, and wounded him, and departed, leaving him half dead.
>
> And by chance there came down a certain priest that way: and when he saw him, he passed by on the other side.
>
> And likewise a Levite, when he was at the place, came and looked on him, and passed by on the other side.
>
> But a certain Samaritan, as he journeyed, came where he was, and when he saw him he had compassion on him.
>
> And went to him, and bound up his wounds, pouring in oil and wine, and set him on his own beast, and brought him to an inn, and took care of him.
>
> And on the morrow, when he departed, he took out two pence, and gave them to the host, and said unto him, "Take care of him; and whatsoever thou spendest more, when I come again, I will repay thee." (Luke 10:30–35)

The Good Samaritan went out of his way, at some cost to himself, to help one in need of it. We are not told what the options were, that is, whether or not the priest and the Levite could have helped by doing less than the Good Samaritan did, but assuming they could have, then the fact they did nothing at all shows they were not even Minimally Decent Samaritans, not because they were not Samaritans, but because they were not even minimally decent.

These things are a matter of degree, of course, but there is a difference, and it comes out perhaps most clearly in the story of Kitty Genovese, who, as you will remember, was murdered while thirty-eight people watched or listened, and did nothing at all to help her. A Good Samaritan would have rushed out to give direct assistance against the murderer. Or perhaps we had better allow that it would have been a Splendid Samaritan who did this, on the ground that it would have involved a risk of death for himself. But the thirty-eight not only did not do this, they did not even trouble to pick up a phone to call the police. Minimally Decent Samaritanism would call for doing at least that, and their not having done it was monstrous.

After telling the story of the Good Samaritan, Jesus said, "Go, and do thou likewise." Perhaps he meant that we are morally required to act as the Good Samaritan did. Perhaps he was urging people to do more than is morally required of them. At all events it seems plain that it was not morally required of any of the thirty-eight that he rush out to give direct assistance at the risk of his own life, and that it is not morally required of anyone that he give long stretches of his life—nine years or nine months—to sustaining the life of a person who has no special right (we were leaving open the possibility of this) to demand it.

Indeed, with one rather striking class of exceptions, no one in any country in the world is legally required to do anywhere near as much as this for anyone else. The class of exceptions is obvious. My main concern here is not the state of the law in respect to abortion, but it is worth drawing attention to the fact that in no state in this country is any man compelled by law to be even a Minimally Decent Samaritan to any person; there is no law under which charges could be brought against the thirty-eight who stood by while Kitty Genovese died. By contrast, in most states in this country women are compelled by law to be not merely Minimally Decent Samaritans, but Good Samaritans to unborn persons inside them. This doesn't by itself settle anything one way or the other, because it may well be argued that there should be laws in this country as there are in many European countries—compelling at least Minimally Decent Samaritanism. But it does show that there is a gross injustice in the existing state of the law. And it shows also that the groups currently working against liberalization of abortion laws, in fact working toward having it declared unconstitutional for a state to permit abortion, had better start working for the adoption of Good Samaritan laws generally, or earn the charge that they are acting in bad faith.

I should think, myself, that Minimally Decent Samaritan laws would be one thing, Good Samaritan laws quite another, and in fact highly improper. But we are not here concerned with the law. What we should ask is not whether anybody should be compelled by law to be a Good Samaritan, but whether we must accede to a situation in which somebody is being compelled—by nature, perhaps—to be a Good Samaritan. We have, in other words, to look now at third-party interventions. I have been arguing that no person is morally required to make large sacrifices to sustain the life of another who has no right to demand them, and this even where the sacrifices do not include life itself; we are not morally required to be Good Samaritans or anyway Very Good Samaritans to one another. But what if a man cannot extricate himself from such a situation? What if he appeals to us to extricate him? It seems to me plain that there are cases in which we can, cases in which a Good Samaritan would extricate him. There you are, you were kidnapped, and nine years in bed with that violinist lie ahead of you. You have your own life to lead. You are sorry, but you simply cannot see giving up so much of your life to the sustaining of his. You cannot extricate yourself, and ask us to do so. I should have thought that—in light of his having no right to the use of your body—it was obvious that we do not have to accede to your being forced to give up so much. We can do what you ask. There is no injustice to the violinist in our doing so.

7.

Following the lead of the opponents of abortion, I have throughout been speaking of the fetus merely as a person, and what I have been asking is whether or not the argument we began with, which proceeds only from the fetus's being a person, really does establish its conclusion. I have argued that it does not.

But of course there are arguments and arguments, and it may be said that I have simply fastened on the wrong one. It may be said that what is important is not merely the fact that the fetus is a person, but that it is a person for whom the woman has a special kind of responsibility issuing from the fact that she is its mother. And it might be argued that all my analogies are therefore irrelevant— for you do not have that special kind of responsibility for that violinist; Henry Fonda does not have that special kind of responsibility for me. And our attention might be drawn to the fact that men and women both are compelled by law to provide support for their children.

I have in effect dealt (briefly) with this argument in section 4 above; but a (still briefer) recapitulation now may be in order. Surely we do not have any such "special responsibility" for a person unless we have assumed it, explicitly or implicitly. If a set of parents do not try to prevent pregnancy, do not obtain an abortion, but rather take it home with them, then they have assumed responsibility for it, they have given it rights, and they cannot now withdraw support from it at the cost of its life because they now find it difficult to go on providing for it. But if they have taken all reasonable precautions against having a child, they do not simply by virtue of their biological relationship to the child who comes into existence have a special responsibility for it. They may wish to assume responsibility for it, or they may not wish to. And I am suggesting that if assuming responsibility for it would require large sacrifices, then they may refuse. A Good Samaritan would not refuse—or anyway, a Splendid Samaritan, if the sacrifices that had to be made were enormous. But then so would a Good Samaritan assume responsibility for that violinist; so would Henry Fonda, if he is a Good Samaritan, fly in from the West Coast and assume responsibility for me.

> In this last section, Thomson considers it a strength of her argument that it allows for some abortions but not abortion for any reason. She considers late-term abortions. What do you think of her argument?

8.

My argument will be found unsatisfactory on two counts by many of those who want to regard abortion as morally permissible. First, while I do argue that abortion is not impermissible, I do not argue that it is always permissible. There may well be cases in which carrying the child to term requires only Minimally Decent Samaritanism of the mother, and this is a standard we must not fall below. I am inclined to think it a merit of my account precisely that it does not give a general yes or a general no. It allows for and supports our sense that, for example, a sick and desperately frightened fourteen-year-old schoolgirl, pregnant due to rape, may of course choose abortion, and that any law which rules this out is an insane law. And it also allows for and supports our sense that in other cases resort to abortion is even positively indecent. It would be indecent in the woman to request an abortion, and indecent in a doctor to perform it, if she is in her seventh month, and wants the abortion just to avoid the nuisance of postponing a trip abroad. The very fact that the arguments I have been drawing attention to treat all cases of abortion, or even all cases of abortion in which the mother's life is not at stake, as morally on a par ought to have made them suspect at the outset.

Second, while I am arguing for the permissibility of abortion in some cases, I am not arguing for the right to secure the death of the unborn child. It is easy to confuse these two things in that up to a certain point in the life of the fetus it is not able to survive outside the mother's body; hence removing it from her body guarantees its death. But they are importantly different. I have argued that you are not morally required to spend nine months in bed, sustaining the life of that violinist, but to say this is by no means to say that if, when you unplug yourself, there is a miracle and he survives, you then have a right to turn round and slit his throat. You may detach yourself even if this costs him his life; you have no right to be guaranteed his death, by some other means, if unplugging yourself does not kill him. There are some people who will feel dissatisfied by this feature of my argument. A woman may be utterly devastated by the thought of a child, a bit of herself, put out for adoption and never seen or heard of again. She may therefore want not merely that the child be detached from her, but more, that it die. Some opponents of abortion are inclined to regard this as beneath contempt—thereby showing insensitivity to what is surely a powerful source of despair. All the same, I agree that the desire for the child's death is not one which anybody may gratify, should it turn out to be possible to detach the child alive....

Reading 9.2: Francis Beckwith, "Personal Bodily Rights, Abortion, and Unplugging the Violinist"

The strength of Thomson's argument rests on the analogy between aborting a fetus and unplugging a famous violinist. Beckwith questions the strength of this analogy and argues that there are undefended assumptions that weaken Thomson's case.

...

I. Argument from Unplugging the Violinist

In an article, which by 1986 was "the most widely reprinted essay in all of contemporary philosophy," Professor Judith Jarvis Thomson presents a philosophically sophisticated version of the argument from a woman's right to control her body. Thomson argues that even if the unborn entity has a right to life, this does not mean that a woman must be forced to use her bodily organs to sustain its life. Just as one does not have a right to use another's kidney if one's kidney has failed, the unborn entity, although having a basic right to life, does not have a right to life so strong that it outweighs the pregnant woman's right to personal bodily autonomy.

It should be noted that Thomson's argument was not used in any of the landmark Supreme Court decisions which have sided with the abortion-rights position, such as Roe v. Wade (1973) or Doe v. Bolton (1973). Recently, however, Harvard law professor Laurence Tribe, whose influence on the Court's liberal wing is well-known, has suggested that it should have used Thomson's argument. Tribe writes: "... [P]erhaps the Supreme Court's opinion in Roe, by gratuitously insisting that the fetus cannot be deemed a person, needlessly insulted and alienated those for whom the view that the fetus is a person represents a fundamental article of faith or a bedrock personal commitment.... The Court should have instead said: Even if the fetus is a person, our Constitution forbids compelling a woman to carry it for nine months and become a mother."

In this section Beckwith restates what he thinks are the important parts of Thomson's argument for his critique.

1. PRESENTATION OF THE ARGUMENT

This argument is called "the argument from unplugging the violinist" because of a story Thomson uses in order to illustrate her position:

> You wake up in the morning and find yourself back to back in bed with an unconscious violinist. A famous unconscious violinist. He has been found to have a fatal kidney ailment, and the Society of Music Lovers has canvassed all the available medical records and found that you alone have the right blood type to help. They have therefore kidnapped you, and last night the violinist's circulatory system was plugged into yours, so that your kidneys can be used to extract poisons from his blood as well as your own. The director of the hospital now tells you, "Look we're sorry the Society of Music Lovers did this to you—we would never have permitted it if we had known. But still, they did it, and the violinist now is plugged into you. To unplug you would be to kill him. But never mind, it's only for nine months. By then he will have recovered from his ailment, and can safely be unplugged from you." Is it morally incumbent on you to accede to this situation? No doubt it would be very nice of you if you did, a great kindness. But do you have to accede to it? What if it were not nine months, but nine years? Or still longer? What if the director of the hospital says, "Tough luck, I agree, but you've now got to stay in bed, with the violinist plugged into you, for the rest of your life. Because remember this. All persons have a right to life, and violinists are persons. Granted you have a right to decide what happens in and to your body, but a person's right to life outweighs your right to decide what happens in and to your body. So you cannot ever be unplugged from him." I imagine that you would regard this as outrageous....

Thomson concludes that by use of the violinist illustration she is "only arguing that having a right to life does not guarantee having either a right to be given the use of or a right to be allowed continued use of another person's body—even if one needs it for life itself." Thomson anticipates several objections to her argument, and in the process of responding to them further clarifies it. It is not important, however, that we go over these clarifications now, for some are not germane to the prolife position I am defending in this article, and the remaining will be dealt with in the following critique.

Although I believe that it would be difficult to find an ethicist who would seriously defend the position that it is not prima facie wrong to kill innocent human beings, Thomson's argument poses a special difficulty because she believes that since pregnancy constitutes an infringement on the pregnant woman's personal rights by the unborn entity, the ordinary abortion, although it results in the death of an innocent human being, is not prima facie wrong. I believe, however, that there are many flaws in Thomson's use of the violinist analogy.

2. A CRITIQUE OF THOMSON'S ARGUMENT

I believe that there at least six problems with Thomson's argument. These can be put into two categories: ethical and ideological. First, under the ethical category, there are at least four problems with Thomson's argument:

> The four objections seem to stem from what Beckwith calls Thomson's "volunteerism." Do you think his objections are strong or weak? Beckwith relies on several intuitions about "what is natural." Does this weaken or strengthen his argument? Why?

1) Thomson assumes volunteerism. By using the violinist story as a paradigm for all relationships, which implies that moral obligations must be voluntarily accepted in order to have moral force, Thomson mistakenly infers that all true moral obligations to one's offspring are voluntary. But consider the following story. Suppose a couple has a sexual encounter which is fully protected by several forms of birth-control (condom, the Pill, IUD, etc.), but nevertheless results in conception. Instead of getting an abortion, the mother of the conceptus decides to bring it to term although the father is unaware of this decision. After the birth of the child the mother pleads with the father for child support. Because he refuses, she seeks legal action and takes him to court. Although he took every precaution to avoid fatherhood, thus showing that he did not wish to accept such a status, according to nearly all child support laws in this United States he would still be obligated to pay support precisely because of his relationship to this child. As Michael Levin points out, "All child-support laws make the parental body an indirect resource for the child. If the father is a construction worker, the state will intervene unless some of his calories he expends lifting equipment go to providing food for his children."

But this obligatory relationship is not based strictly on biology, for this would make sperm-donors morally responsible for children conceived by their seed. Rather, the father's responsibility for his offspring stems from the fact that he engaged in an act, sexual intercourse, which he fully realized could result in the creation of another human being, although he took every precaution to avoid such a result. This is not an unusual way to frame moral obligations, for we hold drunk people whose driving results in manslaughter responsible for their actions, even if they did not intend to kill someone prior to becoming intoxicated. Such special obligations, although not directly undertaken voluntarily, are necessary in any civilized culture in order to preserve the rights of the vulnerable, the weak, and the young, who can offer very little in exchange for the rights bestowed upon them by the strong, the powerful, and the post-uterine in Thomson's moral universe of the social contract. Thus, Thomson is simply wrong, in addition to ignoring the natural relationship between sexual intercourse and human reproduction when she claims that if a couple has "taken all reasonable precautions against having a child, they do not by virtue of their biological relationship to the child who comes into existence have a special responsibility for it" since "surely we do not have any such 'special responsibility' for a person unless we have assumed it, explicitly or implicitly." Hence, instead of providing reasons for rejecting any special responsibilities for one's offspring, Thomson simply dismisses the concept altogether.

2) Thomson's argument is fatal to family morality. It follows from the first criticism that Thomson's volunteerism is fatal to family morality, which has as one of its central beliefs that an individual has special personal obligations to his offspring and family which he does not have to other persons. Although Thomson may not consider such a fatality as being all that terrible, since she may buy into the feminist dogma that the traditional family is "oppressive" to women, a great number of ordinary men and women, who have found joy, happiness, and love in family life, find Thomson's volunteerism to be counter-intuitive. Philosopher Christina Sommers has come to a similar conclusion:

> For it [the volunteerist thesis] means that there is no such thing as filial [sic] duty per se, no such thing as the special duty of mother to child, and generally no such thing as morality of special family or kinship relations. All of which is contrary to what people think. For most people think that we do owe special debts to our parents even though we have not voluntarily assumed our obligations to them. Most people think that what we owe to our children does not have its origin in any voluntary undertaking, explicit or implicit, that we have made to them. And "preanalytically," many people believe that

we owe special consideration to our siblings even at times when we may not feel very friendly to them.... The idea that to be committed to an individual is to have made a voluntarily implicit or explicit commitment to that individual is generally fatal to family morality. For it looks upon the network of felt obligation and expectation that binds family members as a sociological phenomenon that is without presumptive moral force. The social critics who hold this view of family obligation usually are aware that promoting it in public policy must further the disintegration of the traditional family as an institution. But whether they deplore the disintegration or welcome it, they are bound in principle to abet it.

3) A case can be made that the unborn does have a prima facie right to her mother's body. Assuming that there is such a thing as a special parental obligation, which does not have to be voluntarily accepted in order to have moral weight, it is not obvious that the unborn entity in ordinary circumstances (that is, with the exception of when the mother's life is in significant danger) does not have a natural prima facie claim to her mother's body. There are several reasons to suppose that the unborn entity does have such a natural claim:

a) Unlike Thomson's violinist who is artificially attached to another person in order to save his life and is therefore not naturally dependent on any particular human being, the unborn entity is a human being who is by her very nature dependent on her mother, for this is how human beings are at this stage of their development.

b) This period of a human being's natural development occurs in the womb. This is the journey which we all must take and is a necessary condition for any human being's post-uterine existence. And this fact alone brings out the most glaring disanalogy between the violinist and the unborn: the womb is the unborn's natural environment whereas being artificially hooked-up to a stranger is not the natural environment for the violinist. It would seem, then, that the unborn has a prima facie natural claim upon its mother's body. This brings us to my third point.

c) This same entity, when it becomes a newborn, has a natural claim upon her parents to care for her, regardless of whether her parents "wanted" her (see the above story of the irresponsible father). This is why we prosecute child-abusers, people who throw their babies in trash cans, and parents who abandon their children. Although it should not be ignored that pregnancy and childbirth entail certain emotional, physical, and financial sacrifices on the part of the pregnant woman, these sacrifices are also endemic of parenthood in general (which ordinarily lasts much longer than nine months), and do not seem to justify the execution of troublesome infants and younger children whose existence entails a natural claim to certain financial and bodily goods which are under the ownership of their parents.

d) If the unborn entity is fully human, as Thomson is willing to grant, why should the unborn's natural prima facie claim to her parents' goods differ before birth? Of course, a court will not force a parent to donate a kidney to her dying offspring, but this sort of dependence on the parent's body is highly unusual and is not part of the ordinary obligations associated with the natural process of human development, just as in the case of the violinist's artificial dependency on the reluctant music lover.

As Professor Schwarz points out: "So, the very thing that makes it plausible to say that the person in bed with the violinist has no duty to sustain him; namely, that he is a stranger unnaturally hooked up to him, is precisely what is absent in the case of the mother and her child." That is to say, the mother "does have an obligation to take care of her child, to sustain her, to protect her, and especially, to let her live in the only place where she can now be protected, nourished, and allowed to grow, namely the womb."

> Now Beckwith engages with an imaginary version of Thomson. Do you think he treats Thomson's argument fairly before he criticizes it? Why or why not? Has the author lapsed into sentiment when he questions "how something so human, so natural, so beautiful" is reduced to a brutal caricature? Does this undermine his argument?

Now if Thomson responds to this by saying that birth is the threshold at which parents become fully responsible, then she has begged the question, for her violinist argument was supposed to show us why there is no parental responsibility before birth. That is to say, Thomson can not appeal to birth as the decisive moment at which parents become responsible in order to prove that birth is the time at which parents become responsible.

It is evident that Thomson's violinist illustration undermines the deep natural bond between mother and child by making it seem no different than two strangers artificially hooked-up to each other so that one can "steal" the service of the other's kidneys. Never has something so human, so natural, so beautiful, and so wonderfully demanding of our human creativity and love been reduced to such a brutal caricature.

I am not saying that the unborn entity has an absolute natural claim to her mother's body, but simply that she has a prima facie natural claim. For one can easily imagine a situation in which this natural claim is outweighed by other important prima facie values, such as when a pregnancy significantly endangers the mother's life. Since the continuation of such a pregnancy would most likely entail the death of both mother and child, and since it is better that one human should live rather than two die, I believe that terminating such a pregnancy via abortion is morally justified.

Now someone may respond to the above four criticisms by agreeing that Thomson's violinist illustration may not apply in cases of ordinary sexual intercourse, but only in cases in which pregnancy results from rape or incest; although it should be noted that Thomson herself does not press the rape argument. She writes: "Surely the question of whether you have a right to life at all, or of how you have it, shouldn't turn on the question of whether or not you are the product of rape."

But those who do press the rape argument may choose to argue in the following way. Just as the sperm-donor is not responsible for how his sperm is used or what results from its use (e.g., it may be stolen, or an unmarried woman may purchase it, inseminate herself, and give birth to a child), the raped woman, who did not voluntarily engage in intercourse, cannot be held responsible for the unborn human who is living inside her.

But there is a problem with this analogy: The sperm-donor's relinquishing of responsibility does not result in the death of a human life while the raped woman's does. The following story should help to illustrate the differences and similarities between these two cases.

> Now Beckwith gives his own analogy about a sperm-donor being forced to provide monetary compensation for a child he did not intend to father as analogous to a woman who terminates a pregnancy due to rape. Do you think his analogy is strong or weak? Refer back to Thomson's own claim about lying in bed for nine months after being forced to be hooked up to a violinist.

Suppose that the sperm donated by the sperm-donor was stolen by an unscrupulous physician and inseminated into a woman. Although he is not morally responsible for the child which results from such an insemination, he is nevertheless forced by an unjust court to pay a large monthly sum for child support, a sum so large that it may drive him into serious debt, maybe even bankruptcy. This would be similar to the woman who became pregnant as a result of rape. She was unjustly violated and is supporting a human being against her will at an emotional and financial cost. Is it morally right for the sperm-donor to kill the child he is supporting in order to allegedly right the wrong which has been committed against him? Not at all, because such an act would be murder. Now if we assume, as does Thomson, that the raped woman is carrying a being who is fully human, her killing of the unborn entity by abortion, except if the pregnancy has a strong possibility of endangering her life, would be as unjust as the sperm-donor killing the child he is unjustly forced to support. As the victimized man may rightly refuse to pay the child support, the raped woman may rightly refuse to bring up her child after the pregnancy has to come to term. She can choose to put the child up for adoption. But in both cases, the killing of the child is not morally justified. Although neither the sperm-donor nor the rape victim has the same special obligation to their biological offspring as does the couple who voluntarily engaged in intercourse with no direct intention to produce a child, it seems that the more general obligation not to kill directly another human being does apply, which is supported by my fourth ethical objection.

In this last ethical objection, Beckwith argues that Thomson wrongly assumes that withholding a kidney from the violinist is the same as aborting a fetus. It is not the kidney match's fault that the violinist is dependent on the kidney she provides, Beckwith says. However, an abortion is not just withholding treatment, he says; it is killing. Do you agree? (It might be helpful to read about this distinction in Jeff McMahan's article on killing and letting die in Chapter 5.)

4) Thomson ignores the fact that abortion is indeed killing and not merely the withholding of treatment. Thomson makes an excellent point in her use of the violinist story, namely, that there are times when withholding and/or withdrawing of medical treatment is morally justified. For instance, I am not morally obligated to donate my kidney to Fred, my next door neighbor, simply because he needs a kidney in order to live. In other words, I am not obligated to risk my life so that Fred may live a few years longer. Fred should not expect that of me. If, however, I donate one of my kidneys to Fred, I will have acted above and beyond

the call of duty, since I will have performed a supererogatory moral act. But this case is not analogous to pregnancy and abortion.

Levin argues that there is an essential disanalogy between abortion and the unplugging of the violinist. In the case of the violinist (as well as my relationship to Fred's welfare), "the person who withdraws [or withholds] his assistance is not completely responsible for the dependency on him of the person who is about to die, while the mother is completely responsible for the dependency of her fetus on her. When one is completely responsible for dependence, refusal to continue to aid is indeed killing." For example, "if a woman brings a newborn home from the hospital, puts it in its crib and refuses to feed it until it has starved to death, it would be absurd to say that she simply refused to assist it and had done nothing for which she should be criminally liable." In other words, just as the withholding of food kills the child after birth, in the case of abortion, it is the abortion which kills the child. In neither case is there any ailment from which the child suffers and which highly invasive medical treatment, with the cooperation of another's bodily organs, is necessary in order to cure this ailment and save the child's life.

Or consider a case parallel to rape. Suppose a person returns home after work to find a baby at his doorstep (like in the film with Tom Selleck, Ted Danson, and Steve Guttenberg, *Three Men and a Baby*). Suppose that no one else is able to take care of the child, but this person only has to take care of the child for nine months (after that time a couple will adopt the child). Imagine that this person will have some bouts with morning sickness, water retention, and other minor ailments. If we assume with Thomson that the unborn child is as much a person as you or I, would "withholding treatment" from this child and its subsequent death be justified on the basis that the homeowner was only "withholding treatment" of a child he did not ask for in order to benefit himself? Is any person, born or unborn, obligated to sacrifice his life because his death would benefit another person? Consequently, there is no doubt that such "withholding" of treatment (and it seems totally false to call ordinary shelter and sustenance "treatment") is indeed murder.

But is it even accurate to refer to abortion as the "withholding of support or treatment"? Professors Schwarz and R.K. Tacelli make the important point that although "a woman who has an abortion is indeed 'withholding support' from her unborn child ... abortion is far more than that. It is the active killing of a human person—by burning him, by crushing him, by dismembering him." Euphemistically calling abortion the "withholding of support or treatment" makes about as much sense as calling suffocating someone with a pillow the withdrawing of oxygen.

In summary, then, of the four problems with Thomson's argument under the ethical category, I agree with Professor Brody when he concludes that "Thomson has not established the truth of her claim about abortion, primarily because she has not sufficiently attended to the distinction between our duty to save X's life and our duty not to take it." But "once one attends to that distinction, it would seem that the mother, in order to regain control over her body, has no right to abort the fetus from the point at which it becomes a human being."

ETHICS COMMITTEE

Botched Abortion

At a rural hospital annex, a 17-year-old girl, Jennifer, is admitted to the emergency department complaining of vaginal bleeding. She doesn't remember when her last period was but shows early signs of pregnancy. She admits to nursing staff that she tried to use a folk abortion cure by inserting some tablets given to her by her boyfriend. She assumed this was the reason for the bleeding. Upon examination, the tablets are identified as misoprostol, and the fetus is between eight and ten weeks gestation. The patient continues to have profuse vaginal bleeding and a rapid pulse. The ER attending does not believe the fetus is likely to survive. She believes, however, that a D&C abortion procedure is necessary to save the teen and offers to do the emergency procedure.

"I can't allow it," says the Chief of Medicine. "State law bans abortion after 8 weeks. You know that. We'd have to have a court order."

"This girl could bleed out before you get a court order," responds a nurse.

"Could you authorize an airlift to another hospital? Like one, you know, across state lines?" asks the ER attending physician.

"We could. I could. But it puts the girl at risk. She could die on route," remarks the Chief.

"Well, whatever we do. We better do it fast," says the nurse.

"I need to talk to the ethics committee," says the Chief.

> It seems now that Jennifer's life is at stake. What options are permissible? According to Beckwith, this is a condition that could justify taking the life of the fetus. Do you think Beckwith's argument would condone such a decision?

Permissions Acknowledgments

Allied Control Council, No. 10. "Permissible Medical Experiments," from *Trials of War Criminals Before the Nuremberg Military Tribunals Under Control Council Law No. 10 "Green Series": Volume 2*. 1945. Periodical. Retrieved from the Library of Congress, www.loc.gov/item/2011525364_NT_war-criminals_Vol-II/.

Angell, Marcia. "The Ethics of Clinical Research in the Third World," from *The New England Journal of Medicine*, 337.12 (1997): 847–49 [excerpted]. Copyright © 1990, Massachusetts Medical Society. https://doi.org/10.1056/NEJM199709183371209. Reprinted with permission from Massachusetts Medical Society, conveyed by Copyright Clearance Center, Inc.

Annas, G.J. "The Prostitute, the Playboy, and the Poet: Rationing Schemes for Organ Transplantation," from *American Journal of Public Health*, 75.2 (1985): 187–89. Copyright © 1985 American Journal of Public Health. https://doi.org/10.2105/AJPH.75.2.187. Reprinted by permission of the American Public Health Association.

Arries, E. "Virtue ethics: an approach to moral dilemmas in nursing," from *Curationis*, 28.3 (2005): 64–72 [excerpted]. Copyright © 2005 E. Arries. https://doi.org/10.4102/curationis.v28i3.990. Used under license CC BY 4.0 https://creativecommons.org/licenses/by/4.0/.

Beckwith, Francis J. "Personal Bodily Rights, Abortion, and Unplugging the Violinist," from *International Philosophical Quarterly*, 32.1 (1992): 105–18 [excerpted]. Copyright © 1992 Foundation for International Philosophical Exchange. https://doi.org/10.5840/ipq199232156. Reprinted by permission of the Philosophy Documentation Center, Charlottesville, Virginia.

Briscoe, Rebecca. "Ethical Considerations, Safety Precautions and Parenthood in Legalising Mitochondrial Donation," from *The New Bioethics*, 19.1 (2013): 2–17 [excerpted]. Copyright © 2013 Taylor & Francis Group, LLC. https://doi.org/10.1179/2050287713Z.00000000027. Used by permission of Taylor & Francis Group, LLC https://www.tandfonline.com/.

Brody, Baruch A. "Ethical issues in clinical trials in developing countries," from *Statistics in Medicine*, Special Issue: 9th International Symposium on Long-Term Clinical Trials, 21.19 (2002): 2853–58 [excerpted]. Copyright © 2002 John Wiley & Sons Ltd. https://doi.org/10.1002/sim.1289. Reprinted by permission of John Wiley & Sons Ltd., conveyed by Copyright Clearance Center, Inc.

Callahan, Daniel. "When Self-Determination Runs Amok," from *The Hastings Center Report*, 22.2 (Mar/Apr 1992): 52–55. Copyright © 1992 The Hastings Center. https://doi.org/10.2307/3562566. Reprinted by permission of John Wiley & Sons Ltd., conveyed by Copyright Clearance Center, Inc.

Dworkin, Gerald. "Paternalism," *The Monist*, 56.1 (1972): 64–84. [excerpted]. Copyright © 1972 THE MONIST, La Salle, Illinois. https://doi.org/10.5840/monist197256119. Reprinted by permission of Oxford University Press, conveyed by Copyright Clearance Center, Inc.

Emanuel, Ezekiel J. et al. "Fair Allocation of Scarce Medical Resources in the Time of COVID-19," from *The New England Journal of Medicine*, 382 (2020): 2049–55 [excerpted]. Copyright © 2022 Massachusetts Medical Society. http://dx.doi.org/10.1136/medethics-2020-106320. Reprinted with permission from Massachusetts Medical Society, conveyed by Copyright Clearance Center, Inc.

Grady, Christine. "Money for Research Participation: Does It Jeopardize Informed Consent?," from *The American Journal of Bioethics*, 1.2 (2001): 40–44. Copyright © 2001 Taylor & Francis Group, LLC. https://doi.org/10.1162/152651601300169031. Used by permission of Taylor & Francis Group, LLC https://www.tandfonline.com/.

Groopman, Leonard C., Franklin G. Miller, and Joseph J. Fins. "The Patient's Work," from *Cambridge Quarterly of Healthcare Ethics*, 16.1 (2007): 44–52. Copyright © 2007 Cambridge University Press. https://doi.org/10.1017/S0963180107070053. Reprinted by permission of Cambridge University Press, conveyed by Copyright Clearance Center, Inc.

"Human Clinical Trial Phases: Phase I—IV" [excerpted], from "About Clinical Trials" published by CenterWatch, Falls Church, VA. Copyright © 2022 WCG CenterWatch. Accessed November 7, 2022 https://www.centerwatch.com/clinical-trials/overview/. Reprinted with permission.

Iserson, Kenneth V. "Ethics, Personal Responsibility and the Pandemic: A New Triage Paradigm," from *The Journal of Emergency Medicine*, 62.4 (2022): 508–12. Copyright © 2021 Published by Elsevier Inc. https://doi.org/10.1016/j.jemermed.2021.11.019. Reprinted with permission from Elsevier, conveyed by Copyright Clearance Center, Inc.

Kuczewski, Mark. "Is Informed Consent Enough? Monetary Incentives for Research Participation and the Integrity of Biomedicine," from *The American Journal of Bioethics*, 1.2 (2011): 49–51 [excerpted]. Copyright © 2011 Taylor & Francis Group, LLC. https://doi.org/10.1162/152651601300169086. Used by permission of Taylor & Francis Group, LLC https://www.tandfonline.com/.

Lee, Katarina. "Ethical Implications of Permitting Mitochondrial Replacement," from *The National Catholic Bioethics Quarterly*, 16.4 (2016): 619–31 [excerpted].

Scanlan, Camilla and Ian H. Kerridge. "Autonomy and Chronic Illness: Not Two Components But Many," from *The American Journal of Bioethics*, 9.2 (2009): 40–42 [excerpted]. Copyright © 2009 Taylor & Francis Group, LLC. https://doi.org/10.1080/15265160802663237. Used by permission of Taylor & Francis Group, LLC https://www.tandfonline.com/.

Scheunemann, Leslie P. and Douglas B. White. "The Ethics and Reality of Rationing in Medicine," from *Chest Journal*, 140.6 (2011): 1625–32 [excerpted]. Copyright © 2011 The American College of Chest Physicians. Published by Elsevier Inc. All rights reserved. https://doi.org/10.1378/chest.11-0622. Reprinted by permission of Elsevier Inc., conveyed by Copyright Clearance Center, Inc.

Stoller, Sarah E. "Why We Are Not Morally Required to Select the Best Children: A Response to Savulescu," from *Bioethics*, 22.7 (2008): 364–69 [excerpted]. Copyright © 2008 John Wiley & Sons Ltd. https://doi.org/10.1111/j.1467-8519.2008.00659.x. Reprinted by permission of John Wiley & Sons Ltd., conveyed by Copyright Clearance Center, Inc.

Thomson, Judith Jarvis. "A Defense of Abortion," from *Philosophy & Public Affairs*, 1.1 (1971): 47–66 [excerpted]. Copyright © Philosophy & Public Affairs 1971, Wiley. https://www.jstor.org/stable/2265091. Reprinted by permission of John Wiley & Sons conveyed through Copyright Clearance Center, Inc.

Toulmin, Stephen. "How Medicine Saved the Life of Ethics," from *Perspectives in Biology and Medicine*, 25.4 (1982): 736–50 [excerpted]. Copyright © 1982 The University of Chicago. All rights reserved. https://doi.org/10.1353/pbm.1982.0064. Republished by permission of Project MUSE, Johns Hopkins University Press, conveyed through Copyright Clearance Center, Inc.

United States, Department of Health and Human Services, National Cancer Institute. "Questions to Ask Your Doctor about Treatment Clinical Trials" [excerpted], from "Clinical Trials Information," last update April 11, 2022, https://www.cancer.gov/about-cancer/treatment/clinical-trials/questions.

United States, Department of Health and Human Services, Office for Human Research Protections. "The Belmont Report: Ethical Principles and Guidelines for the Protection of Human Subjects of Research," by the National Commission for the Protection of Human Subjects of Biomedical and Behavioral Research, 1976, https://www.hhs.gov/ohrp/regulations-and-policy/belmont-report/read-the-belmont-report/index.html#xethical.

"WMA Declaration of Helsinki - Ethical Principles for Medical Research Involving Human Subjects," (2013) by the World Medical Association [excerpted]. Copyright © World Medical Association. All Rights Reserved. Reprinted with permission.

Wolf, Susan M. et al. "Sources of Concern about the Patient Self-Determination Act," from *The New England Journal of Medicine*, 325 (1991): 1666–71. Copyright © 1991 Massachusetts Medical Society. https://doi.org/10.1056/NEJM199112053252334. Reprinted with permission from Massachusetts Medical Society, conveyed by Copyright Clearance Center, Inc.

Index

From the Publisher

A name never says it all, but the word "Broadview" expresses a good deal of the philosophy behind our company. We are open to a broad range of academic approaches and political viewpoints. We pay attention to the broad impact book publishing and book printing has in the wider world; for some years now we have used 100% recycled paper for most titles. Our publishing program is internationally oriented and broad-ranging. Our individual titles often appeal to a broad readership too; many are of interest as much to general readers as to academics and students.

Founded in 1985, Broadview remains a fully independent company owned by its shareholders—not an imprint or subsidiary of a larger multinational.

To order our books or obtain up-to-date information, please visit broadviewpress.com.

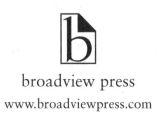

broadview press
www.broadviewpress.com

This book is made of paper from well-managed FSC® - certified
forests, recycled materials, and other controlled sources.

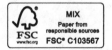